Advances in Experimental Medicine and Biology

Volume 1254

Advances in Experimental Medicine and Biology provides a platform for scientific contributions in the main disciplines of the biomedicine and the life sciences. This series publishes thematic volumes on contemporary research in the areas of microbiology, immunology, neurosciences, biochemistry, biomedical engineering, genetics, physiology, and cancer research. Covering emerging topics and techniques in basic and clinical science, it brings together clinicians and researchers from various fields.

Advances in Experimental Medicine and Biology has been publishing exceptional works in the field for over 40 years, and is indexed in SCOPUS, Medline (PubMed), Journal Citation Reports/Science Edition, Science Citation Index Expanded (SciSearch, Web of Science), EMBASE, BIOSIS, Reaxys, EMBiology, the Chemical Abstracts Service (CAS), and Pathway Studio.

2018 Impact Factor: 2.126.

More information about this series at http://www.springer.com/series/5584

Ji-Yang Wang
Editor

B Cells in Immunity and Tolerance

Springer

Editor
Ji-Yang Wang
Department of Immunology
School of Basic Medical Sciences
Fudan University
Shanghai, China

ISSN 0065-2598 ISSN 2214-8019 (electronic)
Advances in Experimental Medicine and Biology
ISBN 978-981-15-3531-4 ISBN 978-981-15-3532-1 (eBook)
https://doi.org/10.1007/978-981-15-3532-1

This Springer imprint is published by the registered company Springer Nature Singapore Pte Ltd.
The registered company address is: 152 Beach Road, #21-01/04 Gateway East, Singapore 189721, Singapore

Preface

B cells produce antibodies that are indispensable for host defence against infections, through virus neutralization, opsonization of pathogens for efficient phagocytosis by macrophages and antibody-dependent cellular cytotoxicity. Antibodies are not just effector molecules, but also regulate humoral immune responses, both positively and negatively, through their cellular receptors such as Fc receptors. Moreover, B cells may also function to suppress immune reactions by secreting anti-inflammatory cytokines. This book aims to provide a comprehensive overview of B cell development, maturation, activation and differentiation, and of human diseases caused by B cell abnormalities.

B cell development in the bone marrow is accompanied by immunoglobulin (Ig) gene rearrangements and generates a diverse pool of immature B cells. Those reactive with self-antigens are deleted or functionally inactivated, and the remaining immature B cells migrate to the periphery to mature. In Chap. 1, Ying Wang et al. discuss the mechanisms of Ig gene rearrangement, regulation of B cell development and maturation, the elimination/inactivation of autoreactive B cells (B cell tolerance), and B-1 cell development and function.

Mature B cells in the periphery can be activated by antigen stimulation, toll-like receptor signaling and/or T cell help. Antigen binding to the BCR is a critical step to initiate B cell activation. In Chap. 2, Shinya Tanaka and Yoshihiro Baba provide a current update on positive and negative regulation of BCR signaling, focusing on the coordinated function of tyrosine kinases, adaptor molecules and phosphatases. Another important regulator of BCR signaling is reactive oxygen species (ROS). In Chap. 3, Takeshi Tsubata describes the latest findings on the regulation of ROS generation during BCR signaling and its role in B cell survival and activation.

B cells activated by antigen stimulation and in the presence of T cell help form germinal centres (GCs). Here, they undergo Ig V gene somatic hypermutation (SHM) and class switch recombination (CSR) and finally differentiate into memory B or antibody-secreting plasma cells. In Chap. 4, Chuanxin Huang reviews the regulation of the initiation and maintenance of the GC reaction, mechanisms of Ig gene SHM and CSR, and the selection of high-affinity clones in the GC. In Chap. 5, Saya Moriyama et al. provide a comprehensive overview of the systemic and local memory B cell responses in humoral protective immunity against pathogens. In addition, Wataru Ise and Tomohiro Kurosaki review the latest progress in the cellular and molecular mechanisms of plasma cell differentiation from GC B cells in Chap. 6.

During a humoral immune response, B cells typically produce antigen-specific IgM first and then IgG later. It is well known that the antigen–IgG complex can suppress BCR signaling and B cell activation by co-ligation of the BCR and FcγRIIB. However, it is less clear whether the antigen-specific IgM has any role in B cell activation. In Chap. 7, Jun Liu et al. provide a comprehensive overview on the function of IgM, with emphasis on the role of the IgM Fc receptor (FcμR). They also discuss the relative contribution of IgM–complement and IgM–FcμR pathways in regulating humoral immune responses.

Although there is still some controversy, it is now more appreciated that there exists a population of regulatory B cells (Bregs) that function to suppress immune reactions by secreting anti-inflammatory cytokines such as IL-10. In Chap. 8, Luman Wang et al. summarize the phenotypes and functions of Bregs in both mice and humans.

Among the different classes of antibodies, IgA is the most abundantly produced antibody in the body (40–60 mg/kg body weight/day in humans) and plays an essential role in mucosal immunity. In Chap. 9, Keiichiro Suzuki gives a cutting-edge overview on the role of diverse IgA–bacteria interactions in gut homoeostasis. His chapter also provides the latest information on the dynamics and maintenance of gut IgA, including the regulation of IgA–J chain interaction by a marginal zone B and B-1 cell-specific protein.

Chapters 10–12 focus on human diseases caused by B cell abnormalities. Qing Min et al. provide a detailed overview of different types of primary antibody deficiencies (PADs) caused by abnormalities in the development, survival, activation or differentiation of B cells. They also review the clinical manifestations, the causal genes and the treatments of various PADs. Excessive B cell activation and/or breakdown of B cell tolerance can lead to autoantibody production and autoimmune diseases. In Chap. 11, Xiang Lin and Liwei Lu provide an overview of dysregulated B cell responses and the mechanisms underlying the development of autoimmunity. They also discuss both autoantibody-dependent and autoantibody-independent B cell functions in autoimmune diseases and biological therapies targeting B cells. Finally, abnormalities in the genetic alterations experienced by B cells, including Ig gene rearrangements, SHM and CSR, can lead to chromosomal translocations, gene mutations and B cell malignancies. In Chap. 12, Xin Meng et al. summarize the morphology, immune phenotypes, clinical features, genetic defects, treatments and prognosis of human B cell lymphomas.

This book covers as many aspects of B cells as possible in both mice and humans. We hope that it will become a standard reference for both basic researchers and clinicians. As the editor, I would like to express my sincere thanks to all of the authors, who have spared their precious time to contribute excellent chapters, resulting in the timely completion of this exciting book.

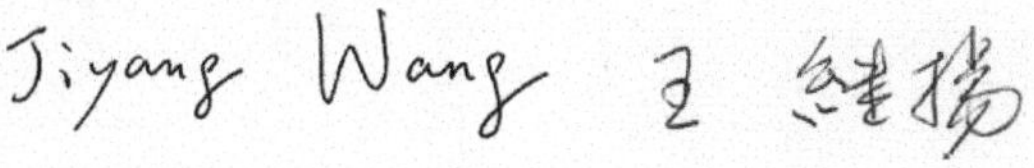

Shanghai, China

Prof. Ji-Yang Wang
wang@fudan.edu.cn

Contents

Contributors

Yu Adachi Department of Immunology, National Institute of Infectious Diseases, Shinjuku, Tokyo, Japan

Yoshihiro Baba Division of Immunology and Genome Biology, Department of Molecular Genetics, Medical Institute of Bioregulation, Kyushu University, Fukuoka, Japan

Peter D. Burrows Department of Microbiology, University of Alabama at Birmingham, Birmingham, AL, USA

Yiwei Chu Department of Immunology, School of Basic Medical Sciences, and Institutes of Biomedical Sciences, Fudan University, Shanghai, China

Ying Fu Department of Immunology, School of Basic Medical Sciences, and Institutes of Biomedical Sciences, Fudan University, Shanghai, China

Birgitta Heyman Department of Medical Biochemistry and Microbiology, Uppsala University, Uppsala, Sweden

Chuanxin Huang Shanghai Jiao Tong University School of Medicine, Shanghai, China

W. Ise Laboratory of Lymphocyte Differentiation, WPI Immunology Frontier Research Center, Osaka University, Osaka, Japan

T. Kurosaki Laboratory of Lymphocyte Differentiation, WPI Immunology Frontier Research Center, Osaka University, Osaka, Japan;
Laboratory for Lymphocyte Differentiation, RIKEN Center for Integrative Medical Sciences (IMS), Yokohama, Kanagawa, Japan

Xiang Lin Department of Pathology and Shenzhen Institute of Research and Innovation, The University of Hong Kong, Hong Kong, China

Jun Liu Department of Immunology, School of Basic Medical Sciences, Fudan University, Shanghai, China

Liwei Lu Department of Pathology, The University of Hong Kong, Pokfulam, Hong Kong, China

Xin Meng Department of Immunology, School of Basic Medical Sciences, Fudan University, Shanghai, China

Qing Min Department of Immunology, School of Basic Medical Sciences, Fudan University, Shanghai, China

Saya Moriyama Department of Immunology, National Institute of Infectious Diseases, Shinjuku, Tokyo, Japan

Keiichiro Suzuki Laboratory for Mucosal Immunity, Center for Integrative Medical Sciences (IMS), RIKEN, Kanagawa, Japan

Yoshimasa Takahashi Department of Immunology, National Institute of Infectious Diseases, Shinjuku, Tokyo, Japan

Shinya Tanaka Division of Immunology and Genome Biology, Department of Molecular Genetics, Medical Institute of Bioregulation, Kyushu University, Fukuoka, Japan

Keisuke Tonouchi Department of Immunology, National Institute of Infectious Diseases, Shinjuku, Tokyo, Japan;
Department of Life Science and Medical Bioscience, Waseda University, Shinjuku, Tokyo, Japan

Takeshi Tsubata Department of Immunology, Medical Research Institute, Tokyo Medical and Dental University, Tokyo, Japan

Ji-Yang Wang Department of Immunology, School of Basic Medical Sciences, Fudan University, Shanghai, China

Luman Wang Department of Immunology, School of Basic Medical Sciences, and Institutes of Biomedical Sciences, Fudan University, Shanghai, China

Ying Wang Department of Immunology, School of Basic Medical Sciences, Fudan University, Shanghai, China

Ermeng Xiong Department of Immunology, School of Basic Medical Sciences, Fudan University, Shanghai, China

B Cell Development and Maturation

1

Ying Wang, Jun Liu, Peter D. Burrows, and Ji-Yang Wang

Abstract

Since the identification of B cells in 1965 (Cooper et al. 1965), three has been tremendous progress in our understanding of B cell development, maturation and function. A number of B cell subpopulations, including B-1, B-2 and regulatory B cells, have been identified. B-1 cells mainly originate from the fetal liver and contain B-1a and B-1b subsets. B-2 cells are derived from the bone marrow (BM) and can be further classified into follicular B (FOB) and marginal zone B (MZB) cells. Regulatory B cells (Bregs) function to suppress immune responses, primarily by production of the anti-inflammatory cytokine IL-10. B cell tolerance is established at several checkpoints, during B cell development in the BM (central tolerance) as well as during B cell maturation and activation in the periphery (peripheral tolerance). This chapter will focus on the regulation of important processes during the development and maturation of B-1 and B-2 cells.

Keywords

Ig gene · V(D)J recombination · Follicular B · Marginal zone B · B-1

1.1 Introduction

B cell development proceeds in an orderly fashion and is regulated by intrinsic genetic programs and by external cues such as cytokines that are present in the specialized microenvironments of fetal liver and BM. One intriguing feature of B cell development is that it is accompanied by immunoglobulin (Ig) gene rearrangements. Progenitor B cells rearrange their Ig heavy chain (HC) genes to differentiate into precursor B (pre-B) cells that express μ HCs. Pre-B cells then rearrange their Ig light chain (LC) genes to differentiate into IgM^+ immature B cells and then become IgM^+IgD^+ mature, resting B cells. Defects in each stage of the B cell development and maturation pathway can lead to primary immunodeficiencies, autoimmune diseases and even B cell malignancies. In this chapter, we will discuss the mechanism of Ig gene rearrangement, regulation of B-2 (FOB and MZB) cell development, the elimination/inactivation of autoreactive B cells

Y. Wang · J. Liu · J.-Y. Wang (✉)
Department of Immunology, School of Basic Medical Sciences, Fudan University, Shanghai, China
e-mail: wang@fudan.edu.cn

P. D. Burrows
Department of Microbiology, University of Alabama at Birmingham, Birmingham, AL, USA

J.-Y. Wang (ed.), *B Cells in Immunity and Tolerance*, Advances in Experimental Medicine and Biology 1254, https://doi.org/10.1007/978-981-15-3532-1_1

(central and peripheral tolerance), regulation of B-1 cell development, fate decision of B-1a vs. B-1b subsets, and the function of B-1 cells.

1.2 Immunoglobulin (Ig) Gene Rearrangement

Antigen receptor gene rearrangement, which is a defining feature of the adaptive immune system, is a unique mechanism to generate diversity in both T and B cells from limited numbers of variable (V) gene segments through genetic recombination. We will focus here on Ig gene rearrangement, which occurs during the early stages of B cell development to generate a diverse repertoire of antibodies.

1.2.1 Structure of Ig Genes

The genome structure of the mouse Ig heavy (H) and light (L) [kappa (*Igκ*) and lambda (*Igλ*)] loci is shown in Fig. 1.1. An antibody is composed of two identical HCs and two identical LCs (either κ or λ), consisting of variable (V) and constant (C) regions linked by disulfide bonds. *Igh*, *Igκ* and *Igλ* genes in mice are located on chromosomes 12, 6 and 16 and in humans on chromosomes 14, 2 and 22, respectively. The V exons of the Ig heavy chains are generated by somatic recombination (rearrangement) of variable (V), diversity (D) and joining (J) gene segments, whereas the V exons of the Ig light chains are generated by rearrangement of V and J but no D segments. During the early stages of B cell development, somatic recombination, known as V(D)J recombination, mediates a physical and permanent juxtaposition of the Ig gene segments at the DNA level that results in a mature V exon and generation of a functional μ HC gene. V(D)J recombination gives rise to a large, diverse repertoire of Ig proteins. In mice, there are 97 V, 14 D and 4 J segments located in the *Igh* locus, 94–96 V and 4 J segments located in the *Igκ* locus, and 3 (laboratory mice) or 8 (wild mice) V and 3 J segments located in the *Igλ* locus.

Downstream of these rearranging gene segments are exons to encode the constant (C) regions of the antibody heavy and light chains. The C exons are not formed by the rearrangement of smaller gene segments and in the *Igh* locus encode several antibody classes and subclasses. Although the *Igκ* locus contains a single $C_κ$ exon, the mouse *Igλ* locus contains four $C_λ$ exons. Moreover, the *Igh* locus contains eight C_H exons, namely Cμ, Cδ, Cγ3, Cγ1, Cγ2b, Cγ2a (BALB/c)/Cγ2c (C57BL/6), Cε and Cα. Each C_H exon encodes a particular Ig isotype. For H and L chains, the most V-proximal C exon is joined to the mature V exon at the RNA level by conventional splicing, which is then translated to generate the H or L protein.

Because of this specific gene structure and mechanism, B cells can generate about 10^{11} different BCR or antibodies by V(D)J

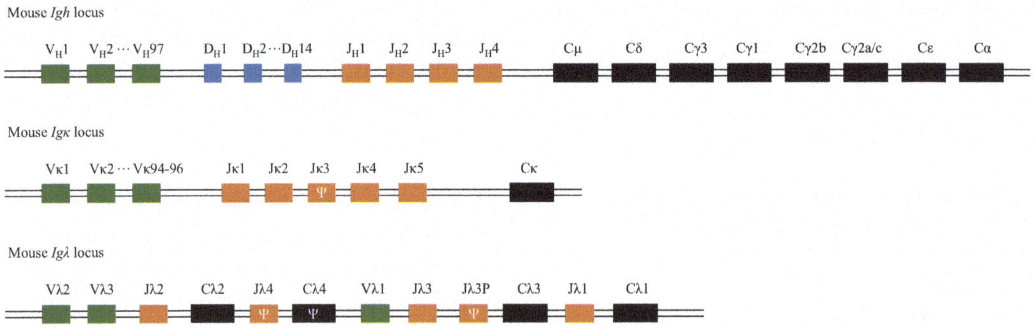

Fig. 1.1 Immunoglobulin loci of mouse (*Notes* The organization of mouse *Igh* locus, *Igκ* locus and *Igλ* locus. Ψ, pseudogene. Not all gene segments and pseudogenes are shown)

recombination (Nussenzweig and Alt 2004). Ig V genes also undergo somatic hypermutation during the germinal center reaction, which further increases the diversity and can change the affinity and sometimes the specificity of antibodies. Such a vast number of different antibodies, the "repertoire," are essential for neutralizing a universe of pathogenic bacteria and viruses.

1.2.2 The Mechanism of V(D)J Recombination

V(D)J recombination can be divided into two processes, i.e., DNA cleavage and DNA repair. The DNA cleavage is a site-specific reaction initiated by the lymphoid-specific proteins recombination-activating gene (RAG) 1 and RAG2 and the ubiquitously expressed DNA-binding protein high-mobility group box protein 1 or 2 (HMGB1 or HMGB2) (van Gent et al. 1997). These proteins bind to the recombination signal sequences (RSSs) that flank each gene segment and introduce a double-strand break (DSB) between the RSS and the flanking coding DNA. Then, joining of the DSB is mediated by the non-homologous end-joining (NHEJ) DNA repair pathway (reviewed by Lieber 2010; Chang et al. 2017).

RSSs flank germ line V_H segments on their 3′ sides, J_H segments on their 5′ sides and D_H segments on both sides. Similarly, the V_L and J_L segments of both the *Igκ* and *Igλ* loci are flanked by RSSs on their 3′ sides and 5′ sides, respectively. The RSS is a short DNA sequence containing a conserved heptamer (consensus sequence 5′-CACAGTG-3′) and nonamer (consensus sequence 5′-ACAAAAACC-3′) separated by either 12 or 23 base pairs (±1 bp), namely the 12 RSSs and 23 RSSs, respectively (Ramsden et al. 1994). The first three positions in the heptamer are the most conserved and are necessary for guiding the RAGs to the correct site of cleavage at the border between the heptamer and the coding segment. Similarly, the tract of adenines is the most invariant portion of the nonamer and is known to guide RAG1 binding at the RSS (Yin et al. 2009). While the sequence of the spacer is less well conserved, the length of the spacer is important as the 12 and 23 RSSs differ by one turn of the DNA helix, placing the heptamers and nonamers of the two RSSs in the same rotational phase and ensuring mutually complementary binding (Ciubotaru et al. 2015). Therefore, only when one gene segment is flanked on one side by a 12 RSSs and the other gene segment is flanked by a 23 RSSs can the pair interact and be recognized by the RAG complex and undergo V(D)J recombination. Such a mechanism has been called the 12/23 rule. The V(D)J recombinases first assemble on a single 12 or 23 RSSs, creating a signal complex (SC) in which nicking can occur (Fig. 1.2). Synapsis with a partner leads to the formation of the paired complex (PC) in which cleavage can occur. Several lines of evidence suggest that the PC is formed by the "capture model," in which one SC captures the appropriate partner RSS to form the PC, maintaining the same protein content in both the SC and the PC (Curry et al. 2005; Jones and Gellert 2002; Mundy et al. 2002; Swanson 2002). However, the capture model is not universally accepted. Some studies support the "association mode," in which two preformed SCs associate to form the PC (Shlyakhtenko et al. 2009; Landree et al. 2001). Under physiological conditions, the DSB is generated only by "coupled cleavage" in the PC. In a two-step transesterification reaction of "coupled cleavage," the free 3′ hydroxyl attacks the phosphate on the bottom strand of the DNA directly (McBlane et al. 1995). Then, hairpin formation in the PC generates two DNA DSBs and yields a pair of blunt DNA ends and two sealed DNA hairpins, all of which are held together by the RAGs (Hiom and Gellert 1998). Both the blunt ends, termed the signal ends, and the DNA hairpins, termed coding ends, are then handed over to the NHEJ DNA repair pathway. After repair, the blunt ends are joined to form the discarded product, a DNA deletion circle. Once opened, the hairpin ends are processed and ligated, yielding the coding joint that contains the newly joined antigen receptor gene segments. In the *Igh* locus, the recombination of D_H and J_H segments occurs first, and then the D_HJ_H recombines with V_H segment to form the complete $V_HD_HJ_H$ exon. In both the *Igκ* and *Igλ* loci, there is only one recombination step between a V_L and a J_L gene segment. Importantly, the fusion of V, D and J segments is not always precise, which leads to junctional diversity at the site of rearrangement, including the deletion of nucleotides in the joint region and the addition of the so-called P- or N-nucleotides. In the last steps of V(D)J recombination, if the DNA ends of the rearranging gene segments are digested by an exonuclease prior to ligation, there will be deletion of a few nucleotides in the D to J and/or V to D junctions. If the hairpin is not opened symmetrically, a single-stranded extension is created, resulting in palindromic insertions (P-nucleotides). Extra nucleotides can also be created by the terminal dideoxynucleotidyl transferase (TdT), which can randomly add "non-templated" N-nucleotides onto the ends of these strands before their final ligation. N-nucleotide addition occurs almost exclusively in the *Igh* locus because TdT is preferentially expressed in pro-B cells undergoing VDJ_H rearrangement. Although this imprecision can introduce diversity in the CDR3 regions of the antibody heavy and light chains, it can also lead to frameshift mutations if deleted or added nucleotides are not in multiples of three (one codon). As a result, 2/3 V(D)J rearrangements are non-functional, aka nonproductive.

The rearrangement of the Ig loci occurs at particular developmental stages in a temporally ordered and allele-exclusive manner. The *Igh* locus is rearranged first, followed by *Igκ* and *Igλ*. After a productive VDJ_H rearrangement is completed on chromosome 12 in a developing mouse B cell, the now functional VDJ-Cμ gene is transcribed and translated. Expression of this μ chain marks an important checkpoint in Ig gene rearrangement and B cell development. Any further V(D)J recombination in the *Igh* locus on the other chromosome 12 is blocked. This outcome is called allelic exclusion, because only one chromosome contributes the H chain gene product (Schatz and Ji 2011; Vettermann and Schlissel 2010). Similarly, only one of the L chain genes, κ or λ, is expressed during normal B cell

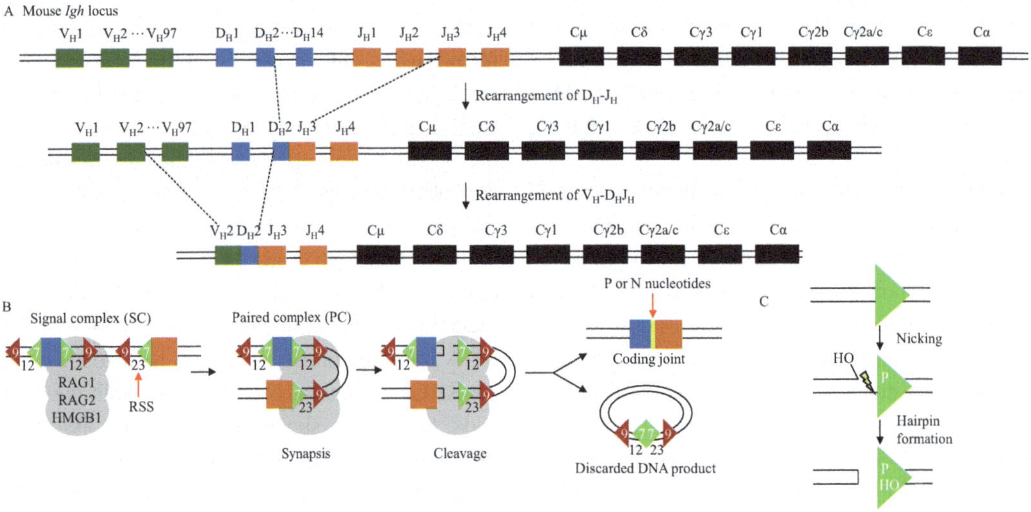

Fig. 1.2 Schematic representation of V(D)J recombination in the mouse *Igh* locus. **a**. In this hypothetical example, D_H2 has joined to J_H3, and then V_H2 has joined to D_H2J_H3. **b**. A single recombination signal sequence (RSS) can be recognized by a RAG1/RAG2/HMGB1 complex and form a signal complex (SC), which then captures another RSS to form the paired complex (PC). Nicking can occur in the SC or PC, but hairpin formation can occur only in the context of the PC. After cleavage, hairpin coding ends and blunt signal ends are processed by the non-homologous end-joining pathway, creating an imperfectly joined coding joint (imperfect joining contains P- or N-nucleotides indicated by the yellow section between coding gene segments) and a discarded DNA product. **c**. Two steps of RAG-mediated DNA cleavage including nicking and hairpin formation. The triangle depicts RSS, and the flanking coding gene segment is omitted for clarity. HO, hydroxyl group

development. (Some exceptional situations will be discussed in the section on B cell central tolerance.)

1.2.3 B Cell Receptor Expression and Tonic Signaling

After $V_HD_HJ_H$ recombination of the *Igh* locus is successfully completed, an intact μ HC protein can be synthesized. Such a free μ HC would usually be retained in the endoplasmic reticulum (ER) as part of the ER quality control system. However, the μ HC in pre-B cells can be expressed at low levels on the cell surface because it associates with a surrogate light chain (SLC), which is composed of two proteins, VpreB and λ5. Two μ HCs and two SLCs plus the Igα/Igβ signaling heterodimer form the pre-BCR, which is expressed transiently to test the functionality of this particular $V_HD_HJ_H$-Cμ combination. The pre-BCR triggers an intracellular signal to inform the cell that the μ HC protein is successfully expressed and associated with the SLCs. If the Ig HC gene rearrangement is unsuccessful or the μ HC fails to associate with the SLC, $V_HD_HJ_H$ recombination will ensue on the other *Igh* allele. This newly generated μ HC protein undergoes the same process of quality testing through the pre-BCR. Failure of Ig HC rearrangement on both chromosomes occurs in about half of the pre-B cells, which will be eliminated by apoptotic death. If the pre-B cell generates a functional pre-BCR, it will promote proliferation and *Igκ* or *Igλ* rearrangement; typically, the *Igκ* locus rearranges first. Only B cells with fully functional H and L chains can survive to become immature B cells. A BCR complex on the B cell surface, which contains two functional H and L chains plus the Igα/Igβ signaling heterodimer, delivers an intracellular signal that terminates all Ig locus rearrangements and mediates central tolerance at the same time. Moreover, both pre-BCR and mature BCR can also generate low-level tonic survival signals through a ligand-independent pathway, termed tonic (pre-)BCR signaling, to support (pre-)B cell survival and further development. Furthermore, the tonic (pre-)BCR signal also plays an important role in B cell carcinogenesis. However, the mechanisms for the initiation of tonic (pre-)BCR signaling are still not fully understood. Based on the existing data, three models have been suggested, namely the homotypic pre-BCR-binding model, lipid raft compartmentalization model and equilibrium model (reviewed in Monroe 2004).

1.3 B-2 Cell Development and Maturation

The majority of B-2 cells originate from the multipotent hematopoietic stem cells (HSCs) in the BM; therefore, the BM microenvironment has a major influence on their development. When an immature B cell starts migrating into the periphery via the bloodstream, it first becomes a transitional B cell and finally differentiates into a FOB or MZB. Only a fraction of BM transitional B cells differentiate into B-1 cells.

1.3.1 BM Microenvironment

BM stromal cells create distinct microenvironments, known as niches, which provide support for self-renewal and differentiation of HSCs into mature blood cells. Although B cell development is known to occur in the niches, their functional organization remains unclear. Some important environmental factors supplied by the cellular niches maintain B cell development.

The adult BM niches contain several cell types associated with HSC development. Osteoblasts generate bone and control the differentiation of HSCs, endothelial cells line the blood vessels and also regulate HSC differentiation, reticular cells mediate processes connecting cells to bone and blood vessels, and sympathetic neurons control the release of hematopoietic cells from the BM. The BM is densely packed with stromal cells and hematopoietic cells of every BM lineage and at every stage of differentiation. With age, however, fat cells gradually replace

50% or more of the BM compartment, and the efficiency of hematopoiesis decreases. The lineage choices that an HSC makes depend largely on the environmental signals it receives. Several microenvironmental components that act on B cell precursors have been identified. CXC chemokine ligand 12 (CXCL12), FLT3 ligand (FLT3L), interleukin-7 (IL-7), stem cell factor (SCF) and receptor activator of nuclear factor-κB ligand (RANKL) have each been shown to be essential for B cell development in vivo.

The main physiological receptor for CXCL12 is CXC chemokine receptor 4 (CXCR4). The CXCL12–CXCR4 axis is essential for the earliest stages of B cell development in the fetus and adult (Nagasawa 2006; Nagasawa et al. 1996; Tokoyoda et al. 2004). FLT3L is a ligand for FTL3, which is essential for the development of pre-pro-B cells (Sitnicka et al. 2002; Sitnicka et al. 2003; Hunte et al. 1996). The receptor for IL-7 is comprised of two chains: IL-7Rα and the cytokine receptor common γ-chain. IL-7 can induce the expression of MCL1 to mediate the survival of B cell precursors (Opferman et al. 2003). IL-7Rα has been shown to deliver a signal that specifically induces VDJ recombination at the *Igh* locus (Corcoran et al. 1998). SCF is a ligand for the class III receptor tyrosine kinase KIT and is encoded by a gene that maps to the steel locus of mice. Cells expressing membrane-bound SCF might function as a niche for pro-B and pre-B cells (Driessen et al. 2003). The transmembrane protein RANKL is a tumor necrosis factor (TNF) family member that is essential for the development of osteoclasts and for bone remodeling. The receptor for RANKL is RANK, which belongs to TNF receptor (TNFR) family and is expressed by DCs, T cells and osteoclast precursors. RANKL expression by lymphoid cells is important for the development of pre-B cells and immature B cells (Kong et al. 1999; Anderson et al. 1997).

It is worth noting that most of the preceding information about the BM microenvironment is derived from studies done in mice. Although its general features are likely also true for humans, the requirements for B cell development are not completely identical in the two species. For example, IL-7 is essential for both T and B cell developments in mice, but only for T cell development in humans (Prieyl and LeBien 1996).

1.3.2 Stages of B Cell Development and Important Transcription Factors

The major stages of B cell development in the BM include the HSC, the multipotent progenitor (MPP), the common lymphoid progenitor (CLP), and then the progenitor B cell (pro-B cell), the precursor B cell (pre-B cell) and the immature B cell. Hardy et al. have elegantly shown that B cell developmental stages can be divided into fractions A, B, C, C′, D and E. Ig gene

Cell stage		Status of Ig genes	Surface Ig	AA4.1	B220	CD43	HSA	BP-1	C-Kit	IL-7Ra	CD19	CD25
Pre-pro B	Fraction A	Germ line arrangement	None	+	+	+	+	-	+	+	-	-
Early pro B	Fraction B	D_HJ_H	None	+	+	+	++	-	++	++	+	-
Late pro B	Fraction C	Some $V_HD_HJ_H$	None	+	+	+	++	-	++	++	+	-
Large pre B	Fraction C'	$V_HD_HJ_H$	Pre-BCR	+	+	+	+++	+	++	++	+	+
Small pre B	Fraction D	$V_HD_HJ_H$ & V_LJ_L arrangement	Decreased Pre-BCR	+	+	-	+++	+	-	++	+	+
Immature B	Fraction E	$V_HD_HJ_H$ & V_LJ_L	IgM-BCR	+	+	-	+++	-	-	-	+	-
Mature B	Fraction F	$V_HD_HJ_H$ & V_LJ_L	IgM-BCR IgD-BCR	-	+	-	+	-	-	-	+	-

Fig. 1.3 Ig gene rearrangements and expression of marker proteins during B cell development

rearrangement status and the expression of several defining cell surface proteins during these stages of B cell development are shown in Fig. 1.3.

With the expression of the B cell lineage-specific marker B220 (CD45R) and the increased expression of the transcription factor EBF1, the developing cell enters pre-pro-B cell stage or fraction A. EBF1, along with E2A, binds to the *Igh* locus, promoting D_HJ_H recombination. Moreover, EBF1 is also essential for the expression of many B cell-associated proteins, including Igα (CD79a), Igβ (CD79b), and the genes encoding the pre-BCR. Pre-pro-B cells remain in contact with CXCL12-secreting stromal cells in the BM. But, after the successful D_HJ_H recombination, which means the cell enters the early pro-B cell stage or fraction B, the developing cell moves within the BM in search of IL-7-secreting stromal cells. Meanwhile, the expression of PAX5, which is one of the EBF1 transcriptional targets, blocks the expression of non-B lineage genes. In addition, many important B cell genes are turned on at this stage, under the control of PAX5 and other transcription factors. During this stage, one of the defining markers of B lineage cells and an important component of the (pre-)B cell co-receptor, CD19, is expressed. In addition, PAX5 promotes V_H to D_H recombination by contracting the *Igh* locus, bringing the V_H gene segments and the D_HJ_H region into closer proximity. Then, the developing B cell enters the late pro-B cell stage or fraction C and most cells have initiated V_H to D_HJ_H Ig gene segment recombination, which is completed by the onset of the early pre-B cell stage. During the pro-B-cell stage or fractions A-C, Igα and Igβ, which are signaling components of the BCR, begin to be expressed, and the expression of c-Kit enables the cell to receive signals from stem cell factor. However, by the beginning of the pre-B cell stage, the expression of c-Kit is irreversibly turned off.

After successful $V_HD_HJ_H$ recombination, the cell expresses a pre-BCR, which is composed of the rearranged μ heavy chain, complexed with VpreB and λ5 plus Igα and Igβ. The developing B cell enters the large proliferating pre-B cell stage or fraction C′. This is an important checkpoint, and only cells with a productively rearranged heavy chain can be selected into the next stage. The pre-BCR is then lost from the surface, and this signals entry into the small/late pre-B cell stage or fraction D. At this stage, light chain rearrangement is initiated with the re-expression of the *Rag1/2* genes. In the mouse, light chain rearrangement begins on one of the κ chain chromosomes, followed by the other. If neither κ chain rearrangement is successful, rearrangement is then attempted on each of the λ chain chromosomes. At the same time, there is very little expression of TdT and therefore N region addition occurs less frequently in light chains than in heavy chains. After successful light chain gene rearrangement and expression, the integrated IgM receptor (BCR) is expressed on the cell surface, which means the developing B cell enters the immature B cell stage or fraction E.

Throughout B cell development, PU.1 sets the stage for lymphoid and myeloid development, and lineage priming in lymphoid progenitors is mediated by Ikaros. In addition, E2A regulates the chromatin landscape to promote gene expression during B cell development and EBF1 plays an important role as a central coordinator of B cell development, collaborating with FOXO1.

1.3.3 B Cell Central Tolerance

There are three mechanisms of central B cell tolerance, clonal deletion, receptor editing and anergy. If an immature B cell recognizes a self-antigen that is present at high concentration in the BM, its BCRs are cross-linked, delivering a strong signal to the cell. In this case, the B cell may undergo apoptosis, a process called clonal deletion. Alternatively, such a B cell may reactivate RAG1 and RAG2 expression and initiate a new round of V_LJ_L recombination. A Vκ segment upstream of the originally rearranged VκJκ unit is joined to a downstream Jκ. As a result, the former rearranged VκJκ exon in the self-reactive immature B cell is deleted and a new Ig light chain is expressed, thus creating a B cell receptor with a new, potentially no longer autoreactive, specificity. This process is called receptor editing. If the edited light chain rearrangement is nonproductive, rearrangement may proceed at the other κ locus, and if that is also nonproductive, rearrangements at the λ light chain loci may follow. Finally, if the receptors on the developing B cell recognize self-antigens with low affinity, the cells may become functionally unresponsive or anergic, due to downregulation of BCR expression and BCR signaling. In principle, receptor editing at the *Igh* locus is not possible, since there are no germ line D_H gene segments available for further VDJ rearrangement; all were deleted during the original V→DJ rearrangement step. However, a "cryptic" RSS heptamer is present in many V_H genes and can be used in a process called V_H gene replacement, in which an upstream V_H gene segment recombines with the cryptic heptamer, replacing most of the V region in a preexisting VDJ exon. Whether this process is more important for diversification than for central B cell tolerance is somewhat controversial, since it appears to occur mainly in pre-B cells that have not yet undergone light chain gene rearrangement and thus their antigen specificity has not yet been defined (Kumar et al. 2015; Sun et al. 2015; Kelsoe 2015).

David Nemazee and colleagues generated mice transgenic for both a heavy and a light chain specific for the H-$2K^k$ MHC molecule. In mice with H-$2K^d$ but no H-$2K^k$ MHC molecules, the transgenic BCR was expressed on B cells and a high concentration of transgenic antibody could be measured in the serum. However, in mice with H-$2K^k$ but no H-$2K^d$ MHC molecule, no anti-H-$2K^k$ B cells or secreted antibodies could be detected, suggesting that all immature B cells bearing the potentially autoimmune BCR had been deleted in the BM. Interestingly, in mice with both H-$2K^d$ and H-$2K^k$ MHC, not all B cells bearing the autoimmune transgenes were deleted, and some of them underwent light chain receptor editing and no longer bound the H-$2K^k$ antigen (Nemazee and Bürki 1989; Tiegs et al. 1993).

Goodnow and colleagues developed double-transgenic mice carrying transgenes encoding membrane hen egg white lysozyme (mHEL) driven by a class I MHC promoter and anti-HEL BCR, which mimics the situation of a self-antigen and a corresponding autoreactive BCR. B cells in double-transgenic mice were arrested at the pre-B stage and underwent efficient clonal deletion, with few B cells reaching the periphery (Hartley et al. 1993). However, when the mHEL transgene in double-transgenic mice was replaced by a soluble HEL (sHEL) transgene linked to a metallothionein promoter and sHEL was expressed in the periphery, but not in the BM, the double-transgenic mice were able to generate mature, peripheral B cells bearing the anti-HEL BCR. However, these B cells were functionally nonresponsive, or anergic, a mechanism called B cell peripheral tolerance (Cyster et al. 1994). Based on these results, it appears that in normal animals, not all self-reactive B cells are deleted in the BM. Some are released to the periphery but are inactivated. It has been suggested that such cells could be abnormally reactivated by non-BCR-mediated signals, resulting in their differentiation into plasma cells and resultant antibody-mediated autoimmune diseases.

1.3.4 B-2 Cell Maturation in the Periphery

1.3.4.1 Transitional B Cells

Immature B cells have a short half-life and are ready for export to the peripheral lymphoid organs, usually the spleen, where they complete their developmental program. During B-2 cell maturation in the periphery, transitional B cells play an important role in linking BM immature and peripheral mature B cells. Moreover, transitional B cells express similar defining cell surface markers, such as AA4.1, HSA and IgM, as immature B cells, and are still susceptible to negative selection.

Newly generated immature B cells that have yet to acquire the ability to recirculate throughout the body are known as T1 B cells. They are found in the BM and the periarteriolar lymphoid sheath (PALS) of spleen and are $AA4.1^+$ IgM^{high} IgD^- $CD21^-$ $CD23^-$. After entering spleen follicles, they acquire cell surface IgD, CD21 and CD23 and the ability to recirculate, but still carry markers of immaturity and are known as T2 B cells. T3 is a third non-proliferating transitional population, which resembles T2 with the exception of a lower level of surface IgM. Recent experiments have suggested that the T3 population may represent B cells that have been rendered anergic by contact with soluble self-antigen but have not yet been eliminated from the B cell repertoire. These transitional B cells can be distinguished by different combinations of surface markers (Allman and Pillai 2008). Studies of the signal transduction pathways in the transitional B cells compared to mature B cells after BCR ligation have identified significant functional differences. T1 and T2 B cells do not proliferate or upregulate the co-stimulatory molecule CD86 in response to BCR stimulation and are susceptible to apoptosis. Thus, the early transitional stages comprise an important peripheral tolerance checkpoint. Despite their muted response to BCR stimulation, gene knockout studies, such as in mice lacking BLNK, PLCγ or BAFF, provide convincing evidence for the importance of intact BCR-mediated signals to drive progression from the transitional B cell stages to the mature B cell stage (Chung et al. 2003).

1.3.4.2 Follicular and Marginal Zone B Cells

The different BCR signaling pathways integrated with BAFFR and Notch2 signaling, as well as signals that mediate their migration and retention, determine the commitment of B cells from the transitional B cell to the mature FOB or MZB cell fate (Pillai and Cariappa 2009; Cerutti et al. 2013). The phenotype and function of FOB and MZB are summarized in Fig. 1.4.

Tonic or even strong BCR signaling, a BAFF survival signal and NF-κB signaling are necessary for the transitional B cell to develop into FOB, which are located in primary follicles and also recirculate via blood and lymphatics into secondary lymphoid organs and back into the BM. FOB tend to have more diversity of Ig V(D)J genes than do MZB. In addition, the main function of FOB is to mediate adaptive Ab production. FOB interact with helper T cells to form germinal centers, undergo class switch recombination (CSR) and somatic hypermutation (SHM) and eventually produce high-affinity antibodies to eliminate pathogens or give rise to memory B cells that function to prevent the reinfection with the same pathogen.

Weak BCR signaling (above and beyond tonic signaling), NF-κB signals and Notch2 signaling are important for the transitional B cell to develop into the MZB, which reside in the outer white pulp of the spleen between the marginal sinus and the red pulp. In the spleen, the Notch2 ligand delta-like 1 (DL1), which is present at high concentrations in venules but is not found in the BM, is a key activator accounting for MZB development. In addition, migration and retention of MZB to the follicles are mediated by the sphingosine 1-phosphate receptor (S1PR1) and CXC chemokine ligand 13 (CXCL13). Although MZB cells seem to primarily express nonmutated Ig V(D)J genes, some other cells, such as DCs, macrophages and iNKT cells, can trigger CSR in MZB. Unlike FOB, MZB constitutively express elevated levels of MHC class

Subsets	Surface markers	Location	Functions
Follicular B	$CD19^{+}$ $B220^{+}$ IgM^{dull} IgD^{hi} $CD21^{mid}$ $CD23^{+}$	Recirculating cell, which can be found in spleen, lymph node and bone marrow and other tissues	1. Main component of the T cell-dependent B cell adaptive immune response 2. Give rise to high affinity antibody-producing PC
Marginal zone B	$CD19^{+}$ $B220^{+}$ IgM^{hi} IgD^{dull} $CD1d^{hi}$ $CD21^{hi}$ $CD23^{-}$	Lining outside the marginal sinus and bordering the red pulp	1. Natural Ab secretion 2. T cell-dependent and -independent responses to blood-borne pathogens

Fig. 1.4 Phenotypes and function of follicular B and marginal zone B cells

II and CD80 and CD86 molecules and display a robust antigen-presenting activity, which is required for the activation of T follicular helper (TFH) cells. Moreover, MZB can also rapidly respond to blood-borne antigens and differentiate into short-lived plasmablasts that produce large amounts of IgM. Therefore, the MZB is considered as a gatekeeper to perform surveillance between the conventional boundaries of innate and adaptive immunity.

1.3.5 B Cell Peripheral Tolerance

In peripheral tissues, mature B lymphocytes that recognize self-antigens in the absence of specific helper T cells may become anergic and/or die by apoptosis. However, most of the mechanisms of peripheral tolerance are reversible because of the potential need for mature B cells to respond to viruses and microorganisms that may carry similar epitopes to self-antigens.

If a self-reactive B cell is repeatedly stimulated by self-antigens, it becomes anergic to further activation. Such cells require high levels of the growth factor BAFF for survival and thus cannot compete efficiently with less BAFF-dependent normal naive B cells for survival in lymphoid follicles. Therefore, these B cells that have encountered self-antigens have a shortened life span and are rapidly eliminated. B cells that bind with high avidity to self-antigens in the periphery may also undergo apoptotic death by the mitochondrial pathway independent of growth factor dependence. The risk of generating peripheral self-reactivity is higher for B cells than T cells because B cells, uniquely, can undergo a high rate of somatic mutation of Ig V genes in germinal centers. These B cells may be actively eliminated via the interaction of Fas on the activated B cells with FasL on helper T cells. Failure of peripheral B cell tolerance may lead to autoimmunity, as observed in Fas- and FasL-deficient mice. On the other hand, B cells that recognize self-antigens with low affinity may be prevented from activation by the engagement of various inhibitory receptors. These inhibitory receptors act to set a threshold for B cell activation, which allows responses to foreign antigens with T cell help or innate immune responses but does not allow responses to self-antigens. This mechanism of peripheral tolerance was revealed by studies showing that mice with defects in the SHP-1 tyrosine phosphatase or the CD22 inhibitory receptor develop autoimmunity. Immunoreceptor tyrosine-based inhibitory motifs (ITIM) in the cytoplasmic tail of CD22 are phosphorylated by LYN, and this inhibitory receptor then recruits SHP-1, thus attenuating B cell receptor signaling. Moreover, foreign antigens systemically administered at high doses also preferentially induce tolerance rather than immune responses (Klinman 1996).

1.4 Development of B-1 Cells

B-1 cells, which are considered to be an innate-like B cell population, have distinct developmental process, unique phenotype, anatomic location, self-renewing capacity and functional characteristics from conventional B-2 cells (Hoffmann et al. 2007; Witt et al. 2003; Berland and Wortis 2002). It has been nearly 40 years since B-1 cells were first identified in mouse spleen in the early 1980s; these cells expressed Ly-1 (now known as CD5), a pan T cell surface glycoprotein (Hayakawa et al. 1983). Later studies found a second subset of B-1 cells, now termed B-1b cells, which did not express CD5 but showed similar phenotypic and histologic features as the $CD5^+$ B-1a cells (Stall et al. 1992; Kantor et al. 1992). B-1 cells mainly reside in pleural and peritoneal cavities, whereas there are few B-1 cells in peripheral lymph nodes (LNs), and the frequency of B-1 cells in spleen is low (Hayakawa et al. 1985; Hardy et al. 1984). We can now use a combination of different cell surface markers to distinguish B-1a and B-1b: $CD5^+$ $CD11b^{+/-}B220^{lo}$ IgM^{hi} IgD^{lo} $CD23^-$ $CD43^+$ for B-1a cells and $CD5^-$ $B220^{lo}$ IgM^{hi} IgD^{lo} $CD23^-$ $CD43^+$ for B-1b cells (reviewed in Prieto and Felippe 2017).

1.4.1 B-1 Cell Developmental Model

B-1 cells function in natural antibody secretion, cytokine production and maintenance of tissue homeostasis, and therefore it is important and essential to understand their development during ontogeny. Yolk sac is the first site of hematopoiesis at day 7 in mouse embryo, while HSCs first emerge in the aorta-gonado-mesonephros (AGM) region at embryonic day 10.5 (Weissman et al. 1977; Moore and Metcalf 1970; Müller et al. 1994; Yoshimoto et al. 2011). HSCs migrate to the fetal liver, where they dramatically expand, and finally they settle in spleen and BM before birth (Morrison et al. 1995; Ikuta and Weissman 1992). It is well known that HSCs in BM are able to differentiate into the common myeloid progenitors (CMPs) and CLPs. The CMPs give rise to neutrophils, basophils, eosinophils, monocyte/macrophages, erythrocytes and myeloid dendritic cells. The CLPs further develop into B lymphocytes, T lymphocytes, innate lymphoid cells and lymphoid dendritic cells (Seita and Weissman 2010; Kondo et al. 1997; Akashi et al. 2000). An increasing number of studies have revealed that there are several waves of hematopoietic cell emergence during embryogenesis including primitive hematopoietic progenitors and HSCs (Yoshimoto 2015). The first wave is termed primitive hematopoiesis, during which red blood cells are produced to provide oxygen for embryonic growth. However, the primitive hematopoietic system is transient and is rapidly replaced upon HSC emergence (Yoshimoto 2015; Orkin and Zon 2008). In essence, the origin of B-1 cells has been a controversy for decades and has centered on two hypotheses regarding their origin and their developmental relationship with B-2 cells: lineage model and selection model.

1.4.2 Lineage Model

In 1989, Herzenberg et al. put forward the lineage model, in which distinct progenitors generate B-2 and B-1 cells, respectively, at different times during development (Herzenberg and Herzenberg 1989). Many experiments support this conjecture. Studies have suggested that an "ontological switch" occurs during B cell development, and a similar process has been described for the development of erythrocytes and γδT cells (Hardy and Hayakawa 1991; Ikuta et al. 1990).

Transfer experiments demonstrated that B cell progenitors in fetal liver were able to give rise to both B-1 and B-2 cells while adult BM transplant failed to repopulate the B-1a cell compartment of lethally irradiated mice (Hayakawa et al. 1985; Ghosn et al. 2012). Similarly, in chimeric mice made by reconstitution with a mix of adult BM and fetal liver, B-1 cells were almost exclusively derived from fetal liver, while B-2 cells were derived from either BM or fetal liver (Herzenberg 2000). Subsequent studies indicated that B-1a progenitors were found mainly in fetal liver, while B-1b progenitors were found principally in adult BM (Kantor et al. 1992; Montecino-Rodriguez et al. 2006; Hardy and Hayakawa 1991). Moreover, in B cell depletion chimeras, endogenous progenitor cells were able to develop into B-2 cells but only a small number of B-1 cells (mainly B-1b) (Hamilton and Kearney 1994; Lalor et al. 1989a, b). Solvason and Godin et al. have shown that embryonic para-aortic splanchnopleura and fetal omentum contained progenitors that could give rise to B-1a and B-1b cells but not conventional B cells (Godin et al. 1993; Solvason et al. 1991, 1992). However, further research made clear that some B-1 progenitor cells originated from primitive B-2 progenitor cells in adult BM (Esplin et al. 2009).

While these results indirectly suggested the independent origin of B-1 and B-2 cells, the most direct evidence supporting the lineage hypothesis was the discovery of B-1 cell precursors. In 2006, abundant B-1 B cell progenitors phenotypically distinct from progenitors for B-2 cells were identified in fetal BM. These Lin^{-} $CD45R^{lo-neg}$ $CD19^{+}$ cells emerged during the late stage of embryonic development (Montecino-Rodriguez et al. 2006). Further study demonstrated that B-1a precursors with the phenotype $CD5^+$ $CD45R^{lo}$ IgM^{hi} were found at day 8.5–9.0 in the mouse embryo, but not B-1b or B-2 cell precursors (Godin et al. 1993).

Additional evidence supporting the lineage model is that B-1 cells display much more limited diversity than B-2 cells. In contrast to B-2 cells, Ig repertoires of B-1 cells tend to be more restricted and autoreactive (Tornberg and Holmberg 1995). Studies showed that B-1 cells preferred to use certain V(D)J genes in their Igs (Mercolino et al. 1989; Kantor et al. 1997). About 50% of B-1 cells derived from fetal liver progenitors had no N-nucleotide insertions at either the D_H or J_H junction because of low expression of TdT, whereas N-nucleotide insertions increased in B-1a and B-1b cells derived from B cell progenitors in adult BM (Holodick et al. 2014; Prieto and Felippe 2017). The biological consequences of these differences in N addition were shown in studies where TdT expression in fetal liver was forced by transgenesis. Compared to WT mice, the TdT transgenic mice with more N-nucleotide insertions in fetal B cells were more sensitive to pneumococcal infection (Benedict and Kearney 1999). This study indicated that B-1 cells with lower Ig diversity in fetal life are essential for the normal adult immune response to infection.

1.4.3 Selection Model

Unlike the lineage model, which postulates that B-1 cells and B-2 cells are derived from distinct progenitors, the selection model proposes that all B cells originate from the same progenitor cells but that the antigen specificity of the B cell receptor determines the B cell differentiation fate (Baumgarth 2011; Ratcliffe 2016).

It is well known that the Ig repertoires of B-1 and B-2 cells are clearly different (Lalor and Morahan 1990). B-1a cells are known to produce autoantibodies, such as antibodies against single-stranded DNA, Thy-1, red blood cells, oxidized lipids including phosphatidyl choline (PtC) and rheumatoid factor, whereas such autoantibodies are rarely produced by B-2 cells (Casali et al. 1987; Hardy et al. 1987; Mercolino et al. 1988). These lines of evidence suggest that autoantigens might be the major driving force for repertoire selection of B-1 cells. In addition, B-1 cells that specifically recognize PtC account for a large proportion of B-1 cells in the peritoneal cavity of adult mice (Mercolino et al. 1986, 1988; Arnold and Haughton 1992). Further studies showed that these cells utilize a restricted set of Ig variable genes (in C57BL/6 mice, B-1 cells mainly use V_H12 paired with $V_\kappa 4$ or V_H11 with $V_\kappa 9$) (Mercolino et al. 1988; Arnold and Haughton 1992; Hardy et al. 1989; Arnold et al. 1994). Moreover, Hayakawa et al. showed that there were no Thy-1-specific B-1 cells or anti-Thy-1 antibodies in Thy-1 knockout mice (Hayakawa et al. 1999, 2003). These observations provided very strong evidence that B-1 cells were selected for self-reactivity.

As discussed above, the strength of the BCR signal can affect the development of B-1 cells. The number of B-1 cells is significantly reduced in mice with impaired BCR signaling. On the other hand, mutations of negative regulators such as CD22 or CD72, which lead to increased BCR signaling, in general promote B-1 cell development and inhibit the development of B-2 cells (reviewed in Berland and Wortis 2002).

Mice transgenic for B-1-derived BCR (V_H12 alone or in combination with $V\kappa 4$) developed mostly B-1 cells, which is consistent with the hypothesis that BCR specificity plays an important role in the development of B-1 cells (Arnold et al. 1994). In addition, Lam and Rajewsky reported that BCR specificity and surface density influenced differentiation into these subsets (Lam and Rajewsky 1999). Very recently, by using an inducible mouse model, Graf et al. were able to change BCR specificity in transgenic mice in vivo and elegantly demonstrated that B-2 cells were able to differentiate into B-1 cells upon switching of their BCR to one typical of a self-reactive BCR from B-1 cells (Graf et al. 2019). These induced B-1 cells not only expressed typical surface markers but also obtained the functional characteristics of B-1 cells. However, in their system, B-1 cells could scarcely be transformed into B-2 cells. These results provide concrete evidence that BCR specificity determines the B-1 versus B-2 cell lineage choice.

1.4.4 Two-Pathway Model

Despite accumulating evidence, the origin and development of B-1 cells are still controversial. Studies have shown that there is feedback inhibition of B-1 development. Peripheral B-1 cell pools are generated during late embryonic life and a few weeks after birth, then they are maintained by self-renewal, and further de novo B-1 cell development is inhibited (reviewed in Berland and Wortis 2002, Herzenberg 2000). Furthermore, recent studies revealed that Lin28b is a master regulator of B-1 cell development in fetal but not in adult hematopoiesis. Lin28b, first identified in *Caenorhabditis elegans*, acts to block the maturation of let-7 family microRNAs and the emergence of their active forms (Shyh-Chang and Daley 2013). The data in mice showed that in neonates Lin28b functioned to promote positive selection of self-reactive B-1 cells, similarly in adult mice that overexpress Lin28b (Chung et al. 2012; Poe et al. 2012; Benhamou et al. 2016; Vanhee et al. 2019). BM stem cells overexpressing Lin28b were able to give rise to B-1a cells, but their BCR repertoire was different from that found in conventional B-1a cells (Yuan et al. 2012; Zhou et al. 2015). These results suggested that the reciprocal expression of Lin28b and let-7 (the Lin28b levels are high in fetal and low in adult HSCs) controls the timing of developmental events. Recent studies proposed that the lineage model and selection model both occur to ensure the generation and maintenance of B-1 cells throughout life (Hardy and Hayakawa 2015; Baumgarth 2011). Revealing the origin of B-1 cells is a very interesting area of research that can also help us better understand the role of these cells.

1.4.5 Regulation of B-1a vs B-1b Cell Development

B-1a cells are the main producer of poly-reactive and autoreactive natural IgM antibodies, which are involved in the clearance of apoptotic cells and their nuclear and cytoplasmic components (Jellusova et al. 2010). Failure to eliminate apoptotic cells can lead to autoantibody production (Hanayama et al. 2004). Paradoxically, expansion of B-1a cells was found to be associated with autoimmunity (Duan and Morel 2006; Binder and Silverman 2005). On the other hand, B-1b cells were shown to respond specifically to T-independent antigens. Adoptive transfer experiments showed that B-1b cells mediated long-lasting IgM memory to infection (Cunningham et al. 2014). Both peritoneal B-1a and B-1b cells are important for host defense against pathogens that enter the peritoneum through the gut epithelium (Roy et al. 2013). Despite the functional differences between B-1a and B-1b cells, little is known about the developmental relationship between these two subsets. Hoffmann et al. have demonstrated that Siglec-G is a B-1 cell inhibitory receptor that controls expansion of the B-1a cells (Hoffmann et al. 2007). We have recently found that Kelch-like 14 (KLHL14) promotes B-1a development in mice (Li et al. 2018).

A model has been proposed for the regulation of B-1a and B-1b development (Hardy 2006). In this model, the B-1 progenitor may develop into either a B-1a or a B-1b cell, depending on the strength of BCR signal triggered by self-antigen. B-1 precursors expressing BCR that bind to self-antigen strongly and thus trigger strong BCR signals become B-1a cells, whereas B-1 precursors expressing BCR that bind to self-antigen with intermediate strength develop into B-1b cells. In support of this model, mice overexpressing CD19 generated primarily B-1a cells whereas CD19-deficient mice generated mainly B-1b cells (Haas et al. 2005). In addition, mice lacking NCK, an adaptor protein that recruits

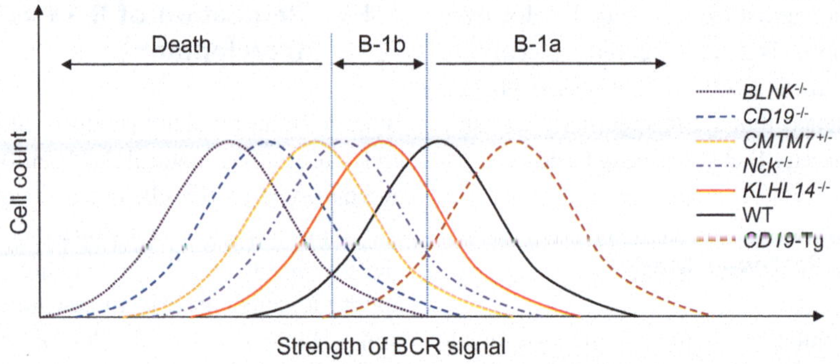

Fig. 1.5 Relationship between the strength of BCR signaling and the development of B-1a and B-1b cells. The graph is based on a previously suggested model for B-1a/B-1b development (Hardy 2006), along with the results of mice deficient for or overexpressing CD19 (Haas et al. 2005), mice deficient for BLNK (Pappu et al. 1999) or NCK (Castello et al. 2013), mice heterozygous for CMTM7 (Zhang et al. 2014) and *KLHL14*$^{-/-}$ mice (Li et al. 2018). *Source* Adapted from Li et al. (2018)

BCAP to the BCR, or mice heterozygous for CMTM7, had reduced B-1a but increased B-1b cells (Castello et al. 2013; Zhang et al. 2014; Liu et al. 2019). Furthermore, mice lacking the B cell linker protein (BLNK) had a severe reduction of both B-1a and B-1b cells (Pappu et al. 1999), suggesting that very weak BCR signal inhibits the development of both B-1a and B-1b cells. Figure 1.5 illustrates the relationship between the strength of BCR signaling and the development of B-1a and B-1b cells (Li et al. 2018).

1.4.6 The Functions of B-1 Cells

1.4.6.1 Natural Antibody Secretion

Antibodies that spontaneously appear without any external antigenic stimulation, such as in antigen-free mice, are referred to as natural antibodies (Tlaskalová-Hogenová et al. 1992; Coutinho et al. 1995). B-1 cells are able to produce natural antibodies, mainly IgM, IgA and IgG3. Actually, B-1 cells produce about 80% of natural IgM, which forms a pentamer and has low affinity but high poly-reactivity and complement activation ability. Several studies revealed that sIgM$^{-/-}$mice (mice that lack secretory IgM) were more sensitive to pathogen infection (Baumgarth et al. 2000; Boes et al. 1998b; Subramaniam et al. 2010). These results demonstrated that IgM, as the first and crucial barrier, plays an important role in protection against pathogen invasion prior to the establishment of adaptive responses (Fearon and Locksley 1996; Baumgarth et al. 1999). Moreover, sIgM$^{-/-}$mice were reported to have low levels of B-2-dependent IgG responses to antigens, consistent with the results reported in FcμR knockout mice (Baumgarth et al. 2000; Boes et al. 1998a; Ouchida et al. 2012). These data suggested that an IgM-FcμR signal might participate in enhancing IgG responses. B-1 cells could be induced to undergo CSR in vitro, preferentially generating IgA and Ig subclasses (Kaminski and Stavnezer 2006; Tarlinton et al. 1995). Natural poly-reactive IgA is abundant in the intestinal mucosa, where it acts to maintain a homeostatic environment between host and microbiota (Smith and Baumgarth 2019). Until now, we know less about the function of natural IgG3, although one study showed that it was able to protect individuals from *P. aeruginosa* infection (Panda et al. 2013).

1.4.6.2 Pathogen Defense

We are surrounded by a variety of pathogens including bacteria, viruses, fungi and parasites. As discussed in 1.4.6.1, B-1 cells are capable of secreting natural antibodies to protect from infection. Upon pathogen invasion, B-1 cells migrate to the secondary lymphoid tissues and then differentiate into antibody-secreting cells (Choi et al. 2012; Kawahara et al. 2003).

However, B-1 cells might have opposite function. For example, during nematode parasite infection, B-1 cell-derived IgE downregulated the degranulation of mast cells, thereby impeding parasite expulsion, which results in part from smooth muscle contraction induced by mediators contained in the mast cell granules (Martin et al. 2018). B-1 cells may have other functions. Recent studies revealed that B-1 cells were able to secrete several kinds of cytokines. Natural or induced IL-10 produced by B-1 cells contributes to control the extent of inflammation (Mosser and Zhang 2008; Gonzaga et al. 2015), and B-1 cells can secrete IL-3 and GM-CSF, which promote inflammatory responses (Weber et al. 2015). Similar to B-2 cells, B-1 cells have the ability to present antigens. For example, B-1 cells could present OVA peptide to OVA-specific $CD4^+$ T cells in vivo (Margry et al. 2013). Furthermore, B-1a cells can promote $CD4^+$ T cells to differentiate into Th17 cells (Zhong et al. 2007). In conclusion, in addition to their ability to secrete natural antibodies, B-1 cells are able to secrete cytokines, as well as uptake and present antigens to T cells during pathogen invasion (Novaes E Brito et al. 2019; Smith and Baumgarth 2019).

1.4.6.3 Tissue Homeostasis Maintenance and Autoimmunity

During the process of apoptosis, dead cells release self-antigens such as single-stranded DNA, which B-1 cells can recognize via their BCR. Antibodies secreted by the plasma cell progeny of these B-1 cells are thought to promote phagocytosis, leading to the removal of self-antigens (Chen et al. 2009). Several features of B-1 cells are considered anti-inflammatory; e.g., they are a major source of IL-10, which can suppress inflammatory responses, and they can secrete IgA, which does not activate complement. Thus, IgA-mediated immune responses could avoid complement-mediated tissue damage in the intestinal mucosa (Smith and Baumgarth 2019). B-1 cells and the IgM antibodies they produce play an important role in immune homeostasis. Compared to control mice, lpr mice without secreted IgM showed elevated levels of IgG autoantibodies and severe symptoms of glomerulonephritis along with increased mortality rates (Boes et al. 2000). In contrast, B-1 cells may instead contribute to the development of autoimmune diseases. Following studies indicating that B-1 cells accumulated in the thymus during the developmental of lupus nephritis, Sato and colleagues speculated that these autoreactive B-1 cells, which expressed high levels of co-stimulatory molecules, activate cognate autoreactive T cells, resulting in the production of autoantibodies (Sato et al. 2004). Moreover, studies found that the number of B-1 cells is increased in patients with Sjogren's syndrome and rheumatoid arthritis (Dauphinée et al. 1988; Youinou et al. 1990). Together, these observations suggest a link between B-1 cells and the development of autoimmune diseases.

1.4.7 Human B-1 Cells

Following the discovery of mouse B-1 cells, several studies also found $CD5^+$ B cells in rheumatoid arthritis patients (Casali et al. 1987; Hardy et al. 1987). However, researchers suspected that CD5 cannot be used as a marker to identify human B-1 cells for two major reasons: (1) CD5 can be detected on almost all types of human B cells from immature to memory B cell, especially on activated, transitional and pre-naive B cells (Lee et al. 2009; Sims et al. 2005; Freedman et al. 1989); (2) it was found that $CD5^-$ human B cells could produce natural antibodies like $CD5^+$ cells (Kasaian et al. 1992). Subsequently, Griffin et al. identified a population of B cells in human umbilical cord and peripheral blood with a phenotype of $CD20^+$ $CD27^+$ $CD43^+$ $CD70^-$, which had similar characteristics and functions to mouse B-1 cells (Griffin et al. 2011). However, there are some differences between human and mouse B-1 cells. For example, antibodies produced by human B-1 cells had N-nucleotide insertions and substantial somatic mutations (Rothstein and Quach 2015). There are studies showing that human B-1 cells might develop from Lin^- $CD34^+$ $CD38^{lo}$ stem cells (Quách et al. 2016). However, the origin and tissue distribution of human B-1 cells are not fully understood.

1.5 Conclusion

Although there has been tremendous progress in our understanding of B cell development, maturation and function, many questions still remain to be answered. It is not fully understood how the function of different B cell subsets, including FOB, MZB, B-1a and B-1b cells, is regulated and coordinated during bacterial and viral infections. It is also less clear what B cell subsets contribute to the production of IgA in the gut. An additional intriguing issue is that impaired B cell development not only results in reduced B cell numbers and immunodeficiencies, but frequently causes autoantibody production. Furthermore, less is known about the regulation of human B cell development and maturation. Further studies are needed to fully understand the regulatory mechanisms of B cell development and function in mice and humans.

Acknowledgements We thank Luming Zhang for secretarial assistance, Fudan University Animal Facility for maintaining the mice and the members in Wang Laboratory for helpful suggestions. This work was supported by the Major Research Plan of the National Natural Science Foundation of China (91942302 to J.Y.W.), the National Key R & D Plan of the Ministry of Science and Technology (SQ2019YFE0100600 to J.Y.W.), the National Natural Science Foundation of China (81571529 and 31870898 to J.Y.W), Projects of International Cooperation and Exchanges NSFC (81811540035 to J.Y.W.), a grant-in-aid for scientific research (C) from Japan Society for the Promotion of Science (17K08878 to J.Y.W), China Postdoctoral Science Foundation Grant (2018M641929 to J.L.) and National Natural Science Foundation for Young Scholar (81901594 to J.L.).

References

Akashi K, Traver D, Miyamoto T, Weissman IL (2000) A clonogenic common myeloid progenitor that gives rise to all myeloid lineages. Nature 404(6774):193–197. https://doi.org/10.1038/35004599

Allman D, Pillai S (2008) Peripheral B cell subsets. Curr Opin Immunol 20(2):149–157. https://doi.org/10.1016/j.coi.2008.03.014

Anderson DM, Maraskovsky E, Billingsley WL, Dougall WC, Tometsko ME, Roux ER et al (1997) A homologue of the TNF receptor and its ligand enhance T-cell growth and dendritic-cell function. Nature 390(6656):175–179. https://doi.org/10.1038/36593

Arnold LW, Haughton G (1992) Autoantibodies to phosphatidylcholine. The murine antibromelain RBC response. Ann N Y Acad Sci 651:354–359. https://doi.org/10.1111/j.1749-6632.1992.tb24635.x

Arnold LW, Pennell CA, McCray SK, Clarke SH (1994) Development of B-1 cells: segregation of phosphatidyl choline-specific B cells to the B-1 population occurs after immunoglobulin gene expression. J Exp Med 179(5):1585–1595. https://doi.org/10.1084/jem.179.5.1585

Baumgarth N (2011) The double life of a B-1 cell: self-reactivity selects for protective effector functions. Nat Rev Immunol 11(1):34–46. https://doi.org/10.1038/nri2901

Baumgarth N, Herman OC, Jager GC, Brown L, Herzenberg LA, Herzenberg LA (1999) Innate and acquired humoral immunities to influenza virus are mediated by distinct arms of the immune system. Proc Natl Acad Sci USA 96(5):2250–2255. https://doi.org/10.1073/pnas.96.5.2250

Baumgarth N, Herman OC, Jager GC, Brown LE, Herzenberg LA, Chen J (2000) B-1 and B-2 cell-derived immunoglobulin M antibodies are nonredundant components of the protective response to influenza virus infection. J Exp Med 192(2):271–280. https://doi.org/10.1084/jem.192.2.271

Benedict CL, Kearney JF (1999) Increased junctional diversity in fetal B cells results in a loss of protective anti-phosphorylcholine antibodies in adult mice. Immunity 10(5):607–617. https://doi.org/10.1016/s1074-7613(00)80060-6

Benhamou D, Labi V, Novak R, Dai I, Shafir-Alon S, Weiss A et al (2016) A c-Myc/miR17-92/Pten axis controls PI3K-mediated positive and negative selection in B cell development and reconstitutes CD19 deficiency. Cell Rep 16(2):419–431. https://doi.org/10.1016/j.celrep.2016.05.084

Berland R, Wortis HH (2002) Origins and functions of B-1 cells with notes on the role of CD5. Annu Rev Immunol 20:253–300. https://doi.org/10.1146/annurev.immunol.20.100301.064833

Binder CJ, Silverman GJ (2005) Natural antibodies and the autoimmunity of atherosclerosis. Springer Semin Immunopathol 26(4):385–404. https://doi.org/10.1007/s00281-004-0185-z

Boes M, Esau C, Fischer MB, Schmidt T, Carroll M, Chen J (1998a). Enhanced B-1 cell development, but impaired IgG antibody responses in mice deficient in secreted IgM. J Immunol (Baltimore, MD: 1950) 160(10): 4776–4787. https://www.ncbi.nlm.nih.gov/pubmed/9590224

Boes M, Prodeus AP, Schmidt T, Carroll MC, Chen J (1998b) A critical role of natural immunoglobulin M in immediate defense against systemic bacterial

infection. J Exp Med 188(12):2381–2386. https://doi.org/10.1084/jem.188.12.2381
Boes M, Schmidt T, Linkemann K, Beaudette BC, Marshak-Rothstein A, Chen J (2000) Accelerated development of IgG autoantibodies and autoimmune disease in the absence of secreted IgM. Proc Natl Acad Sci USA 97(3):1184–1189. https://doi.org/10.1073/pnas.97.3.1184
Casali P, Burastero SE, Nakamura M, Inghirami G, Notkins AL (1987) Human lymphocytes making rheumatoid factor and antibody to ssDNA belong to Leu-1+ B-cell subset. Science (New York, NY) 236 (4797):77–81. https://doi.org/10.1126/science.3105056
Castello A, Gaya M, Tucholski J, Oellerich T, Lu KH, Tafuri A et al (2013) Nck-mediated recruitment of BCAP to the BCR regulates the PI(3)K-Akt pathway in B cells. Nat Immunol 14(9):966–975. https://doi.org/10.1038/ni.2685
Cerutti A, Cols M, Puga I (2013) Marginal zone B cells: virtues of innate-like antibody-producing lymphocytes. Nat Rev Immunol 13(2):118–132. https://doi.org/10.1038/nri3383
Chang HHY, Pannunzio NR, Adachi N, Lieber MR (2017) Non-homologous DNA end joining and alternative pathways to double-strand break repair. Nat Rev Mol Cell Biol 18(8):495–506. https://doi.org/10.1038/nrm.2017.48
Chen Y, Park Y-B, Patel E, Silverman GJ (2009) IgM antibodies to apoptosis-associated determinants recruit C1q and enhance dendritic cell phagocytosis of apoptotic cells. J Immunol (Baltimore, MD: 1950) 182(10):6031–6043. https://doi.org/10.4049/jimmunol.0804191
Choi YS, Dieter JA, Rothaeusler K, Luo Z, Baumgarth N (2012) B-1 cells in the bone marrow are a significant source of natural IgM. Eur J Immunol 42(1):120–129. https://doi.org/10.1002/eji.201141890
Chung EY, Psathas JN, Yu D, Li Y, Weiss MJ, Thomas-Tikhonenko A (2012) CD19 is a major B cell receptor-independent activator of MYC-driven B-lymphomagenesis. J Clin Investig 122(6):2257–2266. https://doi.org/10.1172/JCI45851
Chung JB, Silverman M, Monroe JG (2003) Transitional B cells: step by step towards immune competence. Trends Immunol 24(6):343–349. https://doi.org/10.1016/s1471-4906(03)00119-4
Ciubotaru M, Surleac MD, Metskas LA, Koo P, Rhoades E, Petrescu AJ et al (2015) The architecture of the 12RSS in V(D)J recombination signal and synaptic complexes. Nucleic Acids Res 43(2):917–931. https://doi.org/10.1093/nar/gku1348
Cooper MD, Peterson RD, Good RA (1965) Delineation of the thymic and bursal lymphoid systems in the chicken. Nature 205:143–146. https://doi.org/10.1038/205143a0
Corcoran AE, Riddell A, Krooshoop D, Venkitaraman AR (1998) Impaired immunoglobulin gene rearrangement in mice lacking the IL-7 receptor. Nature 391 (6670):904–907. https://doi.org/10.1038/36122
Coutinho A, Kazatchkine MD, Avrameas S (1995) Natural autoantibodies. Curr Opin Immunol 7 (6):812–818. https://doi.org/10.1016/0952-7915(95)80053-0
Cunningham AF, Flores-Langarica A, Bobat S, Dominguez Medina CC, Cook CN, Ross EA et al (2014) B1b cells recognize protective antigens after natural infection and vaccination. Front Immunol 5:535. https://doi.org/10.3389/fimmu.2014.00535
Curry JD, Geier JK, Schlissel MS (2005) Single-strand recombination signal sequence nicks in vivo: evidence for a capture model of synapsis. Nat Immunol 6 (12):1272–1279. https://doi.org/10.1038/ni1270
Cyster JG, Hartley SB, Goodnow CC (1994) Competition for follicular niches excludes self-reactive cells from the recirculating B-cell repertoire. Nature 371 (6496):389–395. https://doi.org/10.1038/371389a0
Dauphinée M, Tovar Z, Talal N (1988) B cells expressing CD5 are increased in Sjögren's syndrome. Arthritis Rheum 31(5):642–647. https://doi.org/10.1002/art.1780310509
Driessen RL, Johnston HM, Nilsson SK (2003) Membrane-bound stem cell factor is a key regulator in the initial lodgment of stem cells within the endosteal marrow region. Exp Hematol 31(12):1284–1291. https://doi.org/10.1016/j.exphem.2003.08.015
Duan B, Morel L (2006) Role of B-1a cells in autoimmunity. Autoimmun Rev 5(6):403–408. https://doi.org/10.1016/j.autrev.2005.10.007
Esplin BL, Welner RS, Zhang Q, Borghesi LA, Kincade PW (2009) A differentiation pathway for B1 cells in adult bone marrow. Proc Natl Acad Sci USA 106 (14):5773–5778. https://doi.org/10.1073/pnas.0811632106
Fearon DT, Locksley RM (1996) The instructive role of innate immunity in the acquired immune response. Science (New York, NY) 272(5258):50–53. https://doi.org/10.1126/science.272.5258.50
Freedman AS, Freeman G, Whitman J, Segil J, Daley J, Nadler LM (1989). Studies of in vitro activated CD5+ B cells. Blood 73(1):202–208. https://www.ncbi.nlm.nih.gov/pubmed/2462935
Ghosn EEB, Yamamoto R, Hamanaka S, Yang Y, Herzenberg LA, Nakauchi H et al (2012) Distinct B-cell lineage commitment distinguishes adult bone marrow hematopoietic stem cells. Proc Natl Acad Sci USA 109(14):5394–5398. https://doi.org/10.1073/pnas.1121632109
Godin IE, Garcia-Porrero JA, Coutinho A, Dieterlen-Lièvre F, Marcos MA (1993) Para-aortic splanchnopleura from early mouse embryos contains B1a cell progenitors. Nature 364(6432):67–70. https://doi.org/10.1038/364067a0
Gonzaga WFKM, Xavier V, Vivanco BC, Lopes JD, Xander P (2015) B-1 cells contribute to susceptibility in experimental infection with Leishmania (Leishmania) chagasi. Parasitology 142(12):1506–1515. https://doi.org/10.1017/S0031182015000943
Graf R, Seagal J, Otipoby KL, Lam K-P, Ayoub S, Zhang B et al (2019) BCR-dependent lineage

plasticity in mature B cells. Science (New York, NY) 363(6428):748–753. https://doi.org/10.1126/science.aau8475

Griffin DO, Holodick NE, Rothstein TL (2011) Human B1 cells in umbilical cord and adult peripheral blood express the novel phenotype CD20+ CD27+ CD43+ CD70. J Exp Med 208(1):67–80. https://doi.org/10.1084/jem.20101499

Haas KM, Poe JC, Steeber DA, Tedder TF (2005). B-1a and B-1b cells exhibit distinct developmental requirements and have unique functional roles in innate and adaptive immunity to *S. pneumoniae*. Immunity 23(1):7–18. https://doi.org/10.1016/j.immuni.2005.04.011

Hamilton AM, Kearney JF (1994) Effects of IgM allotype suppression on serum IgM levels, B-1 and B-2 cells, and antibody responses in allotype heterozygous F1 mice. Dev Immunol 4(1):27–41. https://doi.org/10.1155/1994/45728

Hanayama R, Tanaka M, Miyasaka K, Aozasa K, Koike M, Uchiyama Y et al (2004) Autoimmune disease and impaired uptake of apoptotic cells in MFG-E8-deficient mice. Science (New York, NY) 304(5674):1147–1150. https://doi.org/10.1126/science.1094359

Hardy RR (2006) B-1 B cell development. J Immunol 177(5):2749–2754. https://doi.org/10.4049/jimmunol.177.5.2749

Hardy RR, Carmack CE, Shinton SA, Riblet RJ, Hayakawa K (1989). A single VH gene is utilized predominantly in anti-BrMRBC hybridomas derived from purified Ly-1 B cells. Definition of the VH11 family. J Immunol (Baltimore, MD: 1950), 142(10):3643–3651. https://www.ncbi.nlm.nih.gov/pubmed/2497178

Hardy RR, Hayakawa K (1991) A developmental switch in B lymphopoiesis. Proc Natl Acad Sci USA 88(24):11550–11554. https://doi.org/10.1073/pnas.88.24.11550

Hardy RR, Hayakawa K (2015) Perspectives on fetal derived CD5+ B1 B cells. Eur J Immunol 45(11):2978–2984. https://doi.org/10.1002/eji.201445146

Hardy RR, Hayakawa K, Parks DR, Herzenberg LA, Herzenberg LA (1984) Murine B cell differentiation lineages. J Exp Med 159(4):1169–1188. https://doi.org/10.1084/jem.159.4.1169

Hardy RR, Hayakawa K, Shimizu M, Yamasaki K, Kishimoto T (1987) Rheumatoid factor secretion from human Leu-1+ B cells. Science (New York, NY) 236(4797):81–83. https://doi.org/10.1126/science.3105057

Hartley SB, Cooke MP, Fulcher DA, Harris AW, Cory S, Basten A et al (1993) Elimination of self-reactive B lymphocytes proceeds in two stages: arrested development and cell death. Cell 72(3):325–335. https://doi.org/10.1016/0092-8674(93)90111-3

Hayakawa K, Asano M, Shinton SA, Gui M, Allman D, Stewart CL et al (1999) Positive selection of natural autoreactive B cells. Science (New York, NY) 285(5424):113–116. https://doi.org/10.1126/science.285.5424.113

Hayakawa K, Asano M, Shinton SA, Gui M, Wen L-J, Dashoff J et al (2003) Positive selection of anti-thy-1 autoreactive B-1 cells and natural serum autoantibody production independent from bone marrow B cell development. J Exp Med 197(1):87–99. https://doi.org/10.1084/jem.20021459

Hayakawa K, Hardy RR, Herzenberg LA, Herzenberg LA (1985) Progenitors for Ly-1 B cells are distinct from progenitors for other B cells. J Exp Med 161(6):1554–1568. https://doi.org/10.1084/jem.161.6.1554

Hayakawa K, Hardy RR, Parks DR, Herzenberg LA (1983) The "Ly-1 B" cell subpopulation in normal immunodefective, and autoimmune mice. J Exp Med 157(1):202–218. https://doi.org/10.1084/jem.157.1.202

Herzenberg LA (2000). B-1 cells: the lineage question revisited. Immunol. Rev. 175:9–22. https://www.ncbi.nlm.nih.gov/pubmed/10933587

Herzenberg LA, Herzenberg LA (1989) Toward a layered immune system. Cell 59(6):953–954. https://doi.org/10.1016/0092-8674(89)90748-4

Hiom K, Gellert M (1998) Assembly of a 12/23 paired signal complex: a critical control point in V(D)J recombination. Mol Cell 1(7):1011–1019. https://doi.org/10.1016/s1097-2765(00)80101-x

Hoffmann A, Kerr S, Jellusova J, Zhang J, Weisel F, Wellmann U et al (2007) Siglec-G is a B1 cell-inhibitory receptor that controls expansion and calcium signaling of the B1 cell population. Nat Immunol 8(7):695–704. https://doi.org/10.1038/ni1480

Holodick NE, Vizconde T, Rothstein TL (2014) B-1a cell diversity: nontemplated addition in B-1a cell Ig is determined by progenitor population and developmental location. J Immunol. (Baltimore, Md.: 1950) 192(5):2432–2441. https://doi.org/10.4049/jimmunol.1300247

Hunte BE, Hudak S, Campbell D, Xu Y, Rennick D (1996). flk2/flt3 ligand is a potent cofactor for the growth of primitive B cell progenitors. J Immunol (Baltimore, MD: 1950), 156(2):489–496. https://www.ncbi.nlm.nih.gov/pubmed/8543798

Ikuta K, Kina T, MacNeil I, Uchida N, Peault B, Chien YH et al (1990) A developmental switch in thymic lymphocyte maturation potential occurs at the level of hematopoietic stem cells. Cell 62(5):863–874. https://doi.org/10.1016/0092-8674(90)90262-d

Ikuta K, Weissman IL (1992) Evidence that hematopoietic stem cells express mouse c-kit but do not depend on steel factor for their generation. Proc Natl Acad Sci USA 89(4):1502–1506. https://doi.org/10.1073/pnas.89.4.1502

Jellusova J, Duber S, Guckel E, Binder CJ, Weiss S, Voll R et al (2010) Siglec-G regulates B1 cell survival and selection. J Immunol. 185(6):3277–3284. https://doi.org/10.4049/jimmunol.1001792

Jones JM, Gellert M (2002) Ordered assembly of the V(D)J synaptic complex ensures accurate recombination. EMBO J. 21(15):4162–4171. https://doi.org/10.1093/emboj/cdf394

Kaminski DA, Stavnezer J (2006) Enhanced IgA class switching in marginal zone and B1 B cells relative to follicular/B2 B cells. J Immunol (Baltimore, MD: 1950) 177(9):6025–6029. https://doi.org/10.4049/jimmunol.177.9.6025

Kantor AB, Merrill CE, Herzenberg LA, Hillson JL (1997). An unbiased analysis of V(H)-D-J(H) sequences from B-1a, B-1b, and conventional B cells. J Immunol (Baltimore, MD: 1950), 158(3):1175–1186. https://www.ncbi.nlm.nih.gov/pubmed/9013957

Kantor AB, Stall AM, Adams S, Herzenberg LA, Herzenberg LA (1992) Differential development of progenitor activity for three B-cell lineages. Proc Natl Acad Sci USA 89(8):3320–3324. https://doi.org/10.1073/pnas.89.8.3320

Kasaian MT, Ikematsu H, Casali P (1992). Identification and analysis of a novel human surface CD5- B lymphocyte subset producing natural antibodies. J Immunol (Baltimore, MD: 1950), 148(9):2690–2702. https://www.ncbi.nlm.nih.gov/pubmed/1374094

Kawahara T, Ohdan H, Zhao G, Yang Y-G, Sykes M (2003) Peritoneal cavity B cells are precursors of splenic IgM natural antibody-producing cells. J Immunol (Baltimore, MD: 1950) 171(10):5406–5414. https://doi.org/10.4049/jimmunol.171.10.5406

Kelsoe G (2015) Heavy-chain receptor editing unbound. Proc Natl Acad Sci USA 112(8):2297–2298. https://doi.org/10.1073/pnas.1501480112

Klinman NR (1996) The "clonal selection hypothesis" and current concepts of B cell tolerance. Immunity 5 (3):189–195. https://doi.org/10.1016/s1074-7613(00)80314-3

Kondo M, Weissman IL, Akashi K (1997) Identification of clonogenic common lymphoid progenitors in mouse bone marrow. Cell 91(5):661–672. https://doi.org/10.1016/s0092-8674(00)80453-5

Kong YY, Yoshida H, Sarosi I, Tan HL, Timms E, Capparelli C et al (1999) OPGL is a key regulator of osteoclastogenesis, lymphocyte development and lymph-node organogenesis. Nature 397(6717):315–323. https://doi.org/10.1038/16852

Kumar R, Bach MP, Mainoldi F, Maruya M, Kishigami S, Jumaa H., Wakayama T, Kanagawa O, Fagarasan S, Casola S. (2015). Antibody repertoire diversification through VH gene replacement in mice cloned from an IgA plasma cell. Proc Nat Acad Sci USA 112(5): E450–E457. https://doi.org/10.1073/pnas.1417988112

Lalor PA, Herzenberg LA, Adams S, Stall AM (1989a) Feedback regulation of murine Ly-1 B cell development. Eur J Immunol 19(3):507–513. https://doi.org/10.1002/eji.1830190315

Lalor PA, Stall AM, Adams S, Herzenberg LA (1989b) Permanent alteration of the murine Ly-1 B repertoire due to selective depletion of Ly-1 B cells in neonatal animals. Eur J Immunol 19(3):501–506. https://doi.org/10.1002/eji.1830190314

Lalor PA, Morahan G (1990) The peritoneal Ly-1 (CD5) B cell repertoire is unique among murine B cell repertoires. Eur J Immunol 20(3):485–492. https://doi.org/10.1002/eji.1830200305

Lam KP, Rajewsky K (1999) B cell antigen receptor specificity and surface density together determine B-1 versus B-2 cell development. J Exp Med 190(4):471–477. https://doi.org/10.1084/jem.190.4.471

Landree MA, Kale SB, Roth DB (2001) Functional organization of single and paired V(D)J cleavage complexes. Mol Cell Biol 21(13):4256–4264. https://doi.org/10.1128/MCB.21.13.4256-4264.2001

Lee J, Kuchen S, Fischer R, Chang S, Lipsky PE (2009) Identification and characterization of a human CD5+ pre-naive B cell population. J. Immunol (Baltimore, MD: 1950) 182(7):4116–4126. https://doi.org/10.4049/jimmunol.0803391

Li S, Liu J, Min Q, Ikawa T, Yasuda S, Yang Y et al (2018) Kelch-like protein 14 promotes B-1a but suppresses B-1b cell development. Int Immunol 30 (7):311–318. https://doi.org/10.1093/intimm/dxy033

Lieber MR (2010) The mechanism of double-strand DNA break repair by the nonhomologous DNA end-joining pathway. Annu Rev Biochem 79:181–211. https://doi.org/10.1146/annurev.biochem.052308.093131

Liu Z, Liu Y, Li T, Wang P, Mo X, Lv P et al (2019) Cmtm7 knockout inhibits B-1a cell development at the transitional (TrB-1a) stage. Int Immunol 31(11):715–728. https://doi.org/10.1093/intimm/dxz041

Margry B, Wieland WH, van Kooten PJ, van Eden W, Broere F (2013) Peritoneal cavity B-1a cells promote peripheral CD4+ T-cell activation. Eur J Immunol 43 (9):2317–2326. https://doi.org/10.1002/eji.201343418

Martin RK, Damle SR, Valentine YA, Zellner MP, James BN, Lownik JC et al (2018) B1 cell IgE impedes mast cell-mediated enhancement of parasite expulsion through B2 IgE blockade. Cell Rep 22 (7):1824–1834. https://doi.org/10.1016/j.celrep.2018.01.048

McBlane JF, van Gent DC, Ramsden DA, Romeo C, Cuomo CA, Gellert M et al (1995) Cleavage at a V(D)J recombination signal requires only RAG1 and RAG2 proteins and occurs in two steps. Cell 83 (3):387–395. https://doi.org/10.1016/0092-8674(95)90116-7

Mercolino TJ, Arnold LW, Haughton G (1986) Phosphatidyl choline is recognized by a series of Ly-1+ murine B cell lymphomas specific for erythrocyte membranes. J Exp Med 163(1):155–165. https://doi.org/10.1084/jem.163.1.155

Mercolino TJ, Arnold LW, Hawkins LA, Haughton G (1988) Normal mouse peritoneum contains a large population of Ly-1+ (CD5) B cells that recognize phosphatidyl choline. Relationship to cells that secrete hemolytic antibody specific for autologous erythrocytes. J Exp Med 168(2):687–698. https://doi.org/10.1084/jem.168.2.687

Mercolino TJ, Locke AL, Afshari A, Sasser D, Travis WW, Arnold LW et al (1989) Restricted immunoglobulin variable region gene usage by normal Ly-1 (CD5+) B cells that recognize phosphatidyl choline. J Exp Med 169(6):1869–1877. https://doi.org/10.1084/jem.169.6.1869

Monroe JG (2004) Ligand-independent tonic signaling in B-cell receptor function. Curr Opin Immunol 16 (3):288–295. https://doi.org/10.1016/j.coi.2004.03.010

Montecino-Rodriguez E, Leathers H, Dorshkind K (2006) Identification of a B-1 B cell-specified progenitor. Nat Immunol 7(3):293–301. https://doi.org/10.1038/ni1301

Moore MA, Metcalf D (1970) Ontogeny of the haemopoietic system: yolk sac origin of in vivo and in vitro colony forming cells in the developing mouse embryo. Br J Haematol 18(3):279–296. https://doi.org/10.1111/j.1365-2141.1970.tb01443.x

Morrison SJ, Hemmati HD, Wandycz AM, Weissman IL (1995) The purification and characterization of fetal liver hematopoietic stem cells. Proc Natl Acad Sci USA 92(22):10302–10306. https://doi.org/10.1073/pnas.92.22.10302

Mosser DM, Zhang X (2008) Interleukin-10: new perspectives on an old cytokine. Immunol Rev 226:205–218. https://doi.org/10.1111/j.1600-065X.2008.00706.x

Müller AM, Medvinsky A, Strouboulis J, Grosveld F, Dzierzak E (1994) Development of hematopoietic stem cell activity in the mouse embryo. Immunity 1 (4):291–301. https://doi.org/10.1016/1074-7613(94)90081-7

Mundy CL, Patenge N, Matthews AGW, Oettinger MA (2002) Assembly of the RAG1/RAG2 synaptic complex. Mol Cell Biol 22(1):69–77. https://doi.org/10.1128/mcb.22.1.69-77.2002

Nagasawa T (2006) Microenvironmental niches in the bone marrow required for B-cell development. Nat Rev Immunol 6(2):107–116. https://doi.org/10.1038/nri1780

Nagasawa T, Hirota S, Tachibana K, Takakura N, Nishikawa S, Kitamura Y et al (1996) Defects of B-cell lymphopoiesis and bone-marrow myelopoiesis in mice lacking the CXC chemokine PBSF/SDF-1. Nature 382(6592):635–638. https://doi.org/10.1038/382635a0

Nemazee DA, Bürki K (1989) Clonal deletion of B lymphocytes in a transgenic mouse bearing anti-MHC class I antibody genes. Nature 337(6207):562–566. https://doi.org/10.1038/337562a0

Novaes E Brito RR, Dos Santos Toledo M, Labussiere GM, Dupin TV, de Campos Reis NF, Perez EC et al (2019) B-1 cell response in immunity against parasites. Parasitol Res 118(5):1343–1352. https://doi.org/10.1007/s00436-019-06211-2

Nussenzweig MC, Alt FW (2004) Antibody diversity: one enzyme to rule them all. Nat Med 10(12):1304–1305. https://doi.org/10.1038/nm1204-1304

Opferman JT, Letai A, Beard C, Sorcinelli MD, Ong CC, Korsmeyer SJ (2003) Development and maintenance of B and T lymphocytes requires antiapoptotic MCL-1. Nature 426(6967):671–676. https://doi.org/10.1038/nature02067

Orkin SH, Zon LI (2008) Hematopoiesis: an evolving paradigm for stem cell biology. Cell 132(4):631–644. https://doi.org/10.1016/j.cell.2008.01.025

Ouchida R, Mori H, Hase K, Takatsu H, Kurosaki T, Tokuhisa T et al (2012) Critical role of the IgM Fc receptor in IgM homeostasis, B-cell survival, and humoral immune responses. Proc Natl Acad Sci USA 109(40):E2699–E2706. https://doi.org/10.1073/pnas.1210706109

Panda S, Zhang J, Tan NS, Ho B, Ding JL (2013) Natural IgG antibodies provide innate protection against ficolin-opsonized bacteria. EMBO J 32(22):2905–2919. https://doi.org/10.1038/emboj.2013.199

Pappu R, Cheng AM, Li B, Gong Q, Chiu C, Griffin N et al (1999) Requirement for B cell linker protein (BLNK) in B cell development. Science 286 (5446):1949–1954. https://doi.org/10.1126/science.286.5446.1949

Pillai S, Cariappa A (2009) The follicular versus marginal zone B lymphocyte cell fate decision. Nat Rev Immunol 9(11):767–777. https://doi.org/10.1038/nri2656

Poe JC, Minard-Colin V, Kountikov EI, Haas KM, Tedder TF (2012) A c-Myc and surface CD19 signaling amplification loop promotes B cell lymphoma development and progression in mice. J Immunol (Baltimore, MD: 1950) 189(5):2318–2325. https://doi.org/10.4049/jimmunol.1201000

Prieto JMB, Felippe MJB (2017) Development, phenotype, and function of non-conventional B cells. Comp Immunol Microbiol Infect Dis 54:38–44. https://doi.org/10.1016/j.cimid.2017.08.002

Prieyl JA, LeBien TW (1996) Interleukin 7 independent development of human B cells. Proc Natl Acad Sci USA 93(19):10348–10353. https://doi.org/10.1073/pnas.93.19.10348

Quách TD, Hopkins TJ, Holodick NE, Vuyyuru R, Manser T, Bayer R-L et al (2016) Human B-1 and B-2 B cells develop from Lin-CD34+ CD38lo stem cells. J Immunol (Baltimore, MD: 1950) 197(10):3950–3958. https://doi.org/10.4049/jimmunol.1600630

Ramsden DA, Baetz K, Wu GE (1994) Conservation of sequence in recombination signal sequence spacers. Nucleic Acids Res 22(10):1785–1796. https://doi.org/10.1093/nar/22.10.1785

Ratcliffe MJH (2016) Encyclopedia of immunobiology, 1st edn. Academic Press, UK

Rothstein TL, Quach TD (2015) The human counterpart of mouse B-1 cells. Ann NY Acad Sci 1362:143–152. https://doi.org/10.1111/nyas.12790

Roy B, Agarwal S, Brennecke AM, Krey M, Pabst O, Duber S et al (2013) B-1-cell subpopulations contribute differently to gut immunity. Eur J Immunol 43 (8):2023–2032. https://doi.org/10.1002/eji.201243070

Sato T, Ishikawa S, Akadegawa K, Ito T, Yurino H, Kitabatake M et al (2004) Aberrant B1 cell migration into the thymus results in activation of CD4 T cells through its potent antigen-presenting activity in the development of murine lupus. Eur J Immunol 34

(12):3346–3358. https://doi.org/10.1002/eji.200425373

Schatz DG, Ji Y (2011) Recombination centres and the orchestration of V(D)J recombination. Nat Rev Immunol 11(4):251–263. https://doi.org/10.1038/nri2941

Seita J, Weissman IL (2010) Hematopoietic stem cell: self-renewal versus differentiation. Wiley Interdisc Rev. Syst Biol Med 2(6):640–653. https://doi.org/10.1002/wsbm.86

Shlyakhtenko LS, Gilmore J, Kriatchko AN, Kumar S, Swanson PC, Lyubchenko YL (2009) Molecular mechanism underlying RAG1/RAG2 synaptic complex formation. J Biol Chem 284(31):20956–20965. https://doi.org/10.1074/jbc.M109.028977

Shyh-Chang N, Daley GQ (2013) Lin28: primal regulator of growth and metabolism in stem cells. Cell Stem Cell 12(4):395–406. https://doi.org/10.1016/j.stem.2013.03.005

Sims GP, Ettinger R, Shirota Y, Yarboro CH, Illei GG, Lipsky PE (2005) Identification and characterization of circulating human transitional B cells. Blood 105 (11):4390–4398. https://doi.org/10.1182/blood-2004-11-4284

Sitnicka E, Brakebusch C, Martensson I-L, Svensson M, Agace WW, Sigvardsson M et al (2003) Complementary signaling through flt3 and interleukin-7 receptor alpha is indispensable for fetal and adult B cell genesis. J Exp Med 198(10):1495–1506. https://doi.org/10.1084/jem.20031152

Sitnicka E, Bryder D, Theilgaard-Mönch K, Buza-Vidas N, Adolfsson J, Jacobsen SEW (2002) Key role of flt3 ligand in regulation of the common lymphoid progenitor but not in maintenance of the hematopoietic stem cell pool. Immunity 17(4):463–472. https://doi.org/10.1016/s1074-7613(02)00419-3

Smith FL, Baumgarth N (2019) B-1 cell responses to infections. Curr Opin Immunol 57:23–31. https://doi.org/10.1016/j.coi.2018.12.001

Solvason N, Chen X, Shu F, Kearney JF (1992) The fetal omentum in mice and humans. A site enriched for precursors of CD5 B cells early in development. Ann NY Acad Sci 651:10–20. https://doi.org/10.1111/j.1749-6632.1992.tb24589.x

Solvason N, Lehuen A, Kearney JF (1991) An embryonic source of Ly1 but not conventional B cells. Int Immunol 3(6):543–550. https://doi.org/10.1093/intimm/3.6.543

Stall AM, Adams S, Herzenberg LA, Kantor AB (1992) Characteristics and development of the murine B-1b (Ly-1 B sister) cell population. Ann NY Acad Sci 651:33–43. https://doi.org/10.1111/j.1749-6632.1992.tb24591.x

Subramaniam KS, Datta K, Quintero E, Manix C, Marks MS, Pirofski L-A (2010) The absence of serum IgM enhances the susceptibility of mice to pulmonary challenge with Cryptococcus neoformans. J Immunol (Baltimore, MD: 1950) 184(10):5755–5767. https://doi.org/10.4049/jimmunol.0901638

Sun A, Novobrantseva TI, Coffre M, Hewitt SL, Jensen K, Skok JA, Rajewsky K, Koralov SB. (2015). V_H replacement in primary immunoglobulin repertoire diversification. Proc Nat Acad Sci USA 112 (5):E458–E466. https://doi.org/10.1073/pnas.1418001112

Swanson PC (2002) A RAG-1/RAG-2 tetramer supports 12/23-regulated synapsis, cleavage, and transposition of V(D)J recombination signals. Mol Cell Biol 22 (22):7790–7801. https://doi.org/10.1128/mcb.22.22.7790-7801.2002

Tarlinton DM, McLean M, Nossal GJ (1995) B1 and B2 cells differ in their potential to switch immunoglobulin isotype. Eur J Immunol 25(12):3388–3393. https://doi.org/10.1002/eji.1830251228

Tiegs SL, Russell DM, Nemazee D (1993) Receptor editing in self-reactive bone marrow B cells. J Exp Med 177(4):1009–1020. https://doi.org/10.1084/jem.177.4.1009

Tlaskalová-Hogenová H, Mandel L, Stěpánková R, Bártová J, Barot R, Leclerc M., et al. (1992). Autoimmunity: from physiology to pathology. Natural antibodies, mucosal immunity and development of B cell repertoire. Folia Biol 38(3–4):202–215. https://www.ncbi.nlm.nih.gov/pubmed/1426416

Tokoyoda K, Egawa T, Sugiyama T, Choi B-I, Nagasawa T (2004) Cellular niches controlling B lymphocyte behavior within bone marrow during development. Immunity 20(6):707–718. https://doi.org/10.1016/j.immuni.2004.05.001

Tornberg UC, Holmberg D (1995). B-1a, B-1b and B-2 B cells display unique VHDJH repertoires formed at different stages of ontogeny and under different selection pressures. EMBO J. 14(8):1680–1689. https://www.ncbi.nlm.nih.gov/pubmed/7737121

van Gent DC, Hiom K, Paull TT, Gellert M (1997) Stimulation of V(D)J cleavage by high mobility group proteins. EMBO J 16(10):2665–2670. https://doi.org/10.1093/emboj/16.10.2665

Vanhee S, Åkerstrand H, Kristiansen TA, Datta S, Montano G, Vergani S et al (2019) Lin28b controls a neonatal to adult switch in B cell positive selection. Sci Immunol 4(39):eaax4453. https://doi.org/10.1126/sciimmunol.aax4453

Vettermann C, Schlissel MS (2010) Allelic exclusion of immunoglobulin genes: models and mechanisms. Immunol Rev 237(1):22–42. https://doi.org/10.1111/j.1600-065X.2010.00935.x

Weber GF, Chousterman BG, He S, Fenn AM, Nairz M, Anzai A et al (2015) Interleukin-3 amplifies acute inflammation and is a potential therapeutic target in sepsis. Science (New York, NY) 347(6227):1260–1265. https://doi.org/10.1126/science.aaa4268

Weissman IL, Baird S, Gardner RL, Papaioannou VE, Raschke W (1977) Normal and neoplastic maturation of T-lineage lymphocytes. Cold Spring Harb Symp Quant Biol 41(Pt 1):9–21. https://doi.org/10.1101/sqb.1977.041.01.005

Witt CM, Won W-J, Hurez V, Klug CA (2003) Notch2 haploinsufficiency results in diminished B1 B cells and a severe reduction in marginal zone B cells. J Immunol (Baltimore, MD: 1950) 171(6):2783–2788. https://doi.org/10.4049/jimmunol.171.6.2783

Yin FF, Bailey S, Innis CA, Ciubotaru M, Kamtekar S, Steitz TA et al (2009) Structure of the RAG1 nonamer binding domain with DNA reveals a dimer that mediates DNA synapsis. Nat Struct Mol Biol 16 (5):499–508. https://doi.org/10.1038/nsmb.1593

Yoshimoto M (2015) The first wave of B lymphopoiesis develops independently of stem cells in the murine embryo. Ann NY Acad Sci 1362:16–22. https://doi.org/10.1111/nyas.12612

Yoshimoto M, Montecino-Rodriguez E, Ferkowicz MJ, Porayette P, Shelley WC, Conway SJ et al (2011) Embryonic day 9 yolk sac and intra-embryonic hemogenic endothelium independently generate a B-1 and marginal zone progenitor lacking B-2 potential. Proc Natl Acad Sci USA 108(4):1468–1473. https://doi.org/10.1073/pnas.1015841108

Youinou P, Mackenzie L, Katsikis P, Merdrignac G, Isenberg DA, Tuaillon N et al (1990) The relationship between CD5-expressing B lymphocytes and serologic abnormalities in rheumatoid arthritis patients and their relatives. Arthritis Rheum 33(3):339–348. https://doi.org/10.1002/art.1780330306

Yuan J, Nguyen CK, Liu X, Kanellopoulou C, Muljo SA (2012) Lin28b reprograms adult bone marrow hematopoietic progenitors to mediate fetal-like lymphopoiesis. Science (New York, NY) 335 (6073):1195–1200. https://doi.org/10.1126/science.1216557

Zhang Y, Wang JY, Han W (2014) A role for CMTM7 in BCR expression and survival in B-1a but not B-2 cells. Int Immunol 26(1):47–57. https://doi.org/10.1093/intimm/dxt042

Zhong X, Gao W, Degauque N, Bai C, Lu Y, Kenny J et al (2007) Reciprocal generation of Th1/Th17 and T (reg) cells by B1 and B2 B cells. Eur J Immunol 37 (9):2400–2404. https://doi.org/10.1002/eji.200737296

Zhou Y, Li Y-S, Bandi SR, Tang L, Shinton SA, Hayakawa K et al (2015) Lin28b promotes fetal B lymphopoiesis through the transcription factor Arid3a. J Exp Med 212(4):569–580. https://doi.org/10.1084/jem.20141510

B Cell Receptor Signaling

2

Shinya Tanaka and Yoshihiro Baba

Abstract

Signaling through the B cell receptor (BCR) plays a critical role at multiple checkpoints of B cell biology. BCR acts as a gatekeeper of the progression of their early development in bone marrow (BM). It is also essential in triggering mechanisms such as clonal deletion and receptor editing to eliminate autoreactive B cells. In the periphery, it most importantly functions as a receptor that recognizes various extracellular antigens in response to bacterial and viral infections for conferring host defense. The recognition of antigens by BCR is the first step to receive T cell help for the functional differentiation of naive B cells toward plasma cells, germinal center (GC) B cells and memory B cells. In addition, similar to the role of BCR in the early stages of B cell development, BCR signaling plays a crucial role in the prevention of dysregulated activation of autoreactive B cells which can induce autoimmunity in the secondary lymphoid organs. Thus, since BCR is essential for the proper elicitation of immune responses by B cells, signaling through the BCR is tightly controlled by the intracellular positive and negative regulators. In this chapter, the mechanisms of activation and repression of BCR signaling are reviewed on the basis of the recent findings.

Keywords

B cell receptor · Calcium signal · NF-kB · MAPK · PI3K · SHP · SHIP

2.1 Introduction

B cell receptor (BCR) is one of the most important receptors for B cells to sense their environment. In viral and bacterial infections, recognition of antigens derived from these pathogens induces proliferation and functional differentiation of B cells to effector subsets in periphery, which is essential process for host defense. On the other hand, antibodies against host cells can be pathogenic and the major risk factors for many autoimmune diseases, such as systemic lupus erythematosus (SLE), rheumatoid arthritis and diabetes. Clinical depletion of B cells often provides a therapeutic effect on these diseases, suggesting that the elimination of self-reactive B cells reduces antigen presentation to self-reactive T cells as well as the production of harmful autoantibodies. To prevent self-reactive B cell activation and ultimate

S. Tanaka (✉) · Y. Baba
Division of Immunology and Genome Biology, Department of Molecular Genetics, Medical Institute of Bioregulation, Kyushu University, Higashi-Ku, Fukuoka 812-8582, Japan
e-mail: stanaka@bioreg.kyushu-u.ac.jp

J.-Y. Wang (ed.), *B Cells in Immunity and Tolerance*, Advances in Experimental Medicine and Biology 1254, https://doi.org/10.1007/978-981-15-3532-1_2

autoimmune responses, the immunological tolerance must be induced against self-reactive B cells by the recognition of self-antigens by the BCR. Thus, qualitative and quantitative differences in antigen recognition by B cells play a major role in determining the B cell fate. The B cell fate is determined by the intracellular gene expression patterns which in turn is shaped up by the differential activation of distinct signaling pathways upon stimulation of B cells by different types of antigens. Since the B cell signal transduction is regulated by various proteins such as kinases, phosphatases and scaffold proteins, a comprehensive study of functions of these signal molecules and their interaction within the B cells are required for the better understanding of the B cell biology.

BCR signaling is initiated upon antigen recognition by the phosphorylation of BCR-associating CD79 molecules, which activates proximal signaling molecules, leading to the formation of central signaling complex, called signalosome (Fig. 2.1). Then, the downstream branches such as nuclear factor of activated T cells (NFAT), nuclear factor κ B (NFκB) and Ras-extracellular-signal-regulated kinase (ERK) signaling cascades are activated. A co-receptor, CD19 plays an important role in the activation of PI3K–AKT pathway. On the other hand, the BCR signal is regulated by multiple inhibitory molecules. Although phosphatases, which inhibit the proximal BCR signaling, are well-studied, other factors that negatively regulate the downstream pathways of BCR signaling have also been explored and add further layers of complexities by enabling the spatiotemporal fine-tuning of the BCR signaling.

2.2 BCR Signaling Pathways

2.2.1 Proximal B Cell Receptor Signaling Events

BCR consists of a pair of identical immunoglobulin heavy (IgH) and light (IgL) chains. These Ig chains possess a unique variable region which recognizes diverse antigens in the surrounding environment. Although membrane BCR per se is not able to transduce downstream signaling, it does so by making BCR complex with CD79. The extracellular portion of the BCR is non-covalently coupled to a disulfide-linked heterodimer of the CD79A and CD79B. This association allows expression of BCR on the plasma membrane and BCR internalization after antigen recognition (Gazumyan et al. 2006; Hou et al. 2006). Although the BCR internalization was suggested to suppress BCR-mediated positive signaling (Stoddart et al. 2005), a study using a specific inhibitor against dynamin1 and dynamin2 to prevent clathrin-mediated BCR endocytosis demonstrated that the treatment of B cells with the inhibitor after BCR crosslinking resulted in hyperphosphorylation of mitogen-activated protein (MAP) kinases and AKT as well as its downstream target, forkhead box protein (FOXO), causing dysregulated gene expression. Therefore, the intracellular localization of BCR after antigen recognition was suggested to be crucial for appropriate outcomes (Chaturvedi et al. 2011). The CD79 molecules contain signaling molecules called immunoreceptor tyrosine-based activation motifs (ITAMs) in their intracellular portion. ITAMs are bound by the SRC kinases such as LYN, FYN and B-lymphoid tyrosine kinase (BLK). The crosslinking of BCR by specific antigens induces phosphorylation of ITAM tyrosines by these SRC kinases (Saijo et al. 2003). In the early stage of B cell development, the stochastic recombination of gene segments encoding the immunoglobulin variable regions generates tremendous amount of diversified BCRs, which also include autoreactive ones. It is estimated that up to 50% of these naturally arising BCR undergo receptor editing to rescue autoreactive B cells from clonal deletion (Retter and Nemazee 1998). A recent report suggests that a membrane protein caveolin-1 recruits IgM into ganglioside GM1-enriched lipid domain, upon phosphorylation by SRC kinase following BCR stimulation and functions as a crucial regulator of receptor editing (Minguet et al. 2017). Indeed, caveolin-1-deficient mice developed autoimmune disease due to defective central tolerance. The core amino acid sequence of the ITAM in CD79

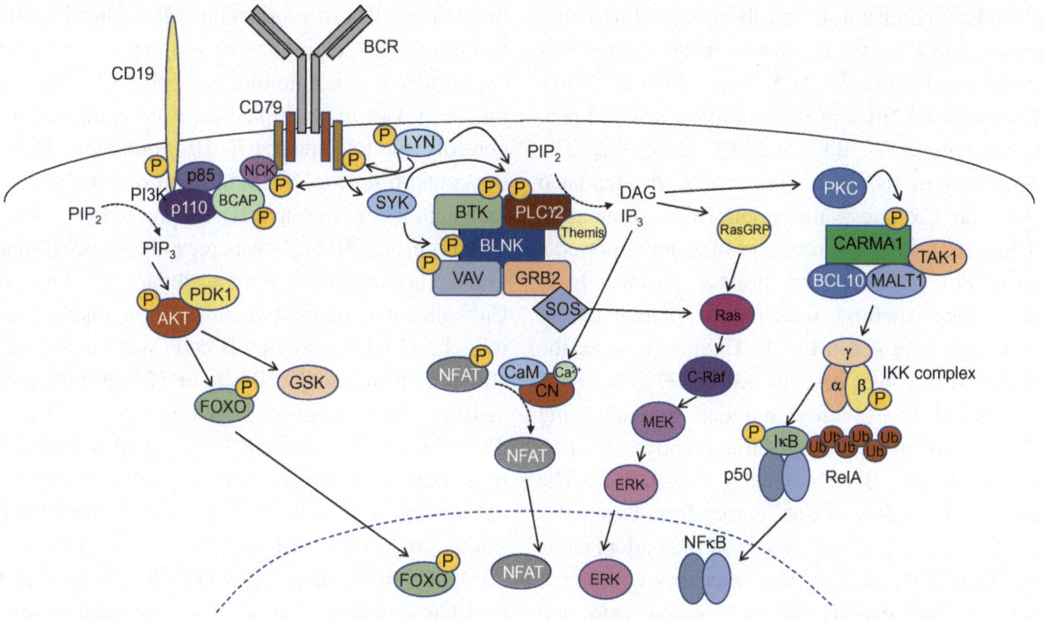

Fig. 2.1 B cell signaling pathway. The recognition of antigen by the BCR initiates BCR signaling cascade by phosphorylation of CD79, resulting in SRC and non-SRC kinase activation. These kinases in proximal BCR signaling phosphorylate signal molecules such as BTK, PCLγ2 and BLNK, which form signalosome. DAG produced by PCLγ2 activates both Ras-ERK and IKK–NFκB pathways. Another product of PCLγ2, IP_3 activates calcium–NFAT pathway. Upon the phosphorylation co-stimulatory molecule, CD19, the activation of PI3K–AKT pathway is initiated

comprises two tyrosine residues which are separated by 11 residues and followed by leucine or isoleucine. A mutagenesis study demonstrated the requirement of these structures for proper initiation of the BCR signaling (Sanchez et al. 1993; Flaswinkel and Reth 1994). The tyrosine phosphorylation of the ITAM of CD79 promotes the activation of the non-SRC family tyrosine kinase, spleen tyrosine kinase (SYK), which becomes a key part of a signalosome formed by many other kinases and adaptor proteins (Fig. 2.1). The SYK which is recruited to the phosphorylated CD79-ITAM facilitates the complex formation of B-cell linker protein (BLNK), leading to activation of Bruton's tyrosine kinase (BTK), phospholipase Cγ2 (PLCγ2) and VAV, growth factor receptor-bound protein 2 (GRB2). It is well established that BCR-derived constitutive but low "tonic" signaling and BAFFR signaling are required for B cell survival (Lam et al. 1997; Thompson et al. 2001; Gross et al. 2001; Miller and Hayes 1991; Mackay et al. 2010), and the signaling is propagated through SYK activation in the majority of follicular B cells (Schweighoffer et al. 2013). Surprisingly, the ligation of BAFF and its receptor leads to the direct phosphorylation of both CD79A and SYK, turning on activation of PI3K and ERK signaling pathways, indicating a crosstalk between two different receptors for B cell survival (Schweighoffer et al. 2013). It has been recently reported that the Fc μ receptor (FcμR) interacts with membrane-type IgM in the trans-Golgi network (TGN), and this interaction controls the BCR surface expression, affecting the tonic signaling (Nguyen et al. 2017).

2.2.2 PLCγ2-Calcium-NFAT Pathway

The phosphorylated adaptor BLNK binds to PLCγ2 and BTK following which then PLCγ2 is phosphorylated by SYK/BTK and thus gets activated to produce the second messenger, diacylglycerol (DAG) and inositol-1, 4,5-triposphate (IP_3) from phosphatidylinositol-4,5-bisphosphate (PIP_2) and thus to transduce the downstream signaling events (Hikida and Kurosaki 2005; Kurosaki et al. 2010). Therefore, BLNK serves as a critical scaffold protein to bring SYK, BTK and PLCγ2 together. The deficiency of these proteins results in attenuated cytosolic Ca^{2+} response upon BCR stimulation (Ishiai et al. 1999). A recent publication reported a novel PLCγ2 associating protein Themis2 in B cells. Like Themis1 which is a Themis family molecule expressed in T cells, Themis2 lowered the threshold of lower limit to activate B cells when recognized low avidity antigens by enhancing PLCγ2 activation, thus enabling positive selection of B1 and GC B cells (Cheng et al. 2017). The intracellular inflow of Ca^{2+} comes from two major sources: Ca^{2+} that outflows from the endoplasmic reticulum (ER) and Ca^{2+} that enters from outside of the cells. The ligation of IP_3 to IP_3 receptors located in the ER membrane leads to the quick and temporal release of Ca^{2+} from the ER. This triggers an initial increase in the cytoplasmic Ca^{2+} concentration, followed by opening of the Ca^{2+} channels at the plasma membrane. Then, extracellular Ca^{2+} flows into the cells and further prolongs the intracellular Ca^{2+} rise, a process known as store-operated Ca^{2+} entry (SOCE), which is regulated by two major proteins: stromal interaction molecule (STIM: STIM1 and STIM2) and Orai (Orai1, Orai2 and Orai3) (Roos et al. 2005; Liou et al. 2005; Feske et al. 2006; Vig et al. 2006). Orai is as a store-operated Ca^{2+} channel for SOCE, whose function is activated by STIM1 and STIM2 that sense ER-stored Ca^{2+} depletion (Baba and Kurosaki 2011). The released Ca^{2+} is recognized by a cytosolic Ca^{2+} sensor, calmodulin. Calcineurin is a Ca^{2+}-calmodulin-dependent serine/threonine phosphatase, composed of a catalytic subunit and regulatory subunit. The binding of the calcineurin regulatory subunit with Ca^{2+} leads to its association with the activated calmodulin, turning on dephosphorylation of NFAT by calcineurin. Although Ca^{2+} influx is critical for the appropriate activation of B cells, it may be harmful when dysregulated. The genetic ablation of STIM1/2 in B cells provides an evidence of STIM-dependent Ca^{2+} signaling in B cell regulatory function. The ablation of STIM1/2 in B cells caused defects in NFAT activation and interleukin (IL)-10 production. Mice with B cells lacking STIM1/2 proteins develop an exacerbated experimental autoimmune encephalomyelitis, a mouse model of multiple sclerosis, compared to controls due to impaired IL-10 production. Thus, the calcium sensors STIM1/2 control B cell regulatory function through IL-10 production (Matsumoto et al. 2011). It was recently reported that gradual accumulation of intracellular Ca^{2+} through Ca^{2+} channel after BCR stimulation resulted in mitochondrial damage of B cells without second stimulation such as T cell help or TLR stimulation, causing their apoptosis (Akkaya et al. 2018). Therefore, BCR-mediated Ca^{2+} signal imposes a time frame for fate decision of cell survival or elimination of B cells. B cells express the NFAT family molecules such as NFAT1, NFAT2 and NFAT4 (Timmerman et al. 1997), that are activated by BCR signaling. The deletion of regulatory subunit B1 (CnB1) of calcineurin specifically in B cells resulted in the reduced plasma cell development and B1 cell number although the development of follicular and marginal zone (MZ) B cells was normal (Winslow et al. 2006). A study suggested that mice deficient in NFAT molecules has reduced B cell proliferation (Peng et al. 2001). It is possible that this may partially account for the compromised phenotype with plasma cells and reduced B1 cell numbers in B cell-specific CnB1 deficient mice.

2.2.3 IKK/NFκB Pathway

As described above, DAG generated by PLCγ2 activates protein kinase Cβ (PKCβ), which phosphorylates the downstream adaptor protein, caspase recruitment domain-containing membrane-associated guanylate kinase protein-1 (CARMA1). The phosphorylated CARMA1 recruits another kinase, TGFβ-activated kinase 1 (TAK1) which associates with the inhibitor of κB (IκB) kinase (IKK) complex (IKKα, IKKβ and IKKγ), letting the TAK1 phosphorylate IKKβ (Shinohara et al. 2005). Moreover, it forms a complex with mucosa-associated lymphoid tissue lymphoma translocation protein 1 (MALT1) and B-cell lymphoma 10 (BCL10) (CBM complex), which function as a scaffold to facilitate IKK activation. Then, the activated IKK phosphorylates IκB for ubiquitin-mediated degradation. Followed by IκB ubiquitination and degradation, NFκB which is usually retained in cytoplasm by IκB in steady state translocated to the nucleus for gene regulation. The NFκB activity is further reinforced by positive feedback regulation. The activated IKKβ phosphorylates CARMA1 on Ser578, which is a different Ser from the Ser that is phosphorylated by PKCβ. This feedback regulation contributes to the facilitation and/or stabilization of the interaction of CARMA1 with MALT1 and BCL10, enhancing IKK activation (Shinohara et al. 2007).

2.2.4 Ras/ERK Pathway

As is the case with other key signaling pathways, BCR stimulation also activates the extracellular signal-regulated kinase (ERK) mitogen-activated protein (MAP) kinase pathway (Nagaoka et al. 2000; Yasuda et al. 2008; Rowland et al. 2010). The ERK–MAP kinase pathway is regulated by the small G protein, Ras, whose activity is controlled by two functionally opposite regulatory proteins: the guanine nucleotide exchange factor (GEF) activating Ras by replacing Ras-bound GDP for GTP and the GTPase-activating protein (GAP) setting Ras back to its GDP-bound inactivate state. The Ras guanine-nucleotide releasing proteins (RasGRP) family molecules such as RasGRP1 and RasGRP3 are expressed in mouse models and B cell lines and play a major roles as GEFs. The C1 subdomain of RasGRP3 binds to DAG (a product of PLCγ2 activation), controls Ras activation and the ERK–MAP signaling pathway (Oh-hora et al. 2003; Coughlin et al. 2005). In addition, the phosphorylation of RasGRP3 on Thr133 by PKCβ is required for its full activation (Aiba et al. 2004; Zheng et al. 2005). Therefore, these kinases activated by BCR stimulation may contribute to the ERK–MAP pathway. In contrast to these observations, a recent paper reported that only small amount of RasGRP isoforms is expressed in mature human B cells and an alternative mechanism of Ras activation by son of sevenless (SOS) functions to transduce the ERK–MAP kinase pathway in the human system (Vanshylla et al. 2018).The GTP-bound Ras subsequently activates the Raf-1/B-Raf, which phosphorylates MEK1 and MEK2, followed by ERK activation. In addition, GRB2 has been reported to activate Ras in class-switched B cells such as IgG and IgE-bearing B cells by association of GRB2 on their cytoplasmic tail of the heavy chains (Engels et al. 2009). The dimerization of ERK phosphorylated by MEKs allows them to translocate to nucleus for the activation of the downstream transcription factors such as Fos, Jun and Ets family proteins for transcriptional gene regulation (Hollenhorst 2012; Dong et al. 2002).

2.2.5 PI3K Pathway

The activation of PI3K is thought to be mediated mainly by CD19, which is a B cell-specific membrane protein having multiple tyrosine residues on its cytoplasmic tail. Upon the BCR stimulation, the tail of CD19 is phosphorylated by LYN, providing a binding site for the PI3K subunit, p85α. The association of LYN with tyrosine-phosphorylated CD19 prevented the autoinhibitory function of LYN, amplifying its activity (Fujimoto et al. 2000). Double deficiency of CD19 and BCAP in B cells resulted in the almost complete loss of PI3K activation upon BCR stimulation suggesting that even though CD19 has a crucial role in PI3K activation (Okada et al. 2000), another cytoplasmic adaptor molecule, B cell adaptor for PI3K (BCAP) is also required for its activation (Aiba et al. 2008). To initiate the PI3K pathway, another adaptor protein, NCK (NCK1 and NCK2) is required, which directly binds to phosphorylated Tyr204 on CD79A, dependent on LYN, and phosphorylates BCAP for its recruitment to the signalosome (Castello et al. 2013). In addition, it has been reported that a small GTPase, TC21 is necessary for PI3K activation (Delgado et al. 2009). The activated PI3K converts phosphatidylinositol-4,5-bisphosphate (PIP_2) to phosphatidylinositol-3,4,5-triphosphate (PIP_3), a secondary lipid messenger by phosphorylation. The PIP_3 recruits AKT and phosphoinositide-dependent protein kinase1 (PDK1) to the plasma membrane, enabling the PDK1 and the mammalian target of rapamycin complex 2 (mTORC2) (Limon and Fruman 2012) to phosphorylate AKT on its threonine residue. The phosphorylated AKT has multiple targets related to B cell activity. Also, the AKT was reported to inhibit mTOR signaling by phosphorylating TSC complex (Dengler et al. 2008; Amin and Schlissel 2008; Srinivasan et al. 2009; Dominguez-Sola et al. 2015; Sander et al. 2015; Lin et al. 2010; Mansson et al. 2012). The glycogen synthase kinase 3 (GSK3) phosphorylated by AKT contributes to activation of multiple molecules regulating cell growth such as c-Myc and cyclin D3 (Gregory et al. 2003; Cato et al. 2011). The study with B cell-specific deletion of GSK3 isoforms (GSK3α and GSK3β) demonstrated that GSK3 is required for quiescence, long-term survival of mature B cells and growth and proliferation of GC B cells by regulating metabolic status (Jellusova et al. 2017). Also, the AKT was reported to inhibit mTOR signaling via TSC complex phosphorylation (Inoki et al. 2002).

For the initiation of signal transduction, a dynamic reorganization of actin cytoskeleton is required. (Fleire et al. 2006). In resting B cells, the cortical actin network makes BCR relatively unmovable (defused BCR), which prevents antigen-independent BCR clustering but allows B cells to propagate a weak "tonic" signal for their survival (Treanor et al. 2010a, b). Upon antigen recognition by the BCR, a rapid actin depolymerization occurs, which allows BCR more mobile for the formation of microcluster composed of oligomerized BCR, CD19 and other adaptor proteins and kinases forming signalosome. The protooncogenic protein VAV (VAV1, VAV2, VAV3) interacts with Y391EEP in the cytoplasmic tail of CD19, which is presumably phosphorylated by SYK (O'Rourke et al. 1998), facilitating localization of LYN and SYK within close proximity. Then, VAV is phosphorylated by SYK (Chen et al. 2011) and which then functions as a GEF for Rho GTPases such as Rac2, which are crucial actin-organizer enabling B cell adhesion and microcluster formation (Arana et al. 2008). In addition to the actin cytoskeletal structure, a network of transmembrane proteins, tetraspanin CD81, is crucial for organization of appropriate interaction of BCR and CD19 because CD81-deficient B cells exhibited impaired BCR signaling upon ligation of antigen on cell surface (Miyazaki et al. 1997; Mattila et al. 2013). In the absence of Wiskott–Aldrich syndrome protein-interacting protein (WIP) in B cells, distortion of actin cytoskeleton and tetraspanin networks occur, causing impaired CD19 activation and PI3K signaling. This impairment results in multiple defects in the process of chemotactic homing, survival and differentiation, suggesting a central role for WIP in cytoskeletal actin dynamics-mediated PI3K activation (Keppler et al. 2015).

2.3 Negative Regulators of BCR Signaling

The magnitude and duration of the BCR signaling are controlled by a balance between activating and inhibitory mechanisms. The positive signals are normally counterbalanced by negative signals that limit B cell activation and prevent spontaneous self-reactive B cell response. The negative regulatory mechanisms of the BCR signaling cascade target its crucial enzymes by counteracting their activity and by regulating their stability and localization. The mechanisms are often induced by activating signals.

2.3.1 Negative Regulation of the Proximal BCR Signaling

LYN is a BCR-associated SRC kinase involved in the positive regulation of BCR, but it also functions as a negative regulator by phosphorylating the immunoreceptor tyrosine-based inhibitory motifs (ITIMs) of FcγRIIB and CD22. This phosphorylated ITIMs recruit several tyrosine phosphatases including SRC homology region 2 domain-containing phosphatase-1 (SHP-1) to suppress downstream signaling by

BCR (Fig. 2.2). It was recently reported that in the LYN-deficient background, other SRC kinases such as FYN and BLK propagated BCR signaling, but the suppression of the signaling was impaired, balancing the BCR signaling by LYN and FYN (Mkaddem et al. 2017). Indeed, B cell-specific *Lyn*-deficient mice developed autoimmune diseases, which were normalized by further deletion of MyD88 (Lamagna et al. 2014; Hua et al. 2014).

As mentioned above, SHP-1, highly expressed in hematopoietic lineage cells, is recruited by the phosphorylated ITIM-bearing receptors such as FcγRIIB, CD22, PIR-B, CD72 and Siglec-G, and it dephosphorylates proximal BCR signaling molecules such as CD79, SYK, BLNK and VAV (Tsubata 2012, 2017). The B cell-specific deficiency of *protein tyrosine phosphatase non-receptor type (Ptpn) 6* encoding SHP-1 resulted in SLE-like diseases, accompanied by the production of anti-DNA autoantibodies and renal autoantibody deposition in old age (5–8-month old). Of interest, although Ca^{2+} response in B2 cells in young B cell-specific *Ptpn6*-deficient mice is completely normal, the proliferation of the cells is impaired upon anti-IgM stimulation in vitro and both T cell-dependent (TD) and T cell-independent (TI) immunoglobulin production is reduced, probably due to the reduced cell number of B2 and MZ B cells due to the deletion of *Ptpn6* (Pao et al. 2007).

In addition to the ITIM-bearing suppressive receptors described above, CD300d (also called MAIR-II) participates in suppression of B cell activation (Fig. 2.2). Deficiency of either CD300d or DNAX activation protein 12 (DAP12) in B cells enhances B cell proliferation when stimulated by anti-IgM and also enhances TD response as well as autoantibody production. Therefore, CD300d requires an adaptor protein, DAP12, which associates with SHP-1 after BCR stimulation for CD300d-DAP12-dependent suppression (Nakano-Yokomizo et al. 2011). In addition, SHP-2, which is more widely expressed in various cell lineages in comparison with SHP-1, exerts its suppressive function after being recruited to programmed death-1 (PD-1) and/or FcγRIIb. The SHP-2 dephosphorylates BCR-associating key molecules like CD79, SYK, PLCγ and GRAB1 (Okazaki et al. 2001; Koncz et al. 2001). Another *Ptpn* family gene *Ptpn22* is associated with several autoimmune disorders. A single nucleotide polymorphism in the *PTPN22* gene generates a mutant form of

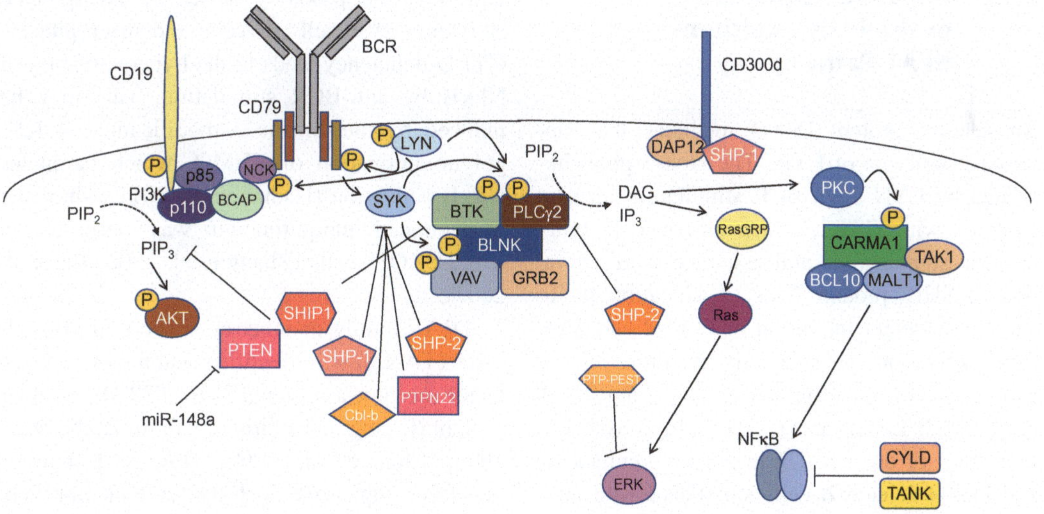

Fig. 2.2 Antagonization of the BCR signaling. SYK which mediates the proximal BCR signaling is inhibited by phosphatases, SHP-1/2 and PTPN22. CD300d-DAP12-SHP-1 complex may contribute to it. PHIP1 and PTEN suppress PI3K–AKT pathway by reduction of PIP_3 production. ERK and NFκB are inhibited by PTP-PEST and CYLD/TANK, respectively

PTPN22 (R620W amino acid substitution) in human. In a knock in mice with an analogous *Ptpn22* mutation (R619W), B cells represent hyperactivation of SYK following BCR stimulation. Furthermore, B cell-specific induction of the R619W mutant is sufficient to develop autoimmune disease (Dai et al. 2013). In line with this observation, carrying of the mutant protein prevents removal of autoreactive human B cells, suggesting a critical role for PTPN22 in B cell tolerance (Menard et al. 2011).

Casitas B-lineage Lymphoma (Cbl) family protein Cbl-b is a E3 ubiquitin ligase which negatively regulates SRC kinases (Thien and Langdon 2001). Upon BCR stimulation, SYK was ubiquitinylated by Cbl-b in B cells, and B cells isolated from Cbl-b KO mice showed the enhanced activation (indicated by CD86 expression) of proximal BCR signaling molecules including SYK, VAV1 and PLCγ2 (Bachmaier et al. 2000; Rao et al. 2001; Sohn et al. 2003; Kitaura et al. 2007). The Cbl null mice in which Cbl-b was additionally deleted only in B cells developed the lupus-like autoimmune disease, suggesting that Cbl proteins may regulate the B cell tolerance (Kitaura et al. 2007).

2.3.2 Negative Regulation of the PLCγ2-Calcium-NFAT Pathway

An adaptor protein Dok-3 mediates the suppressive function of LYN. The Dok-3 phosphorylated by LYN upon BCR stimulation forms a complex with GRB2, which allows it to enter into the signalosome and associate with activation of SHIP protein. This translocation facilitates the efficient inhibition of PLCγ2 and SYK from activation, subsequently resulting in the suppression of downstream Ca^{2+} signaling (Stork et al. 2007; Losing et al. 2013). In consistence with this, TI but not TD response is enhanced, and Dok-3-deleted B cells stimulated with anti-BCR show advanced proliferation and activation (Ng et al. 2007).

2.3.3 Negative Regulation of the IKK/NFκB Pathway

A20, encoded by *Tnfaip3*, is a cytoplasmic zinc finger protein which downregulates NFκB signaling by cooperative action with two different ubiquitin-regulating domains; deubiquitinating (DUB) that removes lysine-63 (K63)-linked ubiquitin chains and ubiquitin ligase domain that polyubiquitinate target proteins with K48-linked ubiquitin chains (Wertz et al. 2004). In line with observations in germline null A20 KO mice (Lee et al. 2000), B cell-specific *Tnfaip3*-deficient mice developed an autoimmune disease phenotype, which was thought to be caused by aberrant activation of B cells as well as T cells. The A20-deficient B cells represent prolonged NFκB signaling when stimulated by various stimuli including anti-BCR and resistance against programmed cell death, which is presumably caused by enhanced expression of anti-apoptotic protein, Bcl-x (Tavares et al. 2010; Chu et al. 2011; Hovelmeyer et al. 2011).

Cylindromatosis (CYLD) is a ubiquitin-carboxyterminal hydrolase, which removes lysine 63-linked (K63-linked) polyubiquitin chains from various target proteins. CYLD KO mice is susceptible to chronic inflammatory tumorigenesis, probably caused by dysregulated activation of T cells, B cells and macrophages. CYLD deficiency leads to the hyperactivation of NFκB by anti-BCR stimulation. This may be induced by the enhanced modification of K63 polyubiquitination of NEMO, which facilitates NFκB activation (Hadian et al. 2011), since the dysregulated ubiquitination was observed in CYLD KO T cells (Zhang et al. 2006; Jin et al. 2007).

TRAF family member-associated NFκB activator (TANK) was identified as a tumor necrosis factor receptor-associated factor (TRAF)-binding protein (Cheng and Baltimore 1996; Rothe et al. 1996; Chin et al. 1999). TANK KO mice developed lupus-like nephritis with autoantibody production. TANK KO B cells displayed an increased proliferative ability upon BCR stimulation with enhanced NFκB activity and TRAF6 ubiquitination (Kawagoe et al. 2009). However, since TRAF6 seems dispensable for BCR-mediated proliferation (Kobayashi et al. 2009), there may be another target of TANK. Furthermore, introduction of MyD88 deletion in TANK KO mice suppressed autoantibody production (Kobayashi et al. 2009), suggesting that TLR signaling might be a major target of TANK.

2.3.4 Negative Regulation of the Ras/ERK Pathway

An adaptor protein $p62^{dok}$ has been reported to associate with RasGAP upon BCR stimulation (Gold et al. 1993). Upon co-ligation of BCR with FcγRIIb, $p62^{dok}$ is phosphorylated in a SHIP-dependent manner. Then, the phosphorylated $p62^{dok}$ associates with RasGAP, resulting in the suppression of Ras/ERK signaling (Tamir et al. 2000). Therefore, $p62^{dok}$ serves as a SHIP-dependent suppressive adaptor protein upon BCR and FcγRIIb aggregation. In addition, a protein tyrosine phosphatase, PTP-PEST, coded by *Ptpn12*, is expressed in a wide variety of hematopoietic cells and inhibits the phosphorylation of ERK1 and ERK2 in PTP-PEST-overexpressing mature B cell line upon BCR stimulation (Davidson and Veillette 2001).

2.3.5 Negative Regulation of the PI3K Pathway

The inositol polyphosphate 5-phosphatase (SHIP) and phosphatase and tensin homolog (PTEN) serve as negative regulators of PI3K to target PIP_3, which is a second messenger generated by PI3K (Fig. 2.2). In SHIP1 KO mice, B cells show enhanced proliferation and activation when stimulated by anti-BCR and anti-CD40 plus IL-4, accompanied with increased antibody production (Helgason et al. 2000; Brauweiler et al. 2000). The B cell-specific deletion confirmed the above-mentioned result and further demonstrated a B cell-intrinsic role for SHIP1 in SLE-like autoimmune disease (O'Neill et al. 2011; Maxwell et al. 2011; Leung et al. 2013). Since the aggregation of BCR and FcγRIIb inhibits the trophic signal provided by BAFFR (Crowley et al. 2009), the exaggerated survival signals in these conditional SHIP1KO mice may, in part, contribute to the autoimmune disorders. In contrast to SHIP1, little is known about SHIP2. The SHIP2 is induced in LPS-stimulated B cells. The SHIP1 might presumably play a redundant role with SHIP2 in resting B cells (Brauweiler et al. 2001).

PTEN also plays a crucial role in the suppression of AKT activation by hydrolyzation of PIP_3. The B cell-specific *Pten*-deficient mice represents autoantibody production (Suzuki et al. 2003). This may be partly due to advanced proliferation and activation by various stimuli including anti-BCR and persistence of transitional immature B cells because of impaired apoptosis by PTEN deletion (Anzelon et al. 2003; Cheng et al. 2009). In addition, the recent study with in vivo functional screening of microRNA library identified miR-148a as a suppressor of PTEN (Gonzalez-Martin et al. 2016).

2.4 Concluding Remarks

In the past few decades, a number of studies on BCR signaling, in particular with an emphasis on their positive regulators, have been carried out. However, many studies in the early days were performed in cell lines. Therefore, it is necessary to validate their roles and functions under physiological conditions, which is especially important in case the factors are to be considered as a novel therapeutic target. On the other hand, number of molecules that suppress the activity of proximal kinases of BCR signaling have been identified, but suppressors including feedback regulators that dampen distal signaling branches are much less studied. Studies about these regulatory proteins will help in better understanding of immunological disorders and tumor immunity and may contribute to the development of novel strategies for therapy and diagnosis.

Acknowledgements This work was supported by Grant-in-Aid from the Ministry of Education, Culture, Sports, Science and Technology, Japan to S.T. & Y.B. and AMED under Grant Number JP19ek0410044 and JP19gm6110004 to Y.B.

References

Aiba Y, Kameyama M, Yamazaki T, Tedder TF, Kurosaki T (2008) Regulation of B-cell development by BCAP and CD19 through their binding to phosphoinositide 3-kinase. Blood 111:1497–1503

Aiba Y, Oh-hora M, Kiyonaka S, Kimura Y, Hijikata A, Mori Y, Kurosaki T (2004) Activation of RasGRP3 by phosphorylation of Thr-133 is required for B cell receptor-mediated Ras activation. Proc Natl Acad Sci USA 101:16612–16617

Akkaya M, Traba J, Roesler AS, Miozzo P, Akkaya B, Theall BP, Sohn H, Pena M, Smelkinson M, Kabat J, Dahlstrom E, Dorward DW, Skinner J, Sack MN, Pierce SK (2018) Second signals rescue B cells from activation-induced mitochondrial dysfunction and death. Nat Immunol 19:871–884

Amin RH, Schlissel MS (2008) Foxo1 directly regulates the transcription of recombination-activating genes during B cell development. Nat Immunol 9:613–622

Anzelon AN, Wu H, Rickert RC (2003) Pten inactivation alters peripheral B lymphocyte fate and reconstitutes CD19 function. Nat Immunol 4:287–294

Arana E, Vehlow A, Harwood NE, Vigorito E, Henderson R, Turner M, Tybulewicz VL, Batista FD (2008) Activation of the small GTPase Rac2 via the B cell receptor regulates B cell adhesion and immunological-synapse formation. Immunity 28:88–99

Baba Y, Kurosaki T (2011) Impact of Ca2+ signaling on B cell function. Trends Immunol 32:589–594

Bachmaier K, Krawczyk C, Kozieradzki I, Kong YY, Sasaki T, Oliveira-dos-Santos A, Mariathasan S, Bouchard D, Wakeham A, Itie A, Le J, Ohashi PS, Sarosi I, Nishina H, Lipkowitz S, Penninger JM (2000) Negative regulation of lymphocyte activation and autoimmunity by the molecular adaptor Cbl-b. Nature 403:211–216

Brauweiler A, Tamir I, Dal Porto J, Benschop RJ, Helgason CD, Humphries RK, Freed JH, Cambier JC (2000) Differential regulation of B cell development, activation, and death by the src homology 2 domain-containing 5' inositol phosphatase (SHIP). J Exp Med 191:1545–1554

Brauweiler A, Tamir I, Marschner S, Helgason CD, Cambier JC (2001) Partially distinct molecular mechanisms mediate inhibitory FcgammaRIIB signaling in resting and activated B cells. J Immunol 167:204–211

Castello A, Gaya M, Tucholski J, Oellerich T, Lu KH, Tafuri A, Pawson T, Wienands J, Engelke M, Batista FD (2013) Nck-mediated recruitment of BCAP to the BCR regulates the PI(3)K-Akt pathway in B cells. Nat Immunol 14:966–975

Cato MH, Chintalapati SK, Yau IW, Omori SA, Rickert RC (2011) Cyclin D3 is selectively required for proliferative expansion of germinal center B cells. Mol Cell Biol 31:127–137

Chaturvedi A, Martz R, Dorward D, Waisberg M, Pierce SK (2011) Endocytosed BCRs sequentially regulate MAPK and Akt signaling pathways from intracellular compartments. Nat Immunol 12:1119–1126

Chen CH, Martin VA, Gorenstein NM, Geahlen RL, Post CB (2011) Two closely spaced tyrosines regulate NFAT signaling in B cells via Syk association with Vav. Mol Cell Biol 31:2984–2996

Cheng D, Deobagkar-Lele M, Zvezdova E, Choi S, Uehara S, Baup D, Bennett SC, Bull KR, Crockford TL, Ferry H, Warzecha C, Marcellin M, de Peredo AG, Lesourne R, Anzilotti C, Love PE, Cornall RJ (2017) Themis2 lowers the threshold for B cell activation during positive selection. Nat Immunol 18:205–213

Cheng G, Baltimore D (1996) TANK, a co-inducer with TRAF2 of TNF- and CD 40L-mediated NF-kappaB activation. Genes Dev 10:963–973

Cheng S, Hsia CY, Feng B, Liou ML, Fang X, Pandolfi PP, Liou HC (2009) BCR-mediated apoptosis associated with negative selection of immature B cells is selectively dependent on Pten. Cell Res 19: 196–207

Chin AI, Shu J, Shan Shi C, Yao Z, Kehrl JH, Cheng G (1999) TANK potentiates tumor necrosis factor receptor-associated factor-mediated c-Jun N-terminal kinase/stress-activated protein kinase activation through the germinal center kinase pathway. Mol Cell Biol 19:6665–6672

Chu Y, Vahl JC, Kumar D, Heger K, Bertossi A, Wojtowicz E, Soberon V, Schenten D, Mack B, Reutelshofer M, Beyaert R, Amann K, van Loo G, Schmidt-Supprian M (2011) B cells lacking the tumor suppressor TNFAIP3/A20 display impaired differentiation and hyperactivation and cause inflammation and autoimmunity in aged mice. Blood 117:2227–2236

Coughlin JJ, Stang SL, Dower NA, Stone JC (2005) RasGRP1 and RasGRP3 regulate B cell proliferation by facilitating B cell receptor-Ras signaling. J Immunol 175:7179–7184

Crowley JE, Stadanlick JE, Cambier JC, Cancro MP (2009) FcgammaRIIB signals inhibit BLyS signaling and BCR-mediated BLyS receptor up-regulation. Blood 113:1464–1473

Dai X, James RG, Habib T, Singh S, Jackson S, Khim S, Moon RT, Liggitt D, Wolf-Yadlin A, Buckner JH, Rawlings DJ (2013) A disease-associated PTPN22 variant promotes systemic autoimmunity in murine models. J Clin Invest 123:2024–2036

Davidson D, Veillette A (2001) PTP-PEST, a scaffold protein tyrosine phosphatase, negatively regulates lymphocyte activation by targeting a unique set of substrates. EMBO J 20:3414–3426

Delgado P, Cubelos B, Calleja E, Martinez-Martin N, Cipres A, Merida I, Bellas C, Bustelo XR, Alarcon B (2009) Essential function for the GTPase TC21 in homeostatic antigen receptor signaling. Nat Immunol 10:880–888

Dengler HS, Baracho GV, Omori SA, Bruckner S, Arden KC, Castrillon DH, DePinho RA, Rickert RC (2008) Distinct functions for the transcription factor Foxo1 at various stages of B cell differentiation. Nat Immunol 9:1388–1398

Dominguez-Sola D, Kung J, Holmes AB, Wells VA, Mo T, Basso K, Dalla-Favera R (2015) The FOXO1 Transcription Factor Instructs the Germinal Center Dark Zone Program. Immunity 43:1064–1074

Dong C, Davis RJ, Flavell RA (2002) MAP kinases in the immune response. Annu Rev Immunol 20:55–72

Engels N, Konig LM, Heemann C, Lutz J, Tsubata T, Griep S, Schrader V, Wienands J (2009) Recruitment of the cytoplasmic adaptor Grb2 to surface IgG and IgE provides antigen receptor-intrinsic costimulation to class-switched B cells. Nat Immunol 10:1018–1025

Feske S, Gwack Y, Prakriya M, Srikanth S, Puppel SH, Tanasa B, Hogan PG, Lewis RS, Daly M, Rao A (2006) A mutation in Orai1 causes immune deficiency by abrogating CRAC channel function. Nature 441:179–185

Flaswinkel H, Reth M (1994) Dual role of the tyrosine activation motif of the Ig-alpha protein during signal transduction via the B cell antigen receptor. EMBO J 13:83–89

Fleire SJ, Goldman JP, Carrasco YR, Weber M, Bray D, Batista FD (2006) B cell ligand discrimination through a spreading and contraction response. Science 312:738–741

Fujimoto M, Fujimoto Y, Poe JC, Jansen PJ, Lowell CA, DeFranco AL, Tedder TF (2000) CD19 regulates Src family protein tyrosine kinase activation in B lymphocytes through processive amplification. Immunity 13:47–57

Gazumyan A, Reichlin A, Nussenzweig MC (2006) Ig beta tyrosine residues contribute to the control of B cell receptor signaling by regulating receptor internalization. J Exp Med 203:1785–1794

Gold MR, Crowley MT, Martin GA, McCormick F, DeFranco AL (1993) Targets of B lymphocyte antigen receptor signal transduction include the p21ras GTPase-activating protein (GAP) and two GAP-associated proteins. J Immunol 150:377–386

Gonzalez-Martin A, Adams BD, Lai M, Shepherd J, Salvador-Bernaldez M, Salvador JM, Lu J, Nemazee D, Xiao C (2016) The microRNA miR-148a functions as a critical regulator of B cell tolerance and autoimmunity. Nat Immunol 17:433–440

Gregory MA, Qi Y, Hann SR (2003) Phosphorylation by glycogen synthase kinase-3 controls c-myc proteolysis and subnuclear localization. J Biol Chem 278:51606–51612

Gross JA, Dillon SR, Mudri S, Johnston J, Littau A, Roque R, Rixon M, Schou O, Foley KP, Haugen H, McMillen S, Waggie K, Schreckhise RW, Shoemaker K, Vu T, Moore M, Grossman A, Clegg CH (2001) TACI-Ig neutralizes molecules critical for B cell development and autoimmune disease. Impaired B cell maturation in mice lacking BLyS. Immunity 15:289–302

Hadian K, Griesbach RA, Dornauer S, Wanger TM, Nagel D, Metlitzky M, Beisker W, Schmidt-Supprian M, Krappmann D (2011) NF-kappaB essential modulator (NEMO) interaction with linear and lys-63 ubiquitin chains contributes to NF-kappaB activation. J Biol Chem 286:26107–26117

Helgason CD, Kalberer CP, Damen JE, Chappel SM, Pineault N, Krystal G, Humphries RK (2000) A dual role for Src homology 2 domain-containing inositol-5-phosphatase (SHIP) in immunity: aberrant development and enhanced function of b lymphocytes in ship -/- mice. J Exp Med 191:781–794

Hikida M, Kurosaki T (2005) Regulation of phospholipase C-gamma2 networks in B lymphocytes. Adv Immunol 88:73–96

Hollenhorst PC (2012) RAS/ERK pathway transcriptional regulation through ETS/AP-1 binding sites. Small GTPases 3:154–158

Hou P, Araujo E, Zhao T, Zhang M, Massenburg D, Veselits M, Doyle C, Dinner AR, Clark MR (2006) B cell antigen receptor signaling and internalization are mutually exclusive events. PLoS Biol 4:e200

Hovelmeyer N, Reissig S, Xuan NT, Adams-Quack P, Lukas D, Nikolaev A, Schluter D, Waisman A (2011) A20 deficiency in B cells enhances B-cell proliferation and results in the development of autoantibodies. Eur J Immunol 41:595–601

Hua Z, Gross AJ, Lamagna C, Ramos-Hernandez N, Scapini P, Ji M, Shao H, Lowell CA, Hou B, DeFranco AL (2014) Requirement for MyD88 signaling in B cells and dendritic cells for germinal center anti-nuclear antibody production in Lyn-deficient mice. J Immunol 192:875–885

Inoki K, Li Y, Zhu T, Wu J, Guan KL (2002) TSC2 is phosphorylated and inhibited by Akt and suppresses mTOR signalling. Nat Cell Biol 4:648–657

Ishiai M, Kurosaki M, Pappu R, Okawa K, Ronko I, Fu C, Shibata M, Iwamatsu A, Chan AC, Kurosaki T (1999) BLNK required for coupling Syk to PLC gamma 2 and Rac1-JNK in B cells. Immunity 10:117–125

Jellusova J, Cato MH, Apgar JR, Ramezani-Rad P, Leung CR, Chen C, Richardson AD, Conner EM, Benschop RJ, Woodgett JR, Rickert RC (2017) Gsk3 is a metabolic checkpoint regulator in B cells. Nat Immunol 18:303–312

Jin W, Reiley WR, Lee AJ, Wright A, Wu X, Zhang M, Sun SC (2007) Deubiquitinating enzyme CYLD regulates the peripheral development and naive phenotype maintenance of B cells. J Biol Chem 282:15884–15893

Kawagoe T, Takeuchi O, Takabatake Y, Kato H, Isaka Y, Tsujimura T, Akira S (2009) TANK is a negative regulator of Toll-like receptor signaling and is critical for the prevention of autoimmune nephritis. Nat Immunol 10:965–972

Keppler SJ, Gasparrini F, Burbage M, Aggarwal S, Frederico B, Geha RS, Way M, Bruckbauer A, Batista FD (2015) Wiskott-Aldrich Syndrome Interacting Protein Deficiency Uncovers the Role of the Co-receptor CD19 as a Generic Hub for PI3 Kinase Signaling in B Cells. Immunity 43:660–673

Kitaura Y, Jang IK, Wang Y, Han YC, Inazu T, Cadera EJ, Schlissel M, Hardy RR, Gu H (2007) Control of the B cell-intrinsic tolerance programs by ubiquitin ligases Cbl and Cbl-b. Immunity 26:567–578

Kobayashi T, Kim TS, Jacob A, Walsh MC, Kadono Y, Fuentes-Panana E, Yoshioka T, Yoshimura A, Yamamoto M, Kaisho T, Akira S, Monroe JG, Choi Y (2009) TRAF6 is required for generation of the B-1a B cell compartment as well as T cell-dependent and -independent humoral immune responses. PLoS ONE 4:e4736

Koncz G, Toth GK, Bokonyi G, Keri G, Pecht I, Medgyesi D, Gergely J, Sarmay G (2001) Co-clustering of Fcgamma and B cell receptors induces dephosphorylation of the Grb2-associated binder 1 docking protein. Eur J Biochem 268:3898–3906

Kurosaki T, Shinohara H, Baba Y (2010) B cell signaling and fate decision. Annu Rev Immunol 28:21–55

Lam KP, Kuhn R, Rajewsky K (1997) In vivo ablation of surface immunoglobulin on mature B cells by inducible gene targeting results in rapid cell death. Cell 90:1073–1083

Lamagna C, Hu Y, DeFranco AL, Lowell CA (2014) B cell-specific loss of Lyn kinase leads to autoimmunity. J Immunol 192:919–928

Lee EG, Boone DL, Chai S, Libby SL, Chien M, Lodolce JP, Ma A (2000) Failure to regulate TNF-induced NF-kappaB and cell death responses in A20-deficient mice. Science 289:2350–2354

Leung WH, Tarasenko T, Biesova Z, Kole H, Walsh ER, Bolland S (2013) Aberrant antibody affinity selection in SHIP-deficient B cells. Eur J Immunol 43:371–381

Limon JJ, Fruman DA (2012) Akt and mTOR in B Cell Activation and Differentiation. Front Immunol 3:228

Lin YC, Jhunjhunwala S, Benner C, Heinz S, Welinder E, Mansson R, Sigvardsson M, Hagman J, Espinoza CA, Dutkowski J, Ideker T, Glass CK, Murre C (2010) A global network of transcription factors, involving E2A, EBF1 and Foxo1, that orchestrates B cell fate. Nat Immunol 11:635–643

Liou J, Kim ML, Heo WD, Jones JT, Myers JW, Ferrell JE Jr, Meyer T (2005) STIM is a Ca2+ sensor essential for Ca2+-store-depletion-triggered Ca2+ influx. Curr Biol 15:1235–1241

Losing M, Goldbeck I, Manno B, Oellerich T, Schnyder T, Bohnenberger H, Stork B, Urlaub H, Batista FD, Wienands J, Engelke M (2013) The Dok-3/Grb2 protein signal module attenuates Lyn kinase-dependent activation of Syk kinase in B cell antigen receptor microclusters. J Biol Chem 288:2303–2313

Mackay F, Figgett WA, Saulep D, Lepage M, Hibbs ML (2010) B-cell stage and context-dependent requirements for survival signals from BAFF and the B-cell receptor. Immunol Rev 237:205–225

Mansson R, Welinder E, Ahsberg J, Lin YC, Benner C, Glass CK, Lucas JS, Sigvardsson M, Murre C (2012) Positive intergenic feedback circuitry, involving EBF1 and FOXO1, orchestrates B-cell fate. Proc Natl Acad Sci USA 109:21028–21033

Matsumoto M, Fujii Y, Baba A, Hikida M, Kurosaki T, Baba Y (2011) The calcium sensors STIM1 and STIM2 control B cell regulatory function through interleukin-10 production. Immunity 34:703–714

Mattila PK, Feest C, Depoil D, Treanor B, Montaner B, Otipoby KL, Carter R, Justement LB, Bruckbauer A, Batista FD (2013) The actin and tetraspanin networks organize receptor nanoclusters to regulate B cell receptor-mediated signaling. Immunity 38:461–474

Maxwell MJ, Duan M, Armes JE, Anderson GP, Tarlinton DM, Hibbs ML (2011) Genetic segregation of inflammatory lung disease and autoimmune disease severity in SHIP-1-/- mice. J Immunol 186:7164–7175

Menard L, Saadoun D, Isnardi I, Ng YS, Meyers G, Massad C, Price C, Abraham C, Motaghedi R, Buckner JH, Gregersen PK, Meffre E (2011) The PTPN22 allele encoding an R620W variant interferes with the removal of developing autoreactive B cells in humans. J Clin Invest 121:3635–3644

Miller DJ, Hayes CE (1991) Phenotypic and genetic characterization of a unique B lymphocyte deficiency in strain A/WySnJ mice. Eur J Immunol 21:1123–1130

Minguet S, Klasener K, Schaffer AM, Fiala GJ, Osteso-Ibanez T, Raute K, Navarro-Lerida I, Hartl FA, Seidl M, Reth M, Del Pozo MA (2017) Caveolin-1-dependent nanoscale organization of the BCR regulates B cell tolerance. Nat Immunol 18:1150–1159

Miyazaki T, Muller U, Campbell KS (1997) Normal development but differentially altered proliferative responses of lymphocytes in mice lacking CD81. EMBO J 16:4217–4225

Mkaddem SB, Murua A, Flament H, Titeca-Beauport D, Bounaix C, Danelli L, Launay P, Benhamou M, Blank U, Daugas E, Charles N, Monteiro RC (2017) Lyn and Fyn function as molecular switches that control immunoreceptors to direct homeostasis or inflammation. Nat Commun 8:246

Nagaoka H, Takahashi Y, Hayashi R, Nakamura T, Ishii K, Matsuda J, Ogura A, Shirakata Y, Karasuyama H, Sudo T, Nishikawa S, Tsubata T, Mizuochi T, Asano T, Sakano H, Takemori T (2000) Ras mediates effector pathways responsible for pre-B cell survival, which is essential for the developmental progression to the late pre-B cell stage. J Exp Med 192:171–182

Nakano-Yokomizo T, Tahara-Hanaoka S, Nakahashi-Oda C, Nabekura T, Tchao NK, Kadosaki M, Totsuka N, Kurita N, Nakamagoe K, Tamaoka A, Takai T, Yasui T,

Kikutani H, Honda S, Shibuya K, Lanier LL, Shibuya A (2011) The immunoreceptor adapter protein DAP12 suppresses B lymphocyte-driven adaptive immune responses. J Exp Med 208:1661–1671
Ng CH, Xu S, Lam KP (2007) Dok-3 plays a nonredundant role in negative regulation of B-cell activation. Blood 110:259–266
Nguyen TT, Klasener K, Zurn C, Castillo PA, Brust-Mascher I, Imai DM, Bevins CL, Reardon C, Reth M, Baumgarth N (2017) The IgM receptor FcmuR limits tonic BCR signaling by regulating expression of the IgM BCR. Nat Immunol 18:321–333
O'Neill SK, Getahun A, Gauld SB, Merrell KT, Tamir I, Smith MJ, Dal Porto JM, Li QZ, Cambier JC (2011) Monophosphorylation of CD79a and CD79b ITAM motifs initiates a SHIP-1 phosphatase-mediated inhibitory signaling cascade required for B cell anergy. Immunity 35:746–756
O'Rourke LM, Tooze R, Turner M, Sandoval DM, Carter RH, Tybulewicz VL, Fearon DT (1998) CD19 as a membrane-anchored adaptor protein of B lymphocytes: costimulation of lipid and protein kinases by recruitment of Vav. Immunity 8:635–645
Oh-hora M, Johmura S, Hashimoto A, Hikida M, Kurosaki T (2003) Requirement for Ras guanine nucleotide releasing protein 3 in coupling phospholipase C-gamma2 to Ras in B cell receptor signaling. J Exp Med 198:1841–1851
Okada T, Maeda A, Iwamatsu A, Gotoh K, Kurosaki T (2000) BCAP: the tyrosine kinase substrate that connects B cell receptor to phosphoinositide 3-kinase activation. Immunity 13:817–827
Okazaki T, Maeda A, Nishimura H, Kurosaki T, Honjo T (2001) PD-1 immunoreceptor inhibits B cell receptor-mediated signaling by recruiting src homology 2-domain-containing tyrosine phosphatase 2 to phosphotyrosine. Proc Natl Acad Sci USA 98:13866–13871
Pao LI, Lam KP, Henderson JM, Kutok JL, Alimzhanov M, Nitschke L, Thomas ML, Neel BG, Rajewsky K (2007) B cell-specific deletion of protein-tyrosine phosphatase Shp1 promotes B-1a cell development and causes systemic autoimmunity. Immunity 27:35–48
Peng SL, Gerth AJ, Ranger AM, Glimcher LH (2001) NFATc1 and NFATc2 together control both T and B cell activation and differentiation. Immunity 14:13–20
Rao N, Ghosh AK, Ota S, Zhou P, Reddi AL, Hakezi K, Druker BK, Wu J, Band H (2001) The non-receptor tyrosine kinase Syk is a target of Cbl-mediated ubiquitylation upon B-cell receptor stimulation. EMBO J 20:7085–7095
Retter MW, Nemazee D (1998) Receptor editing occurs frequently during normal B cell development. J Exp Med 188:1231–1238
Roos J, DiGregorio PJ, Yeromin AV, Ohlsen K, Lioudyno M, Zhang S, Safrina O, Kozak JA, Wagner SL, Cahalan MD, Velicelebi G, Stauderman KA (2005) STIM1, an essential and conserved component of store-operated Ca2+ channel function. J Cell Biol 169:435–445
Rothe M, Xiong J, Shu HB, Williamson K, Goddard A, Goeddel DV (1996) I-TRAF is a novel TRAF-interacting protein that regulates TRAF-mediated signal transduction. Proc Natl Acad Sci USA 93:8241–8246
Rowland SL, DePersis CL, Torres RM, Pelanda R (2010) Ras activation of Erk restores impaired tonic BCR signaling and rescues immature B cell differentiation. J Exp Med 207:607–621
Saijo K, Schmedt C, Su IH, Karasuyama H, Lowell CA, Reth M, Adachi T, Patke A, Santana A, Tarakhovsky A (2003) Essential role of Src-family protein tyrosine kinases in NF-kappaB activation during B cell development. Nat Immunol 4:274–279
Sanchez M, Misulovin Z, Burkhardt AL, Mahajan S, Costa T, Franke R, Bolen JB, Nussenzweig M (1993) Signal transduction by immunoglobulin is mediated through Ig alpha and Ig beta. J Exp Med 178:1049–1055
Sander S, Chu VT, Yasuda T, Franklin A, Graf R, Calado DP, Li S, Imami K, Selbach M, Di Virgilio M, Bullinger L, Rajewsky K (2015) PI3 Kinase and FOXO1 Transcription Factor Activity Differentially Control B Cells in the Germinal Center Light and Dark Zones. Immunity 43:1075–1086
Schweighoffer E, Vanes L, Nys J, Cantrell D, McCleary S, Smithers N, Tybulewicz VL (2013) The BAFF receptor transduces survival signals by co-opting the B cell receptor signaling pathway. Immunity 38:475–488
Shinohara H, Maeda S, Watarai H, Kurosaki T (2007) IkappaB kinase beta-induced phosphorylation of CARMA1 contributes to CARMA1 Bcl10 MALT1 complex formation in B cells. J Exp Med 204:3285–3293
Shinohara H, Yasuda T, Aiba Y, Sanjo H, Hamadate M, Watarai H, Sakurai H, Kurosaki T (2005) PKC beta regulates BCR-mediated IKK activation by facilitating the interaction between TAK1 and CARMA1. J Exp Med 202:1423–1431
Sohn HW, Gu H, Pierce SK (2003) Cbl-b negatively regulates B cell antigen receptor signaling in mature B cells through ubiquitination of the tyrosine kinase Syk. J Exp Med 197:1511–1524
Srinivasan L, Sasaki Y, Calado DP, Zhang B, Paik JH, DePinho RA, Kutok JL, Kearney JF, Otipoby KL, Rajewsky K (2009) PI3 kinase signals BCR-dependent mature B cell survival. Cell 139:573–586
Stoddart A, Jackson AP, Brodsky FM (2005) Plasticity of B cell receptor internalization upon conditional depletion of clathrin. Mol Biol Cell 16:2339–2348
Stork B, Neumann K, Goldbeck I, Alers S, Kahne T, Naumann M, Engelke M, Wienands J (2007) Subcellular localization of Grb2 by the adaptor protein Dok-3 restricts the intensity of Ca2+ signaling in B cells. EMBO J 26:1140–1149

Suzuki A, Kaisho T, Ohishi M, Tsukio-Yamaguchi M, Tsubata T, Koni PA, Sasaki T, Mak TW, Nakano T (2003) Critical roles of Pten in B cell homeostasis and immunoglobulin class switch recombination. J Exp Med 197:657–667

Tamir I, Stolpa JC, Helgason CD, Nakamura K, Bruhns P, Daeron M, Cambier JC (2000) The RasGAP-binding protein p62dok is a mediator of inhibitory FcgammaRIIB signals in B cells. Immunity 12:347–358

Tavares RM, Turer EE, Liu CL, Advincula R, Scapini P, Rhee L, Barrera J, Lowell CA, Utz PJ, Malynn BA, Ma A (2010) The ubiquitin modifying enzyme A20 restricts B cell survival and prevents autoimmunity. Immunity 33:181–191

Thien CB, Langdon WY (2001) Cbl: many adaptations to regulate protein tyrosine kinases. Nat Rev Mol Cell Biol 2:294–307

Thompson JS, Bixler SA, Qian F, Vora K, Scott ML, Cachero TG, Hession C, Schneider P, Sizing ID, Mullen C, Strauch K, Zafari M, Benjamin CD, Tschopp J, Browning JL, Ambrose C (2001) BAFF-R, a newly identified TNF receptor that specifically interacts with BAFF. Science 293:2108–2211

Timmerman LA, Healy JI, Ho SN, Chen L, Goodnow CC, Crabtree GR (1997) Redundant expression but selective utilization of nuclear factor of activated T cells family members. J Immunol 159:2735–2740

Treanor B, Depoil D, Bruckbauer A, Batista FD (2010a) Dynamic cortical actin remodeling by ERM proteins controls BCR microcluster organization and integrity. J Exp Med 208:1055–1068

Treanor B, Depoil D, Gonzalez-Granja A, Barral P, Weber M, Dushek O, Bruckbauer A, Batista FD (2010b) The membrane skeleton controls diffusion dynamics and signaling through the B cell receptor. Immunity 32:187–199

Tsubata T (2012) Role of inhibitory BCR co-receptors in immunity. Infect Disord Drug Targets 12:181–190

Tsubata T (2017) B-cell tolerance and autoimmunity. *F1000Res* 6:391

Vanshylla K, Bartsch C, Hitzing C, Krumpelmann L, Wienands J, Engels N (2018) Grb2 and GRAP connect the B cell antigen receptor to Erk MAP kinase activation in human B cells. Sci Rep 8:4244

Vig M, Peinelt C, Beck A, Koomoa DL, Rabah D, Koblan-Huberson M, Kraft S, Turner H, Fleig A, Penner R, Kinet JP (2006) CRACM1 is a plasma membrane protein essential for store-operated Ca2+ entry. Science 312:1220–1223

Wertz IE, O'Rourke KM, Zhou H, Eby M, Aravind L, Seshagiri S, Wu P, Wiesmann C, Baker R, Boone DL, Ma A, Koonin EV, Dixit VM (2004) De-ubiquitination and ubiquitin ligase domains of A20 downregulate NF-kappaB signalling. Nature 430:694–699

Winslow MM, Gallo EM, Neilson JR, Crabtree GR (2006) The calcineurin phosphatase complex modulates immunogenic B cell responses. Immunity 24:141–152

Yasuda T, Sanjo H, Pages G, Kawano Y, Karasuyama H, Pouyssegur J, Ogata M, Kurosaki T (2008) Erk kinases link pre-B cell receptor signaling to transcriptional events required for early B cell expansion. Immunity 28:499–508

Zhang J, Stirling B, Temmerman ST, Ma CA, Fuss IJ, Derry JM, Jain A (2006) Impaired regulation of NF-kappaB and increased susceptibility to colitis-associated tumorigenesis in CYLD-deficient mice. J Clin Invest 116:3042–3049

Zheng Y, Liu H, Coughlin J, Zheng J, Li L, Stone JC (2005) Phosphorylation of RasGRP3 on threonine 133 provides a mechanistic link between PKC and Ras signaling systems in B cells. Blood 105:3648–3654

Involvement of Reactive Oxygen Species (ROS) in BCR Signaling as a Second Messenger

3

Takeshi Tsubata

Abstract

Reactive oxygen species (ROS) are not only toxic substances inducing oxidative stress but also play a role in receptor signaling as a second messenger, which augments signaling through various receptors by oxidizing ROS-sensitive signaling molecules. Among ROS, H_2O_2 is suggested to be an important second messenger because of its relative stability. H_2O_2 is generated by superoxide dismutase (SOD)-mediated conversion of superoxide produced by membrane-localized NADPH oxidases (NOXes). Superoxide and H_2O_2 are also produced as a by-product of mitochondrial respiratory chain and various other metabolic reactions. BCR ligation induces ROS production in two phases. ROS production starts immediately after BCR ligation and ceases in 1 h, then re-starts 2 h after BCR ligation and lasts 4–6 h. ROS production in the early phase is mediated by NOX2, a NOX isoform, but does not regulate BCR signaling. In contrast, ROS production at the late phase augments BCR signaling. Although the involvement of mitochondrial respiration was previously suggested in prolonged BCR ligation-induced ROS production, we recently demonstrated that NOX3, another NOX isoform, plays a central role in ROS production at the late phase. NOXes are shown to be a component of ROS-generating signaling endosome called redoxosome together with endocytosed receptors and receptor-associated signaling molecules. In redoxosome, ROS generated by NOXes augment signaling through the endocytosed receptor. The role of NOXes and redoxosome in BCR signaling needs to be further elucidated.

Keywords

Reactive oxygen species · BCR signaling · Second messenger · NADPH oxidases

3.1 Introduction

Reactive oxygen species (ROS) such as superoxide, hydroxyl radical, and hydrogen peroxide (H_2O_2) are produced in eukaryotic cells by various mechanisms (Holmstrom and Finkel 2014; Schieber and Chandel 2014; Reczek and Chandel 2015). Because ROS are chemically reactive, ROS damage proteins, lipids, and DNA resulting in cellular damage in various cell types. ROS are also involved in killing of bacteria by damaging bacterial components in phagocytes such as macrophages and neutrophils (Bedard and Krause 2007). In contrast, accumulating evidence

T. Tsubata (✉)
Department of Immunology, Medical Research Institute, Tokyo Medical and Dental University, Tokyo 113-8510, Japan
e-mail: tsubata.imm@mri.tmd.ac.jp

J.-Y. Wang (ed.), *B Cells in Immunity and Tolerance*, Advances in Experimental Medicine and Biology 1254, https://doi.org/10.1007/978-981-15-3532-1_3

suggests that ROS, especially H_2O_2, play a role in cellular signaling as a second messenger (Schieber and Chandel 2014; Reczek and Chandel 2015; Marinho et al. 2014; Di Marzo et al. 2018). Treatment with ROS scavengers such as N-acetyl cysteine (NAC) has been shown to down-regulate signaling through various cytokine receptors such as PDGF receptor and IL-1 receptor, TLRs and antigen receptors including both T cell receptor (TCR) and B cell receptor (BCR) (Schieber and Chandel 2014; Wheeler and Defranco 2012; Feng et al. 2019). ROS regulate the activity of various transcriptional factors and signaling molecules such as phosphatases by cysteine oxidation (Holmstrom and Finkel 2014; Schieber and Chandel 2014; Reczek and Chandel 2015; Marinho et al. 2014; Prieto-Bermejo and Hernandez-Hernandez 2017). Although the role of ROS in BCR signaling has been studied since the 1990s, a crucial role of ROS in BCR signaling was demonstrated only in the past decade (Wheeler and Defranco 2012; Feng et al. 2019), and still little is known about how ROS regulate BCR signaling. Here, I will first describe mechanisms of ROS production in mammalian cells and then discuss the role of ROS in BCR signaling including our recent findings.

3.2 Mechanisms for Intracellular ROS Production

There are a number of molecular mechanisms in which ROS are produced intracellularly as a by-product. Dependently on the mechanisms, ROS are produced in different organellae (Fig. 3.1). In mitochondria, superoxide is believed to be produced abundantly by complex I and complex III of the electron transport chain (Fig. 3.1b) (Holmstrom and Finkel 2014; Reczek and Chandel 2015). ROS are also produced in endoplasmic reticulum (ER) when disulfide bonds are generated in secretory and membrane proteins by oxidation at the cysteine residues (Zito 2015) (Fig. 3.1c). Electrons generated by protein disulfide isomerases (PDIs) that oxidize proteins are relayed to the endoplasmic reticulum oxireductin 1 (ERO1), which then generates H_2O_2 by reducing O_2. Plasma cells appear to produce a large amount of ROS in ER through biogenesis of immunoglobulins. In peroxisomes, ROS are produced when fatty acids and various other substances such as D-amino acids, polyamines, and glycolate are oxidized by flavin adenine dinucleotide (FAD)- or flavin mononucleotide (FMN)-dependent oxidases such as acyl CoA oxidase (Fig. 3.1d) (Lismont et al. 2019). Oxidation of these substrates generates H_2O_2. Furthermore, ROS are produced as a by-product of various cytosolic enzymes such as xanthine oxidase, cyclooxygenases, cytochrome P450 enzymes, and lipoxygenases (Holmstrom and Finkel 2014).

Unlike other molecular mechanisms in which ROS are produced as a by-product, NADPH oxidases (NOXes) catalyze the production of ROS by electron transfer to molecular oxygen (Fig. 3.1a). NOXes are a family of membrane-bound enzymes consisting of 7 isoforms, i.e., NOX1, NOX2, NOX3, NOX4, NOX5, DUOX1, and DUOX2 (Bedard and Krause 2007; Brandes et al. 2014). Among these isoforms, rodents lack NOX5. Most NOXes require association with interaction partners including both transmembrane and cytoplasmic molecules for their catalytic activity. NOX1-4 interact with the transmembrane molecule $p22^{phox}$ encoded by the Cyba gene, whereas DUOX1 and DUOX2 interact with the transmembrane molecules DUOXA1 and DUOXA2, respectively. By interaction with these transmembrane proteins, NOXes form a catalytic core. NOX5, DUOX1, and DUOX2 contain an EF hand and are activated by Ca^{2+}. NOX1-3 are activated by recruitment of the cytoplasmic subunits together with the small G protein Rac. The cytoplasmic subunits of NOX1 and NOX3 are NOXA1 and NOXO1, whereas those of NOX2 are $p40^{phox}$, $p47^{phox}$, and $p67^{phox}$. Recruitment of these cytosolic subunits is triggered by protein kinase C (PKC)-mediated phosphorylation of $p47^{phox}$ and NOXO1. Rac activation is also involved in activation of NOX1-3. Different NOX isoforms show different tissue distribution and intracellular localization. NOX2 is abundantly expressed in macrophages, neutrophils, and B cells and is

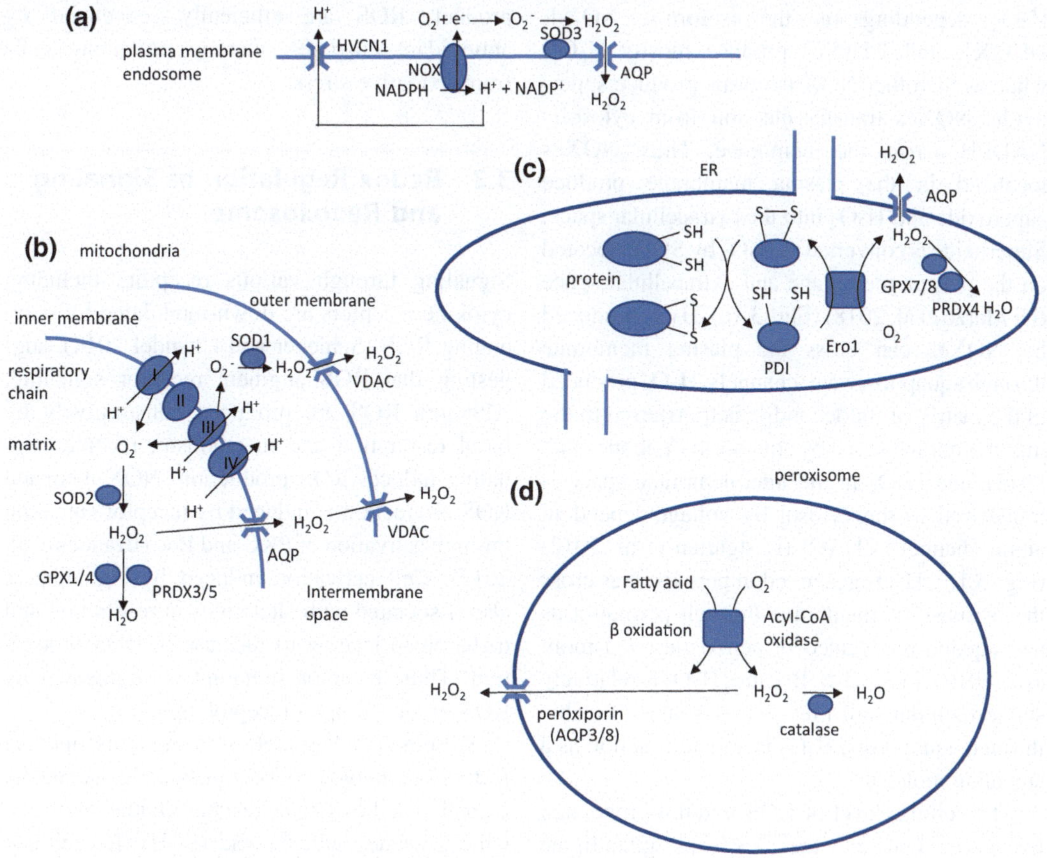

Fig. 3.1 Mechanisms for ROS production. (a) NOX located in the plasma membrane or endosome membrane generates electron (e^-) from cytoplasmic NADPH and transfers electron across the membrane. The electron reacts with molecular oxygen thereby generating superoxide (O_2^-), which is then converted to H_2O_2 by superoxide dismutase (SOD) 3 located in the membrane and extracellular space. H_2O_2 is transferred back to the cytosol through aquaporin (AQP). The proton pump HVCN1 exports H^+ generated by NOX to rebalance the charge level across the membrane for optimal NOX activity. (b) In mitochondria, superoxide is generated from the complex I and III of the respiratory chain. Superoxide is converted to H_2O_2 by SOD2 in the matrix or SOD1 in the intermembrane space. H_2O_2 in the matrix is transferred to the intermembrane space by aquaporin and H_2O_2 in the intermembrane space is transferred to the cytosol by voltage-dependent anion channel (VDAC). H_2O_2 is scavenged by glutaredoxin (GPX) and peroxiredoxin (PRDX) localized in mitochondria. (c) In endoplasmic reticulum (ER), disulfide bonds are generated in secretory and membrane proteins by oxidation at the cysteine residues. Electrons generated by protein disulfide isomerases (PDIs) that oxidize proteins are relayed to the endoplasmic reticulum oxireductin 1 (ERO1), which then generate H_2O_2 by reducing O_2. H_2O_2 is transferred to the cytosol through aquaprorin. H_2O_2 is converted to H_2O by GPX and PRDX. (d) In peroxisome, H_2O_2 is produced when fatty acids and various other substances such as D-amino acids, polyamines, and glycolate are oxidized by flavin adenine dinucleotide (FAD)- or flavin mononucleotide (FMN)-dependent oxidases such as acyl CoA oxidase. H_2O_2 is translocated to cytosol through peroxiporin (aquaporin) or scavenged by catalase

located in both plasma membrane and endosome. In neutrophils and macrophages, NOX2 is involved in the generation of ROS and killing of pathogens in endosome.

Superoxide produced by various mechanisms is converted to H_2O_2 and molecular oxygen by superoxide dismutases (SODs) (Holmstrom and Finkel 2014; Schieber and Chandel 2014; Reczek and Chandel 2015; Di Marzo et al. 2018). Superoxide generated in mitochondria is rapidly converted to H_2O_2 by SOD2 located in mitochondrial matrix (Fig. 3.1b). NOXes produce superoxide or

H_2O_2 depending on the isoforms. NOX4, DUOX1, and DUOX2 produce mostly H_2O_2, whereas the other NOX isoforms produce superoxide. NOXes transfer electron from cytosolic NADPH across the membrane. Thus, NOXes localized in the plasma membrane produce superoxide and H_2O_2 into the extracellular space. Superoxide is converted to H_2O_2 by SOD3 located on the plasma membrane and extracellular space (Di Marzo et al. 2018) (Fig. 3.1a). H_2O_2 produced by NOXes can cross the plasma membrane through aquaporin water channels. H_2O_2 produced in the matrix of mitochondria is transferred to the intermembrane space by aquaporin (Yoboue et al. 2018), and H_2O_2 in the intermembrane space is transferred to the cytosol by voltage-dependent anion channel (VDAC) (Lustgarten et al. 2012) (Fig. 3.1b). H_2O_2 generated in peroxisomes cross the peroxisome membrane through peroxiporins and aquaporins located in peroxisome (Lismont et al. 2019) (Fig. 3.1d). Because H_2O_2 is relatively stable (cellular half-life: $\sim$1 ms) and diffusible through aquaporins, H_2O_2 is able to function as a signaling molecule.

The cellular level of ROS is tightly regulated by antioxidant enzymes such as glutathione peroxidases (GPXs), peroxiredoxins (PRDXs), and catalase (Reczek and Chandel 2015). These enzymes catalyze reduction of H_2O_2 to water. Catalase is preferentially located in peroxisomes (Fig. 3.1d) (Lismont et al. 2019). In contrast, GPXs and PRDXs are located in various organellae depending on isoforms: Mitochondria contain GPX1, GPX4, PRDX3, and PRDX5 (Quijano et al. 2016) (Fig. 3.1b), whereas ER contains GPX7, GPX8, and PRDX4 (Fig. 3.1c) (Zito 2015). Although peroxisomes, ER, and mitochondria actively produce ROS as a by-product, ROS are efficiently scavenged by antioxidant enzymes, thereby protecting cells from oxidative stress.

3.3 Redox Regulation of Signaling and Redoxosome

Signaling through various receptors including cytokine receptors are down-modulated by scavenging ROS (Schieber and Chandel 2014), suggesting that ROS augment receptor signaling. Although ROS are produced constitutively by basal respiration and metabolism, receptor signaling induces ROS production. NOX-mediated ROS production is induced by receptor signaling through activation of PKC and Rac (Brandes et al. 2014). Cell activation induced by signaling is also associated with alterations in respiration and metabolism leading to increase in ROS production. Thus, receptor signaling is augmented by ROS produced upon receptor signaling.

Various signaling molecules and transcriptional factors are known to be functionally altered by oxidation at the cysteine residue. Oxidation of cysteine generates sulfenic acid (SOH) (Reczek and Chandel 2015; Marinho et al. 2014; Prieto-Bermejo and Hernandez-Hernandez 2017). This reaction is called reversible oxidation because sulfenic acid can be reduced. However, further oxidization of cysteine to sulfinic acid (SO_2H) and sulfonic acid (SO_3H) is an irreversible reaction, resulting in permanent alteration. Redox-mediated regulation of signaling molecules was first demonstrated in phosphatases. Various phosphatases were shown to be inactivated by ROS through oxidation of the conserved cysteine residue at the catalytic site (Reczek and Chandel 2015; Prieto-Bermejo and Hernandez-Hernandez

2017). The role of phosphatase oxidation was most extensively studied in cytokine signaling such as signaling generated by EGF and PDGF. When cells are stimulated with these cytokines, NOXes are activated and produce ROS (Sundaresan et al. 1995; Bae et al. 1997), which inactivate phosphatases such as PTP1B (Lee et al. 1998) and SHP-2 (Meng et al. 2002) by oxidation. Phosphatase inactivation augments cytokine signaling including MAPK and Akt pathways by augmenting phosphorylation of signaling molecules. Various other signaling molecules were also shown to be regulated by oxidation although the role of oxidation of these molecules is less clear compared to the redox regulation of phosphatases. Protein kinases including Src family kinases and MAPK are regulated by ROS through cysteine oxidation, resulting in either augmentation or inhibition of kinase activity (Corcoran and Cotter 2013). Cysteine oxidation regulates calcium channels involved in calcium signaling such as STIM1, ORAI1, and ORAI3 (Hempel and Trebak 2017). Various transcription factors such as p53, FOXO, NF-kB, Pax5, Pax8, Egr-1, and AP-1 are also regulated by oxidation (Marinho et al. 2014; Prieto-Bermejo and Hernandez-Hernandez 2017). Oxidation of various signaling molecules especially phosphatases appears to be involved in ROS-mediated augmentation of receptor signaling.

Upon interaction with ligands, membrane receptors are endocytosed, followed by either recycling to the plasma membrane or degradation by lysosomal enzymes in lysosome. Degradation of receptors plays a role in signal desensitization. However, various receptors including BCR are shown to be endocytosed together with receptor-associated signaling molecules, including adaptors, and transmit signaling in endosome (Murphy et al. 2009; Chaturvedi et al. 2011). Receptor signaling activates NOXes in endosome as well as in plasma membrane (Fig. 3.2) (Li et al. 2006, 2009; Miller et al. 2007; Oakley et al. 2009; Tsutsumi et al. 2017). Because NOXes produce ROS across the membrane (Bedard and Krause 2007; Brandes et al. 2014), ROS generated by NOXes in the endosome membrane are released into the endosome lumen, whereas ROS generated by NOXes in the plasma membrane are released into extracellular space. ROS released to the endosome and extracellular

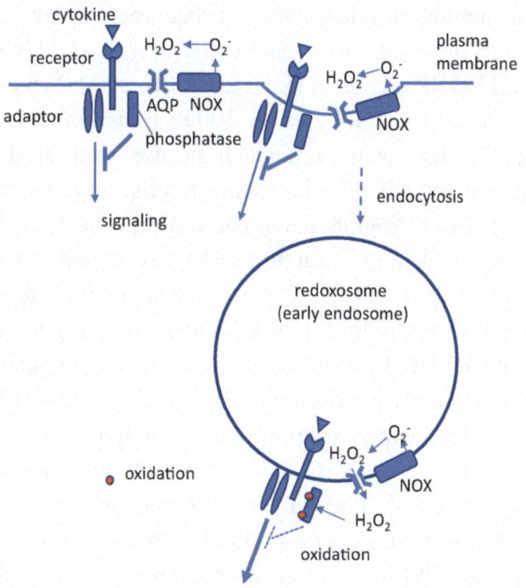

Fig. 3.2 Augmentation of cyokine receptor signaling by ROS in redoxosome. When cytokine interacts with the receptor on the plasma membrane, receptor signaling is generated. Receptor-associated phosphatases down-regulate receptor signaling by counteracting kinases downstream of the receptor. Receptor ligation also activates NOX located in the plasma membrane to generate superoxide into the extracellular space. The receptor is translocated to early endosome together with cytokine and receptor-associated signaling molecules including adaptors by receptor-mediated endocytosis. In the early endosome, cytokine induces receptor signaling, which activates NOX to produce superoxide into the endosome lumen (redoxosome). Superoxide produced in the plasma membrane and endosome is then converted to H_2O_2 and transported to cytosol through aquaporin (AQP). Because the endosome lumen is a closed space, H_2O_2 in the endosome lumen is efficiently transported to the cytosol. H_2O_2 then inactivates phosphatases by cysteine oxidation. Inactivation of phosphatases allows efficient receptor signaling in endosome

space are translocated back to cytosol through aquaporins. ROS transported back to cytosol may oxidize signaling molecules such as phosphatases recruited to the receptors thereby augmenting receptor signaling in endosome (Murphy et al. 2009). As endosome is a closed compartment, ROS in the endosome may be translocated to the cytosol and enhance receptor signaling more efficiently than ROS in the extracellular space do (Fig. 3.2).

ROS-producing signaling endosome, in which ROS augments endosomal signaling, is called redoxosome or redoxisome (Murphy et al. 2009).

Formation of redoxosome has been demonstrated after ligand-induced endocytosis of IL-1, TNF and PDGF receptors (Li et al. 2006, 2009; Miller et al. 2007; Oakley et al. 2009; Tsutsumi et al. 2017). By fractionating cell lysates from IL-1-stimulated MCF7 breast cancer cells, Engelhardt and his colleagues demonstrated that the $Rab5^+$ early endosome fraction contains superoxide, NOX2, and NOX cofactors such as $p47^{phox}$ and $p67^{phox}$ required for NOX2 activation together with IL-1R (Li et al. 2006). This result suggests that the early endosome in these cells contain IL-1R and superoxide-producing active NOX2 complex. They also showed that stimulation of the same cell line with TNFα induces the formation of superoxide-producing endosome containing TNFR (Li et al. 2009). Thus, IL-1R and TNFR endocytosed by ligand-induced endocytosis appear to form redoxosome together with active NOX2 complex. They also demonstrated the presence of adaptor molecules of IL-1R such as MyD88 and TRAF6 or those of TNFR such as TRADD and TRAF2 in redoxosome containing IL-1R and TNFR, respectively (Li et al. 2006, 2009). Among these adaptors, recruitment of TRAF6 and TRAF2 to endosome depends on ROS because these adaptors are no longer recruited when superoxide is scavenged by catalase and SOD. These results suggest that NOX-derived ROS augment receptor signaling in redoxosome, resulting in recruitment of adaptor molecules such as TRAF6 and TRAF2. Recently, Tsutsumi et al. developed proximity ligation assay that detects reversibly oxidized protein phosphatases and demonstrated that oxidized protein phosphatases such as SHP-2 and PTP1B are present in redoxosome generated upon treatment of fibroblasts with PDGF (Tsutsumi et al. 2017). This result suggests that ROS produced in redoxosome augments receptor signaling by inactivating phosphatases by oxidation.

Because ROS are generated in various locations in the cells including plasma membrane, endosome, and mitochondria, role of redoxosome in receptor signaling has been addressed by blocking endocytosis using dominant negative form of dynamin, the dynamin inhibitor Dynasore, and the clathrin inhibitor Pitstop (Li et al. 2006, 2009; Tsutsumi et al. 2017). Inhibition of endocytosis reduces ROS-mediated augmentation of TNFR signaling and PDGF-induced SHP-2 oxidation. These results may suggest a crucial role of redoxosome in ROS-induced augmentation of receptor signaling. However, endocytosis is involved in various cellular processes and is essential for cell survival. Thus, the role of redoxosome in cell activation needs to be further clarified.

3.4 Role of ROS in BCR Signaling

The pioneering work by Wienands and Reth demonstrated that treatment with H_2O_2 alone induces BCR signaling (Wienands et al. 1996), suggesting that BCR signaling is sensitive to ROS. Later studies demonstrated that BCR ligation induces ROS production within one minute (Singh et al. 2005). This immediate ROS production is mediated by NOX2 because $NOX2^{-/-}$ B cells do not show immediate ROS production after BCR ligation (Richards and Clark 2009). A role of NOXes in BCR signaling was suggested by the study on B cells deficient in hydrogen voltage-gated channel 1 (HVCN1). HVCN1 is a proton channel required for optimal NOX-mediated ROS production (Capasso et al. 2011). HVCN1 transport H^+ generated in cytosol as a by-product of NOX-mediated ROS production to rebalance charge across the plasma membrane (Fig. 3.1a). $HVCN1^{-/-}$ B cells show loss of immediate BCR-induced ROS production probably by inhibiting NOX2. $HVCN1^{-/-}$ B cells further show reduction in BCR ligation-induced phosphorylation of Syk and Akt, and slight delay in B cell proliferation (Capasso et al. 2010), suggesting a role of NOXes in BCR signaling. However, $NOX2^{-/-}$ B cells show normal BCR signaling including Ca^{2+} mobilization and phosphorylation of Syk, Erk, and Akt, and normal BCR ligation-induced B cell proliferation (Richards and Clark 2009). Thus, NOX2-mediated immediate ROS production after BCR ligation does not regulate BCR signaling. Because HCNV1 is also involved in NOX-independent function such as histamine release from basophils (Capasso et al. 2011), HCNV1 may regulate phosphorylation of Syk and Akt by a NOX-independent mechanism.

Although immediate ROS production after BCR ligation is not involved in BCR signaling, a role of prolonged ROS production was demonstrated by Wheeler and DeFranco (2012). They detected ROS production in mitochondria using a mitochondria-targeted superoxide indicator 6 h after BCR ligation. They further showed that continuous ROS scavenging markedly inhibit Akt pathway after 12 h and proliferation of B cells at 48 h after BCR ligation. These results suggested a role of prolonged ROS production in mitochondria in BCR ligation-induced B cell activation. Recently, we confirmed the essential role of prolonged ROS production in B cell proliferation induced by BCR ligation (Feng et al. 2019). When BCR is ligated in mouse spleen B cells, ROS is produced in two phases. ROS production starts immediately after BCR ligation and ceases in one hour. Then, ROS production is restarted at 2 h after BCR ligation and lasts for 4–6 h (Fig. 3.3a). ROS scavenging reduced activation of the NF-κB pathway and Akt 6 and 8 h after BCR ligation although the same treatment did not alter activation of these molecules at the early phase up to 2 h after BCR ligation. Moreover, scavenging ROS production at 3 h after BCR ligation and later almost completely inhibited B cell proliferation, clearly indicating that prolonged ROS production is essential for BCR ligation-induced B cell activation. Probably because the magnitude of ROS production at the late phase is much higher than that in the early phase, ROS production at the late phase but not at the early phase regulates BCR signaling.

Unlike the study by Wheeler and DeFranco (2012), we demonstrated that NOXes play a central role in prolonged ROS production after BCR ligation (Feng et al. 2019). Although B cells strongly express NOX2, we found that B cells also express other NOXes such as NOX1, NOX3 and DUOX2, and their interaction partners required for their activity. B cells deficient in both DUOXA1 and DUOXA2 required for activation of DUOX1 and DUOX2, respectively, showed no alteration in BCR ligation-induced

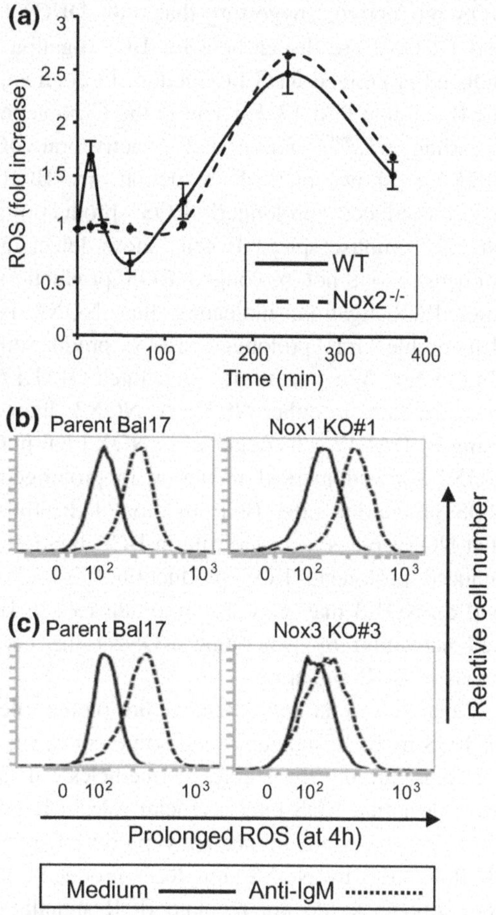

Fig. 3.3 NOX-mediated ROS production is induced by BCR ligation. (a) NOX2 is required for BCR ligation-induced ROS production in the early phase. BCR ligation in spleen B cells from wild-type (WT) mice show ROS production in two phases. ROS production in the early phase at 0-60 min but not in the late phase (120–360 min) is abolished in $NOX2^{-/-}$ B cells. (b and c) NOX3 is involved in BCR ligation-induced ROS production in the late phase. The B cell line BAL17 deficient in NOX3 shows marked reduction in ROS production at 4 h after BCR ligation compared to parent BAL17 cells (c), whereas NOX1-deficient BAL 17 cells show the ROS level similar to parent BAL17 cells (b). ROS production is analyzed by flow cytometry using ROS-sensitive fluorescent dye 2',7'–dichlorofluorescin diacetate (DCFDA). Originally published in *The Journal of Immunology*. Feng Y.-y. et al. 2019. Essential role of NADPH oxidase-dependent production of reactive oxygen species in maintenance of sustained B cell receptor signaling and B cell proliferation. J. Immunol. 202: 2546-2557. Copyright © [2019] The American Association of Immunologists, Inc.

ROS production, suggesting that both DUOX1 and DUOX2 are dispensable for BCR ligation-induced prolonged ROS production. In contrast, the B cell line BAL17 deficient in the *Cyba* gene encoding $p22^{phox}$ required for activation of NOX1-4 show marked reduction in BCR ligation induced prolonged ROS production. $NOX2^{-/-}$ mouse spleen B cells show defect in immediate but not prolonged ROS production after BCR ligation, indicating that NOX2 is dispensable for prolonged ROS production (Fig. 3.3a). We, therefore, generated BAL17 cells deficient in either NOX1 or NOX3. Interestingly, BAL17 cells deficient in NOX3 but not NOX1 showed marked reduction in prolonged ROS production after BCR ligation, indicating that NOX3 plays a central role in BCR ligation-induced prolonged ROS production (Fig. 3.3b and c). NOX3 may play an important role in B cell activation by generating ROS at the late phase in BCR signaling.

There are so far only a few studies on the role of ROS in BCR signaling, and some controversies exist among the studies. Nonetheless, it is now clear that ROS play a crucial role in BCR signaling. ROS are immediately produced after BCR ligation by NOX2, but ROS produced at the early phase do not regulate BCR signaling (Richards and Clark 2009) probably because the level of ROS production is limited. In contrast, BCR ligation induces a higher level of ROS production at the late phase (Feng et al. 2019), which is essential for B cell activation by augmenting BCR signaling. Our recent results suggest that prolonged ROS production involves NOX3 (Feng et al. 2019). Thus, BCR ligation sequentially activates NOX2 and NOX3, resulting in ROS production at the early and late phases, respectively, although molecular mechanism for sequential activation is not known. NOX3 is highly expressed in inner ear and is essential for generation of otoconia required for detection of linear acceleration and gravity by inner ear (Bedard and Krause 2007). Although NOX3 is expressed in B cells at a lower level, low-level expression may be sufficient in regulation of BCR signaling. Indeed, NOXes expressed at a low level play a crucial role in various organs such as cardiovascular system (Gimenez et al. 2016). ROS generated by NOX3 may oxidize signaling molecules such as phosphatases to augment BCR signaling. Although cytokine signaling is augmented by NOX-mediated ROS production in redoxosome, redoxosome is generated transiently in early endosome (Tsutsumi et al. 2017; Spencer and Engelhardt 2014). It is not clear whether persistent redoxosome can be generated to augment prolonged BCR signaling. How BCR ligation induces sequential activation of NOX2 and NOX3, and how NOX3-mediated ROS production augments BCR signaling need to be elucidated.

3.5 Conclusion

Lines of evidence suggest that ROS play a role as a second messenger in signaling through various receptors. ROS are produced upon receptor ligation and enhance signaling by oxidizing ROS-sensitive signaling molecules such as phosphatases. Unlike the other receptor signaling, BCR ligation induces prolonged ROS production in two phases (Feng et al. 2019). ROS production at the early phase up to 1 h after BCR ligation is mediated by NOX2, but does not regulate BCR signaling probably due to a limited level of ROS production. In contrast, NOX3-mediated production of a higher level of ROS starts 2 h after BCR ligation and persists 4–6 h. ROS production at this late phase augments BCR signaling and is essential for B cell proliferation. NOX-mediated ROS production augments receptor signaling in redoxosome by oxidizing redoxosome-associated signaling molecules such as phosphatases (Tsutsumi et al. 2017). However, redoxosome in cytokine signaling is formed transiently from early endosome (Tsutsumi et al. 2017; Spencer and Engelhardt 2014). It is not yet clear whether persistent redoxosome can be generated that allows prolonged BCR signaling.

Although ROS play a crucial role in B cell activation, so far only a few studies have been conducted on the role of ROS in BCR signaling. How ROS are generated by sequential activation of NOX2 and NOX3 after BCR ligation and how ROS augment BCR signaling are not yet clear. Elucidation of the mechanisms for BCR ligation-induced ROS production and the role of ROS in B cell activation may contribute to the understanding of how B cell is activated by antigen stimulation and development of the new therapies of various immunological diseases.

References

Bae YS, Kang SW, Seo MS, Baines IC, Tekle E, Chock PB, Rhee SG (1997) Epidermal growth factor (EGF)-induced generation of hydrogen peroxide. Role in EGF receptor-mediated tyrosine phosphorylation. J Biol Chem 272:217–221

Bedard K, Krause KH (2007) The NOX family of ROS-generating NADPH oxidases: physiology and pathophysiology. Physiol Rev 87:245–313

Brandes RP, Weissmann N, Schroder K (2014) Nox family NADPH oxidases: Molecular mechanisms of activation. Free Radic Biol Med 76:208–226

Capasso M, Bhamrah MK, Henley T, Boyd RS, Langlais C, Cain K, Dinsdale D, Pulford K, Khan M, Musset B et al (2010) HVCN1 modulates BCR signal strength via regulation of BCR-dependent generation of reactive oxygen species. Nat Immunol 11:265–272

Capasso M, DeCoursey TE, Dyer MJ (2011) pH regulation and beyond: unanticipated functions for the voltage-gated proton channel, HVCN1. Trends Cell Biol 21:20–28

Chaturvedi A, Martz R, Dorward D, Waisberg M, Pierce SK (2011) Endocytosed BCRs sequentially regulate MAPK and Akt signaling pathways from intracellular compartments. Nat Immunol 12:1119–1126

Corcoran A, Cotter TG (2013) Redox regulation of protein kinases. FEBS J 280:1944–1965

Di Marzo N, Chisci E, Giovannoni R (2018) The role of hydrogen peroxide in redox-dependent signaling: homeostatic and pathological responses in mammalian cells. Cells 7:156

Feng YY, Tang M, Suzuki M, Gunasekara C, Anbe Y, Hiraoka Y, Liu J, Grasberger H, Ohkita M, Matsumura Y et al (2019) Essential role of NADPH oxidase-dependent production of reactive oxygen species in maintenance of sustained B cell receptor signaling and B cell proliferation. J Immunol 202:2546–2557

Gimenez M, Schickling BM, Lopes LR, Miller FJ Jr (2016) Nox1 in cardiovascular diseases: regulation and pathophysiology. Clin Sci (Lond) 130:151–165

Hempel N, Trebak M (2017) Crosstalk between calcium and reactive oxygen species signaling in cancer. Cell Calcium 63:70–96

Holmstrom KM, Finkel T (2014) Cellular mechanisms and physiological consequences of redox-dependent signalling. Nat Rev Mol Cell Biol 15:411–421

Lee SR, Kwon KS, Kim SR, Rhee SG (1998) Reversible inactivation of protein-tyrosine phosphatase 1B in A431 cells stimulated with epidermal growth factor. J Biol Chem 273:15366–15372

Li Q, Harraz MM, Zhou W, Zhang LN, Ding W, Zhang Y, Eggleston T, Yeaman C, Banfi B, Engelhardt JF (2006) Nox2 and Rac1 regulate H2O2-dependent recruitment of TRAF6 to endosomal interleukin-1 receptor complexes. Mol Cell Biol 26:140–154

Li Q, Spencer NY, Oakley FD, Buettner GR, Engelhardt JF (2009) Endosomal Nox2 facilitates redox-dependent induction of NF-kappaB by TNF-alpha. Antioxid Redox Signal 11:1249–1263

Lismont C, Revenco I, Fransen M (2019) Peroxisomal hydrogen peroxide metabolism and signaling in health and disease. Int J Mol Sci 20:3673

Lustgarten MS, Bhattacharya A, Muller FL, Jang YC, Shimizu T, Shirasawa T, Richardson A, Van Remmen H (2012) Complex I generated, mitochondrial matrix-directed superoxide is released from the mitochondria through voltage dependent anion channels. Biochem Biophys Res Commun 422:515–521

Marinho HS, Real C, Cyrne L, Soares H, Antunes F (2014) Hydrogen peroxide sensing, signaling and regulation of transcription factors. Redox Biol 2: 535–562

Meng TC, Fukada T, Tonks NK (2002) Reversible oxidation and inactivation of protein tyrosine phosphatases in vivo. Mol Cell 9:387–399

Miller FJ Jr, Filali M, Huss GJ, Stanic B, Chamseddine A, Barna TJ, Lamb FS (2007) Cytokine activation of nuclear factor kappa B in vascular smooth muscle cells requires signaling endosomes containing Nox1 and ClC-3. Circ Res 101:663–671

Murphy JE, Padilla BE, Hasdemir B, Cottrell GS, Bunnett NW (2009) Endosomes: a legitimate platform for the signaling train. Proc Natl Acad Sci USA 106:17615–17622

Oakley FD, Smith RL, Engelhardt JF (2009) Lipid rafts and caveolin-1 coordinate interleukin-1beta (IL-1beta)-dependent activation of NFkappaB by controlling endocytosis of Nox2 and IL-1beta receptor 1 from the plasma membrane. J Biol Chem 284:33255–33264

Prieto-Bermejo R, Hernandez-Hernandez A (2017) The importance of NADPH oxidases and redox signaling in angiogenesis. Antioxidants (Basel) 6:32

Quijano C, Trujillo M, Castro L, Trostchansky A (2016) Interplay between oxidant species and energy metabolism. Redox Biol 8:28–42

Reczek CR, Chandel NS (2015) ROS-dependent signal transduction. Curr Opin Cell Biol 33:8–13

Richards SM, Clark EA (2009) BCR-induced superoxide negatively regulates B-cell proliferation and T-cell-independent type 2 Ab responses. Eur J Immunol 39:3395–3403

Schieber M, Chandel NS (2014) ROS function in redox signaling and oxidative stress. Curr Biol 24:R453–R462

Singh DK, Kumar D, Siddiqui Z, Basu SK, Kumar V, Rao KV (2005) The strength of receptor signaling is centrally controlled through a cooperative loop between Ca2+ and an oxidant signal. Cell 121: 281–293

Spencer NY, Engelhardt JF (2014) The basic biology of redoxosomes in cytokine-mediated signal transduction and implications for disease-specific therapies. Biochemistry 53:1551–1564

Sundaresan M, Yu ZX, Ferrans VJ, Irani K, Finkel T (1995) Requirement for generation of H2O2 for platelet-derived growth factor signal transduction. Science 270:296–299

Tsutsumi R, Harizanova J, Stockert R, Schroder K, Bastiaens PIH, Neel BG (2017) Assay to visualize specific protein oxidation reveals spatio-temporal regulation of SHP2. Nat Commun 8:466

Wheeler ML, Defranco AL (2012) Prolonged production of reactive oxygen species in response to B cell receptor stimulation promotes B cell activation and proliferation. J Immunol 189:4405–4416

Wienands J, Larbolette O, Reth M (1996) Evidence for a preformed transducer complex organized by the B cell antigen receptor. Proc Natl Acad Sci USA 93:7865–7870

Yoboue ED, Sitia R, Simmen T (2018) Redox crosstalk at endoplasmic reticulum (ER) membrane contact sites (MCS) uses toxic waste to deliver messages. Cell Death Dis 9:331

Zito E (2015) ERO1: A protein disulfide oxidase and H2O2 producer. Free Radic Biol Med 83:299–304

4 Germinal Center Reaction

Chuanxin Huang

Abstract

Germinal centers (GCs) are transient microstructures formed within the follicles of secondary lymphoid tissues in response to certain types of immunization and foreign pathogens. A mature GC comprises two functionally distinct compartments, a dark zone (DZ) and a light zone (LZ). DZ B cells undergo rapid clonal expansion during which their antibody genes are modified by activation-induced cytidine deaminase (AID)-mediated immunoglobulin variable region (IgV) gene hypermutation to generate a repertoire of antibody mutants with varying affinities to the immunizing antigen. With the help of other immune cells including T follicular helper (Tfh) cells and follicular dendritic cells (FDCs), GC B cells with improved affinity to the antigen are selectively expanded and finally differentiate into memory B cell (MBC) and antibody-producing plasma cell (PC). In the LZ, GC B cells may also undergo AID-mediated class switch recombination. The germinal center reaction involves multiple immune cells and is tightly controlled by lineage-specific transcription factors. In this chapter, I will discuss the cellular and molecular signals, such as key transcription factors, that govern the formation and maintenance and GCs and the selection of GC B cells.

Keywords

Germinal center B · T follicular helper cells · Follicular dendritic cell · Somatic hypermutation · Class switch recombination · Affinity selection

4.1 Introduction

Germinal centers (GCs) were first described by Walther Flemming in 1884 as distinct microanatomical regions of secondary lymphoid organs that contained dividing cells. Although GCs were long believed to be the source of developing lymphocytes, immunization experiments showed that these structures formed only in response to antigen and were the sites of B cell clonal expansion in T cell-dependent antibody responses to infection (Berek et al. 1991; MacLennan 1994; Victora and Nussenzweig 2012). Initiation of the GC reaction occurs via a coordinated cascade involving several different cell types that drive antigen-engaged B cells into the GC reaction (De Silva and Klein 2015; Mesin et al. 2016; Victora and Nussenzweig 2012). Within GCs, B cells express the enzyme activation-induced deaminase (AID), which deaminates cytidine residues in their immunoglobulin gene variable (IgV) and switch

C. Huang (✉)
Shanghai Jiao Tong University School of Medicine, Shanghai 200025, China
e-mail: huangcx@shsmu.edu.cn

J.-Y. Wang (ed.), *B Cells in Immunity and Tolerance*, Advances in Experimental Medicine and Biology 1254, https://doi.org/10.1007/978-981-15-3532-1_4

regions, leading to somatic hypermutation (SHM) and class switch recombination (CSR) (De Silva and Klein 2015; Mesin et al. 2016; Victora and Nussenzweig 2012). GCs were clearly visible by conventional histology techniques, as was their division into "light" and "dark" zones (LZ and DZ, respectively) (MacLennan 1994). Cells were found to proliferate extensively in the GC DZ and move to LZ, where they interact with T follicular helper (Tfh) and follicular dendritic cells (FDCs) (Mesin et al. 2016; Victora and Nussenzweig 2012; Vinuesa et al. 2016). This process leads to the selection of GC B cells that express a highly selected antibody repertoire. GC B cells with higher antigen binding affinity can differentiate into antibody-secreting plasma cell (PC) or memory B cell (MBC) (Suan et al. 2017), to build an immunological memory for future recall responses. The GC reaction is a highly dynamic process and tightly controlled by intrinsic and extrinsic clues (Mesin et al. 2016; Song and Craft 2019; Victora et al. 2010). B cells not only move constantly throughout the entire GC, but also engage in short, dynamic interactions with both T cells and antigen. The aim of the present review is to summarize and discuss the cellular dynamics of the GC reaction, the mechanics of high-affinity B cell selection and the molecular control of these processes.

4.2 Initiation of GC Reaction

GCs form within the center of B cell follicles, which contain a network of FDCs. Upon challenge with T-dependent antigens, antigen-specific naive B cells in the B cell follicles and $CD4^+$ T cells in the T cell zones were activated and migrate toward the T-B border of the follicle or interfollicle, where they proliferate and form cognate interactions (Kerfoot et al. 2011; Kitano et al. 2011; Okada et al. 2005). There, the duration of their interaction depends on their specificity and affinity for the encountered antigen. Then, some activated antigen-specific B cells proliferate extensively, forming extrafollicular foci, and differentiate into short-lived plasmablasts that secrete antibodies with low affinity for the invading pathogen (Fig. 5.1) (Suan et al. 2017). These cells play a crucial protective role by providing a rapid initial response to invading pathogens.

In addition to extrafollicular plasma cells, activated B cells can differentiate into memory B cells or GC B cells. Activated B cells which are destined to the GC pathway change their migratory properties, enabling them to migrate back to the center of the follicle and form nascent GCs. Now it is clear that BCR affinity for the antigen influences the fate choice of B cells. Higher affinity predisposes the activated B cells to differentiate toward plasma cells, whereas lower affinity favors memory B cells or GC B cell development (Paus et al. 2006).

4.3 Establishment of Dark and Light Zones

Nascent GCs within follicles can first be histologically detected at day 4 after immunization. At this time, B cells undergo rapid proliferation and begin to populate the network of FDCs in the center of the follicle. At day 7 after immunization, the GC has been fully established and is polarized into two microenvironments known as the dark zone and the light zone (Victora and Nussenzweig 2012). The dark zone consists almost exclusively of densely packed high proliferating B cells known as centroblasts. The light zone is more sparsely populated by B cells than the dark zone and is characterized by the presence of several cell types, including Tfh cells, Tfr cells, FDCs and macrophages (Fig. 4.1). Centroblasts diversify their IgV genes by SHM and those cells that express newly generated modified antibodies are selected for improved antigen binding in the light zone (De Silva and Klein 2015; Victora and Nussenzweig 2012). A subset of centrocytes undergoes CSR to change their immunoglobulin isotype and to generate antibodies with different effector functions. Some centrocytes eventually differentiate into memory B cells or plasma cells (Fig. 4.1) (Victora and Nussenzweig 2012). Up to half of all GC B cells are lost through

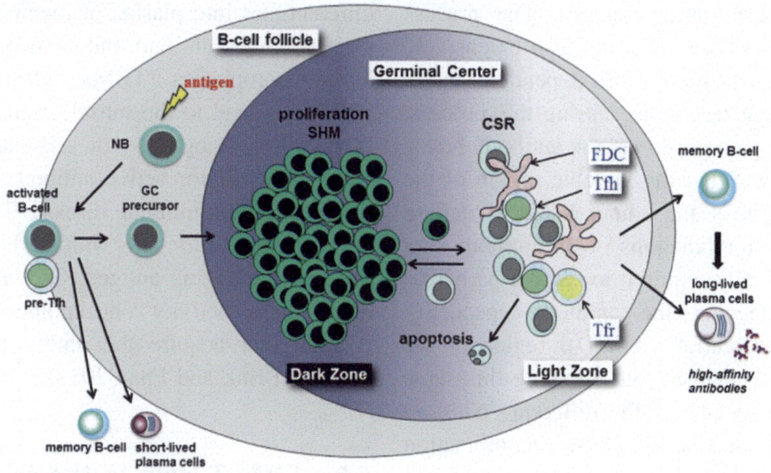

Fig. 4.1 Dynamics of B cells in the GC reaction. In response to T cell-dependent antigen stimulation, antigen-specific B cells are activated and move toward the T-B border and/or interfollicular zones, where they interact with cognate pre-Tfh cells. After that, activated B cells can follow one of three alternative fates; differentiating into extrafollicular short-lived plasma cells which secret low-affinity antibodies, GC precursors or recirculating early memory B cells. GC precursors move into the center of B cell follicles and form nascent GCs. Mature GC is polarized into dark zone and light zone. Dark zone B cells undergo massive clonal expansion and SHM and move to light zone. With the help of T cells (Tfh and Tfr cells) and FDC, light zone B cells may undergo CSR and are positively selected based on their affinity. The high-affinity clones exit GCs and terminally differentiate into memory B cells and long-lived plasma cells

apoptosis every six hours during the GC reaction. Programmed cell death can occur by default for cells that are not positively selected. GC B cells can be poised to undergo apoptosis due to silencing of BCL2 by the BCL6 transcriptional repressor (Basso and Dalla-Favera 2010). GC lifespan can vary greatly depending on the nature of the immune stimulus. Whereas protein model antigens adsorbed in alum usually induce short-lived GCs that collapse within the first month after immunization, certain synthetic vaccines, viral infections, or the gut microbiota can induce GCs that remain active for much longer periods.

4.4 SHM and CSR

SHM is a process that modifies the immunoglobulin variable region (IgV) of both the heavy and light chains, at rates that are about 10^6 fold higher than the background mutation rates observed in other genes. This modification at the V-region genes occurs at the dark zone B cells. The mutations are introduced into the complementarity determining regions (CDRs) of the antibody V genes. The mutations are non-random; transitions dominate over transversions, and mutation hotspots have been identified (e.g., the RGYW motif). Whereas the overall goal of this process is to produce high-affinity antibodies, in the absence of selection, SHM does not distinguish between favorable and unfavorable mutations. The outcome of this process produces antibodies with (1) higher affinity for antigen, (2) lower affinity for antigen and (3) no change in affinity for antigen. SHM can also lead to non-functional antibodies, such as antibodies that cannot fold correctly, or antibody genes that harbor premature stop codons. Whereas SHM of the antibody V-region does not always produce a higher affinity antibody, the selection process for antigen binding that occurs in the light zone of the germinal center selects for B cells that produce the highest affinity antibodies.

CSR is the DNA-level mechanism that mediates antibody isotype switching, a process whereby the heavy chain class of the antibody produced by an activated B cell changes from

IgM and IgD to other isotypes. The process mainly occurs within GCs, but also extensively outside of GCs in both T cell-dependent and T cell-independent responses. During this process, the constant region portion of the antibody heavy chain is changed, but the variable region of the heavy chain stays the same. Class switching alters the effector functions of an antibody that can be specifically required to clear a particular antigen by leaving the antibody specificity defined by the rearranged V(D)J region of the heavy chain unchanged, but allowing this same region to associate with different constant regions. CSR occurs by DNA recombination involving non-homologous end-joining processes between specific repetitive regions of several hundred base pairs (known as switch regions) that precede the immunoglobulin constant region genes. Class switching is controlled by cytokines secreted by Tfh cells within GC. For example, in mouse interleukin-4 (IL-4) promotes antibody switching to IgG^1 and IgE. Both SHM and CSR require the activity of AID.

4.5 Positive Selection of High-Affinity Clones in the GC

Following SHM within the dark zone, high-affinity GC B cell mutants must be selected in the light zone before undergoing further rounds of hypermutation in the dark zone (Victora and Nussenzweig 2012). GC B cells capture antigen on the surface of FDC via their BCR and present the processed antigen on MHC complexes to Tfh cells. Positive selection of GC B cells could occur through either of two mechanisms. Higher affinity cells could receive stronger BCR signals that favor their survival compared to low-affinity cells. Secondly, by acquiring and processing more antigens in a short period of time, higher affinity cells could be more effective in engaging Tfh cells and receiving helper signals. Acquisition of T cell help has been identified as the dominant force behind the selection of high-affinity GC B cells (Wan et al. 2019). Selected clones will reenter into dark zone to under second round expansion and SHM, or terminally differentiates into plasma or memory cells. Unselected clones die and endocytosed by tangible body macrophages (TBMs). Of note, random SHM may lead to the introduction of mutations that lead to recognition of self-antigens, which can generate autoreactive antibodies and potentially cause autoimmune disease. Thus, in addition to selecting for cells with the highest affinity for the immunizing antigen, GCs are thought to rely on autoreactivity “checkpoints” to eliminate B cells that acquire the ability to bind self-antigen (Brink and Phan 2018).

4.6 $CD4^+$ T Help in the GC

During the GC reaction, $CD4^+$ T helper cells play a crucial role in modulating B cell response. Tfh cells, a unique subset of CD4 helper T cells, are specialized in providing cognate help to B cells for the formation of GCs and the development of humoral immunity (Crotty 2011). Tfh cells are generally considered to be of a separate Th cell lineage and arise from naive $CD4^+$ T cells with sequential steps in response to T cell-dependent antigen. Naive $CD4^+$ T cells are primed by dendritic cells and upregulate the chemokine (C-X-C motif) receptor CXCR5, which enables them to migrate into B cell follicles. Tfr cells are derived from thymic regulatory T (Treg) cells co-opt the gene expression program of Tfh cells but limit the GC response (Sage and Sharpe 2015). Within the GCs, GC B cells form cognate interaction with T cells through a pair of co-stimulatory and co-inhibitory molecules, affecting the phenotypes of each other (Papa and Vinuesa 2018; Tangye et al. 2015). The CD40-CD40L axis is crucial for the maintenance of GCs since lack of CD40 or its ligand, or administration of anti-CD40L antibody at any time during the GC reaction, results in complete loss of GC B cells (van Kooten and Banchereau 2000). CD40L, a member of the tumor necrosis factor (TNF) family, is upregulated in Tfh cells, whereas CD40 is constitutively expressed on GC B cells. CD40 engagement renders positive selection via activation of NF-κB-mediated signaling and c-Myc (Luo et al. 2018). Importantly, the interaction between GC B cells and Tfh cells is increased by ICOSL-ICOS signaling within GCs. The CD40L-CD40 signaling transcriptionally activates ICOSL expression. ICOSL on mouse GC B cells induced ICOS signal on Tfh cells and subsequently promote the membrane translocation of CD40L on Tfh cells (a positive feedback loop) (Liu et al. 2015). In humans, CD40 was not found to augment ICOSL expression on GC B cells. Instead, Tfh cells secreted dopamine to augment ICOSL on human GC B cells which expressed dopamine receptor 1 (DRD1). The extent of CD40L-CD40 engagement is thought to impact on the fate decisions of B cells at various stages of differentiation in the context of other extrinsic signals.

Tfh cells are also known to secrete cytokines that profoundly influence B cells (Crotty 2014; Vinuesa et al. 2016). Two of the major cytokines secreted by Tfh cells are IL-4 and IL-21. These cytokines promote B cell proliferation, CSR and differentiation into plasma cells or GC B cells. IL-21 promotes the expression of key genes such as Bcl6 and Aicda in GC B cells. In addition, Tfh cells can secrete other cytokines, such as IL-10 and interferon gamma (IFNγ). The production of IFNγ is associated with CSR to IgG2a or IgG2c.

4.7 Post-GC Cell Fate

In order to exert their effector or memory functions, B cells must differentiate into long-lived PCs or MBCs, respectively (Corcoran and Tarlinton 2016; Suan et al. 2017; Victora and Nussenzweig 2012). PC and MBC differentiation is initiated in the GC. Recent studies have shed the light on how to identify PC and MBC precursors within the GC. PCs leave the second lymphoid tissues and finally locate in the bone marrow. MBCs begin to generate early in the GC reaction and manifest lower immunoglobulin affinity as compared to PCs that egress later (Shinnakasu et al. 2016). Upon antigen recall, MBCs will either differentiate into antibody-producing cells or reseed new GCs to undergo further immunoglobulin affinity mutation. The molecular mechanism underlying GC B cell differentiation into MBCs remains unclear. It is reported that transcription repressor BACH2 is required for the formation of MBC (Shinnakasu et al. 2016). The molecular drivers of B cell differentiation into the PC fate are better understood. The PC master-regulator Blimp1 (Prdm1) and IRF4 are essential for PC differentiation by shutting down expression of transcription factor BCL6 (Basso and Dalla-Favera 2010; Huang et al. 2014a).

4.8 BCL6: A Master Transcriptional Regulator of GC Reaction

GC B cell differentiation is tightly controlled by various transcription regulators including BCL6. BCL6 is a transcriptional repressor identified in 1993 as the target of chromosomal translocations affecting band 3q27 in DLBCL. The transcriptional repression activity of BCL6 is dependent on its binding to co-repressor proteins, and there are many co-repressors that BCL6 can partner with. BCL6 exerts its transcription repression activity by recruiting co-repressors mainly via its conserved N-terminal BTB/POZ domain and a middle unstructured region (often called the second repression domain or "RD2" domain). The transcriptional repression activity of BCL6 requires its binding to specific DNA elements. Recently, whole-genome chromatin immunoprecipitation plus sequencing (ChIP-seq) analysis identified genome-wide BCL6 binding sites and target genes (Hatzi et al. 2013). BCL6 acts as a key regulator of the GC reaction since BCL6 null mice fail to develop GCs and are unable to generate high-affinity antibodies (Dent et al. 1997; Ye et al. 1997).

BCL6 is essential for the initiation of GC reaction and is upregulated in GC-destined GC B cells (Kerfoot et al. 2011; Kitano et al. 2011). BCL6-deficient GC precursor B cells fail to enter the follicle. Mechanistically, BCL6 suppresses G protein-coupled receptor 183 (GPR183; also known as EBI2) (Shaffer et al. 2000), which must be down-regulated by GC precursor B cells to allow their migration toward the center of the follicle, via its RD2 (Huang et al. 2014b). In addition, BCL6-RD2 domain inhibits sphingosine-1-phosphate receptor type 1 (S1PR1) to induce confinement of B cells in the GC.

BCL6 protein is highly expressed in centroblasts, and its expression is maintained in most centrocytes, indicating an essential role of this transcriptional factor in the establishment and/or maintenance of GCs. One of the well-known functions of BCL6 in centroblasts is to facilitate simultaneous rapid proliferation and tolerance of genomic damage occurring during clonal expansion and somatic hypermutation by directly repressing DNA damage sensing and checkpoint genes such as DNA damage sensor ATR, TP53 tumor suppressor and cell cycle arrest gene CDKN1A (Basso and Dalla-Favera 2010). In addition, BCL6 may be important to prevent centroblasts to exit from the GC before they complete the phase of proliferative expansion and of antibody affinity maturation. Finally, BCL6 represses a number of genes required for the differentiation of B cells into plasma cells, including PRDM1, a transcription factor that is crucial for plasma cell development (Basso and Dalla-Favera 2010; Bunting and Melnick 2013). BCL6 must be switched off for GC B cell to exit from the GC and undergo terminal differentiation.

BCL6 is also essential for the generation and effector functions of Tfh cells (Nurieva et al. 2009; Yu et al. 2009). Ectopic BCL6 expression leads to induction of CXCR5, ICOS and PD-1 on $CD4^+$ T cells. BCL6 promotes Tfh differentiation by inhibiting other T cell subset differentiation in a DNA binding-dependent manner. Furthermore, BCL6 directly binds to the transcription factor AP-1 and blocks or subverts downstream TCR signaling of AP-1 and helps in Tfh generation (Hatzi et al. 2015). Interestingly, PRDM1 is a critical negative regulator of Tfh cells and is directly suppressed by BCL6 (Johnston et al. 2009).

4.9 Conclusion

GCs form in secondary lymphoid tissues in response to antigenic challenge and are the site of somatic hypermutation, generating GC B cells with increasing affinity for the inciting agent that are positively selected over time, and providing effective long-lived humoral immunity. The GC reaction is coordinated by multiple immune cells. Considerable progress has been made in understanding the GC reaction. We now have a greatly enhanced picture of the events that follow initial antigen encounter and culminate in the formation of a mature GC that is optimally structured for the selection of high-affinity antibody mutants. Cell-cell crosstalk plays a crucial role in controlling the cell fate decision and affinity selection. However, the GC reaction is complex and highly dynamic. This dynamic system must be instructed by intricate mechanisms of control, which are probably achieved through the integration of transcriptional, post-transcriptional and epigenetic programs.

References

Basso K, Dalla-Favera R (2010) BCL6: master regulator of the germinal center reaction and key oncogene in B cell lymphomagenesis. Adv Immunol 105:193–210

Berek C, Berger A, Apel M (1991) Maturation of the immune response in germinal centers. Cell 67:1121–1129

Brink R, Phan TG (2018) Self-reactive B cells in the germinal center reaction. Annu Rev Immunol 36: 339–357

Bunting KL, Melnick AM (2013) New effector functions and regulatory mechanisms of BCL6 in normal and malignant lymphocytes. Curr Opin Immunol 25:339–346

Corcoran LM, Tarlinton DM (2016) Regulation of germinal center responses, memory B cells and plasma cell formation-an update. Curr Opin Immunol 39:59–67

Crotty S (2011) Follicular helper CD4 T cells (TFH). Annu Rev Immunol 29:621–663

Crotty S (2014) T follicular helper cell differentiation, function, and roles in disease. Immunity 41:529–542

De Silva NS, Klein U (2015) Dynamics of B cells in germinal centres. Nat Rev Immunol 15:137–148

Dent AL, Shaffer AL, Yu X, Allman D, Staudt LM (1997) Control of inflammation, cytokine expression, and germinal center formation by BCL-6. Science 276:589–592

Hatzi K, Jiang Y, Huang C, Garrett-Bakelman F, Gearhart MD, Giannopoulou EG, Zumbo P, Kirouac K, Bhaskara S, Polo JM et al (2013) A hybrid mechanism of action for BCL6 in B cells defined by formation of functionally distinct

complexes at enhancers and promoters. Cell reports 4:578–588
Hatzi K, Nance JP, Kroenke MA, Bothwell M, Haddad EK, Melnick A, Crotty S (2015) BCL6 orchestrates Tfh cell differentiation via multiple distinct mechanisms. J Exp Med 212:539–553
Huang C, Geng H, Boss I, Wang L, Melnick A (2014a) Cooperative transcriptional repression by BCL6 and BACH2 in germinal center B-cell differentiation. Blood 123:1012–1020
Huang C, Gonzalez DG, Cote CM, Jiang Y, Hatzi K, Teater M, Dai K, Hla T, Haberman AM, Melnick A (2014b) The BCL6 RD2 domain governs commitment of activated B cells to form germinal centers. Cell reports 8:1497–1508
Johnston RJ, Poholek AC, DiToro D, Yusuf I, Eto D, Barnett B, Dent AL, Craft J, Crotty S (2009) Bcl6 and Blimp-1 are reciprocal and antagonistic regulators of T follicular helper cell differentiation. Science 325: 1006–1010
Kerfoot SM, Yaari G, Patel JR, Johnson KL, Gonzalez DG, Kleinstein SH, Haberman AM (2011) Germinal center B cell and T follicular helper cell development initiates in the interfollicular zone. Immunity 34:947–960
Kitano M, Moriyama S, Ando Y, Hikida M, Mori Y, Kurosaki T, Okada T (2011) Bcl6 protein expression shapes pre-germinal center B cell dynamics and follicular helper T cell heterogeneity. Immunity 34:961–972
Liu D, Xu H, Shih C, Wan Z, Ma X, Ma W, Luo D, Qi H (2015) T-B-cell entanglement and ICOSL-driven feed-forward regulation of germinal centre reaction. Nature 517:214–218
Luo W, Weisel F, Shlomchik MJ (2018) B cell receptor and CD40 signaling are rewired for synergistic induction of the c-Myc transcription factor in germinal center B cells. Immunity 48:313–326 e315
MacLennan IC (1994) Germinal centers. Annu Rev Immunol 12:117–139
Mesin L, Ersching J, Victora GD (2016) Germinal center B cell dynamics. Immunity 45:471–482
Nurieva RI, Chung Y, Martinez GJ, Yang XO, Tanaka S, Matskevitch TD, Wang YH, Dong C (2009) Bcl6 mediates the development of T follicular helper cells. Science 325:1001–1005
Okada T, Miller MJ, Parker I, Krummel MF, Neighbors M, Hartley SB, O'Garra A, Cahalan MD, Cyster JG (2005) Antigen-engaged B cells undergo chemotaxis toward the T zone and form motile conjugates with helper T cells. PLoS Biol 3:e150
Papa I, Vinuesa CG (2018) Synaptic interactions in germinal centers. Front Immunol 9:1858
Paus D, Phan TG, Chan TD, Gardam S, Basten A, Brink R (2006) Antigen recognition strength regulates the choice between extrafollicular plasma cell and germinal center B cell differentiation. J Exp Med 203:1081–1091
Sage PT, Sharpe AH (2015) T follicular regulatory cells in the regulation of B cell responses. Trends Immunol 36:410–418
Shaffer AL, Yu X, He Y, Boldrick J, Chan EP, Staudt LM (2000) BCL-6 represses genes that function in lymphocyte differentiation, inflammation, and cell cycle control. Immunity 13:199–212
Shinnakasu R, Inoue T, Kometani K, Moriyama S, Adachi Y, Nakayama M, Takahashi Y, Fukuyama H, Okada T, Kurosaki T (2016) Regulated selection of germinal-center cells into the memory B cell compartment. Nat Immunol 17:861–869
Song W, Craft J (2019) T follicular helper cell heterogeneity: time, space, and function. Immunol Rev 288:85–96
Suan D, Sundling C, Brink R (2017) Plasma cell and memory B cell differentiation from the germinal center. Curr Opin Immunol 45:97–102
Tangye SG, Brink R, Goodnow CC, Phan TG (2015) SnapShot: interactions between B cells and T cells. Cell 162:926–926 e921
van Kooten C, Banchereau J (2000) CD40-CD40 ligand. J Leukoc Biol 67:2–17
Victora GD, Nussenzweig MC (2012) Germinal centers. Annu Rev Immunol 30:429–457
Victora GD, Schwickert TA, Fooksman DR, Kamphorst AO, Meyer-Hermann M, Dustin ML, Nussenzweig MC (2010) Germinal center dynamics revealed by multiphoton microscopy with a photoactivatable fluorescent reporter. Cell 143:592–605
Vinuesa CG, Linterman MA, Yu D, MacLennan IC (2016) Follicular helper T cells. Annu Rev Immunol 34:335–368
Wan Z, Lin Y, Zhao Y, Qi H (2019) TFH cells in bystander and cognate interactions with B cells. Immunol Rev 288:28–36
Ye BH, Cattoretti G, Shen Q, Zhang J, Hawe N, de Waard R, Leung C, Nouri-Shirazi M, Orazi A, Chaganti RS et al (1997) The BCL-6 proto-oncogene controls germinal-centre formation and Th2-type inflammation. Nat Genet 16:161–170
Yu D, Rao S, Tsai LM, Lee SK, He Y, Sutcliffe EL, Srivastava M, Linterman M, Zheng L, Simpson N et al (2009) The transcriptional repressor Bcl-6 directs T follicular helper cell lineage commitment. Immunity 31:457–468

Memory B Cells in Local and Systemic Sites

5

Saya Moriyama, Yu Adachi, Keisuke Tonouchi, and Yoshimasa Takahashi

Abstract

Memory B cells are a key cellular component of the protective humoral responses to infectious pathogens. Most of our knowledge of memory B-cell responses comes from studies using mono-epitopic model antigens that elicit systemic humoral responses dominated by canonical B-cell antigen receptors. This approach successfully dissected the systemic responses of memory B cells and greatly advanced our understanding of memory B-cell formation, maintenance, and reactivation to re-invading antigens in the secondary lymphoid organs. However, the canonical memory B-cell responses fail to fully recapitulate the heterogeneity of the protective memory responses. Indeed, accumulating studies using "natural" antigens and live pathogens have uncovered new aspects of memory B-cell responses, which are achieved by memory B cells with different phenotypes, tissue residence, and responsiveness to antigen stimulation. Such non-canonical memory B-cell responses are frequently observed in local sites where live pathogens initially infect and replicate. Importantly, the local memory B-cell responses often serve as the first line of defense against re-infecting pathogens, thereby playing an essential role in controlling the pathogens. Here, we provide a comprehensive overview of the systemic and local memory B-cell responses in the humoral protective immunity against pathogens.

Keywords

Memory B cell · Germinal center · Local tissue-resident memory · Vaccination · Recall response

5.1 Introduction

A fundamental function of adaptive immunity is to remember an initial encounter with invading pathogens and to confer efficient protection against secondary infection. In primary immune responses, activated B cells differentiate into long-lived memory B cells, which are key players in humoral protection. Here, we define memory B cells as antigen-experienced, resting B cells that persist for a durable period in the body and then promptly become effector cells

S. Moriyama (✉) · Y. Adachi · K. Tonouchi · Y. Takahashi
Department of Immunology, National Institute of Infectious Diseases, 1-23-1 Toyama, Shinjuku, Tokyo 162-8640, Japan
e-mail: sayamrym@niid.go.jp

Y. Takahashi
e-mail: ytakahas@niid.go.jp

K. Tonouchi
Department of Life Science and Medical Bioscience, Waseda University, 2-2 Wakamatsucho, Shinjuku, Tokyo 162-8480, Japan

J.-Y. Wang (ed.), *B Cells in Immunity and Tolerance*, Advances in Experimental Medicine and Biology 1254, https://doi.org/10.1007/978-981-15-3532-1_5

upon another encounter with the same antigen. Long-lived plasma cells, another important compartment for humoral protection, will not be covered in this article. Owing to the lack of a single marker for identifying memory B cells, murine memory B cells are detected as CD38^{hi} resting B cells that express antigen-binding B-cell receptors (BCRs) with surface markers (CD80, PD-L2, and so on) at differential levels and/or previous experience with antigen-driven proliferation (Weisel and Shlomchik 2017). Human memory B cells are detected by the combination of surface markers (such as CD27) or the accumulation of dyes representing the absence of ATP-binding cassette B1 transporter expression (Wirths and Lanzavecchia 2005) and the expression of antigen-binding BCRs when the priming antigens are identified. In addition to these classical memory B cells, CD27^{-} memory B cells are detected in human tonsils and are called atypical memory B cells (Ehrhardt et al. 2005). Atypical memory B cells have different gene expression profiles compared to classical memory B cells, mostly show the exhaustion phenotype, and are also found in the circulation of patients with chronic infections such as HIV infection, recurrent malaria, mycobacterium tuberculosis, and hepatitis (Portugal et al. 2017). Thus, there are multiple memory subsets with different phenotypes in humans and mice, and the functions of these subsets are under investigation using model antigens and pathogens.

Efficient containment of viral spread relies on the prompt supply of protective antibodies to the local site of virus infection; therefore, the induction, maintenance, and reactivation of memory B cells in local sites provide a great anatomical advantage to the host. For example, following influenza virus infection in respiratory sites, tertiary lymphoid organs begin to form in the lung tissue where memory B-cell responses are initiated, maintained, and reactivated in response to the infection. Thus, the memory B-cell response in local sites serves as the first line of defense until a sufficient amount of protective antibodies are supplied from humoral memory in secondary lymphoid organs. Here, we comparatively review local and systemic memory B-cell responses with emphasis on the protective function.

5.2 Memory B-Cell Formation

Upon encountering foreign antigens, naïve B cells in the B-cell follicle recognize the antigen through BCR and receive signals from cognate T cells at the B-T border (Fig. 5.1; Okada et al. 2005). Some of the activated B cells upregulate the transcription factor Bcl6, migrate back to the follicle, and form germinal centers (GCs; reviewed elsewhere in this textbook). Other activated B cells differentiate into plasma cells or memory B cells, without entering the GCs. This GC-independent pathway was initially identified in studies using Bcl6-deficient mice that cannot form GCs. Further studies using GC-competent mice confirmed the existence of memory B cells encoding germline BCRs without somatic hypermutations, supporting the hypothesis that GC-independent and -dependent pathways coexist in the immune-competent conditions (Kaji et al. 2012; Shinnakasu et al. 2016; Toyama et al. 2002). Before GC formation, activated B cells rapidly differentiate into memory B cells in the presence of strong CD40 stimulation from helper T cells, but these early memory B cells are gradually replaced by GC-derived, mutated memory B cells at later time points (Taylor et al. 2012; Weisel and Shlomchik 2017). Thus, upon an encounter with T-cell-dependent antigens, memory B cells develop in two waves: the first wave is the GC-independent pathway that promptly recruits germline-encoded, low-affinity memory B cells, and the second wave is the GC-dependent pathway recruiting somatically mutated, affinity-matured memory B cells from GC reactions.

GCs provide a Darwinian microcosm where B cells undergo affinity-driven clonal selection following random diversification of their BCRs through somatic hypermutations. This occurs in two functionally distinct regions. The dark zone (DZ) contains CXCL12 expressing fibroblastic reticular cells and supports rapid cellular division and somatic hypermutation, whereas the light zone (LZ) is the site of antigen-driven selection, achieved by successive interactions of

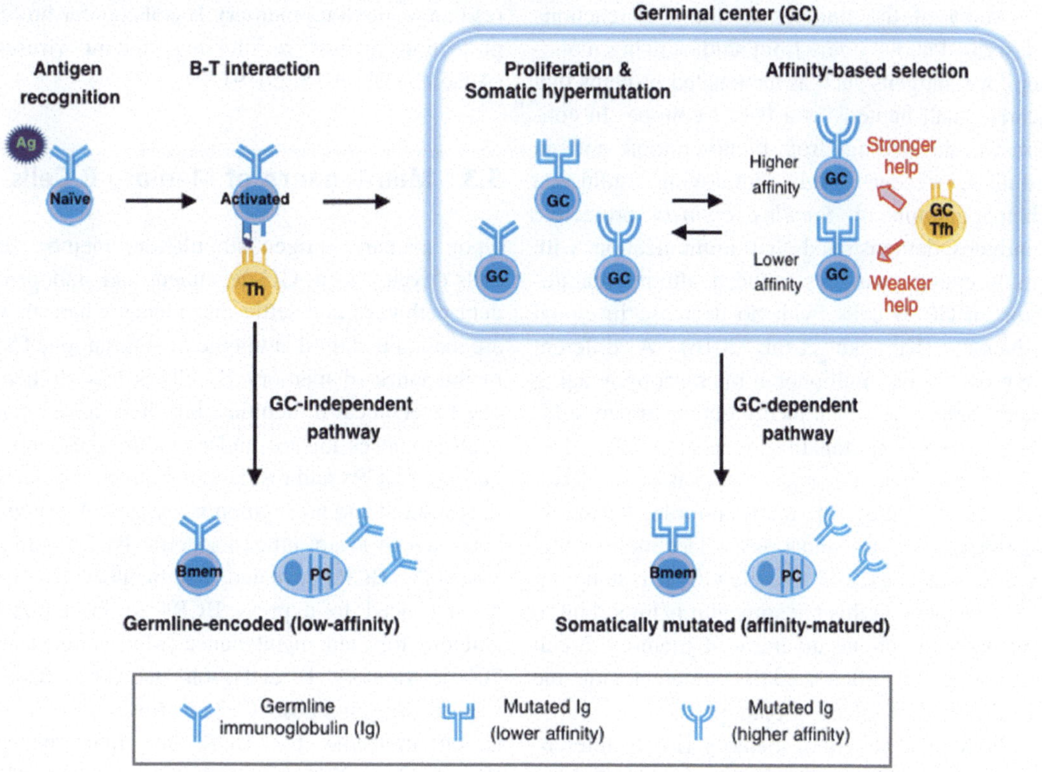

Fig. 5.1 Differentiation of memory B cells during the primary response. Memory B cells are developed through two different pathways. Antigen-specific B cells are primed by antigen recognition and further activated by the secondary signal from cognate T cells. Following B-T interaction, some B cells with germline BCRs differentiate directly into memory B cells or antibody-producing plasma cells (GC-independent pathway). Other activated B cells differentiate to GC B cells and form the GC. In the GC, B cells quickly proliferate, somatically mutated, and are selected through interaction with GC Tfh cells, leading to the affinity maturation. Through GC responses, B cells further differentiate into memory B cells or plasma cells or stay in the GC for further rounds of GC responses (GC-dependent pathway). In most cases, GC-derived memory B cells or plasma cells persist long term and contribute to the quick and robust immune response at antigen re-exposure. Ag, antigen; Th, helper T; GC, germinal center; Tfh, follicular helper T; Bmem, memory B; PC, plasma cell; Ig, immunoglobulin

antigen-bearing follicular dendritic cells (FDCs) and GC follicular helper T (Tfh) cells (Victora and Nussenzweig 2012). LZ B cells with sufficient BCR affinity interact with antigen-bearing FDCs, internalize and process the antigen and then present the antigen to Tfh cells in complex with MHC class II. It is believed that BCR affinity for the antigen determines the amount of antigen presented to the B cells; the consequence being that B cells receive helper signals in proportion to BCR affinity from a limited number of GC Tfh cells. LZ B cells expressing BCRs with a sufficient affinity range is considered to make the following fate decisions based on BCR affinity. (1) Exiting the GC as plasma cells (higher affinity), (2) recycling back to the DZ (medium affinity), or (3) exiting the GC as memory B cells (lower affinity). The fate decision of low-affinity B cells to memory pathway is determined by transcriptional networks; one of the key molecules underlying this process is Bach2 (Kometani et al. 2013). The low-affinity B cells in the LZ have higher levels of Bach2 expression that is inversely correlated with the strength of T cell help, suggesting that low-affinity LZ B cells receive weaker T cell help and become memory precursors due to increased Bach2 expression.

Many of the findings in the GC reactions described above come from studies using mono-epitope antigens such as haptenated proteins that carry small haptens as a B-cell epitope. In contrast to the findings from mono-epitopic antigen studies, recent work employing influenza hemagglutinin or *Bacillus anthrax* protective antigens demonstrated that immunization with multi-epitope antigens induced affinity maturation in GC B cells, with no decrease in clonal diversity (Kuraoka et al. 2016). A different approach using multiphoton microscopy imaging and "brainbow" mice nicely demonstrated similarly diversified clonality, even after GC selection had sufficiently proceeded (Tas et al. 2016). Therefore, following multi-epitopic, "natural" antigens, there are situations where multi-clonal GC B cells coexist in a single GC. It is tempting to speculate that this phenomenon is important to maintain the clonal diversity of memory B-cell repertoires that often need to counteract antigenic variation of re-infecting pathogens.

Following infection, memory B-cell differentiation takes place not only in secondary lymphoid (*e.g.*, the lymph nodes and spleen) but also in non-lymphoid organs. For influenza virus infection, an ectopic lymphoid structure called the inducible bronchus-associated lymphoid tissue (iBALT) is formed in the lung by infiltrated lymphocytes (Randall 2010), the process initiated by type-I interferon production, followed by CXCL13 expression in lung fibroblasts (Denton et al. 2019). iBALTs often contain GC structure, which is able to support mutation and selection cycles for BCR affinity maturation (Adachi et al. 2015). These ectopic GCs are also capable of generating lung-resident IgG^+ and IgA^+ memory B cells with distinct phenotypes, which express CD69, CXCR3, CD80, and PD-L2 more abundantly than canonical memory B cells in secondary lymphoid organs (Allie et al. 2019; Onodera et al. 2012). Of note, the lung-resident memory B cells have distinct function other than the prompt supply of protective antibodies in local sites; their BCRs have increased access to virus vulnerable epitopes which are often protected from BCR access (Adachi et al. 2015, 2019). With the unique BCR specificity and lung residency, the lung memory B cells confer broad protection against re-infecting mutant viruses (Adachi et al. 2015, 2019).

5.3 Maintenance of Memory B Cells

Upon primary antigen stimulation, memory B cells develop from GC-dependent and -independent pathways and settle into niches where they are maintained until antigenic re-stimulation. The maintenance of memory B cells is less studied, due to technical difficulties, but there have been great advances toward understanding the contribution of BCRs and residential maintenance sites in lymphoid and non-lymphoid organs. A genetic approach to swap antigen-specific BCRs with -unspecific BCRs revealed that memory B cells do not need to express BCRs to immunized antigens for their maintenance (Maruyama et al. 2000). Memory B cells, on the other hand, require phospholipase Cγ2, a downstream signaling molecule for BCR, for maintenance (Hikida et al. 2009). Together, it is conceivable that memory B cells require tonic signals from the BCR complex, which does not necessarily recognize the immunizing antigen. This idea is further supported by studies using knockout mice for CD21/CD35, a complement receptor for antigen capture by FDCs, which is required for a long-term B-cell memory persistence (Barrington et al. 2002). In line with this scenario, the lack of a BCR co-receptor molecule, CD19, did not affect GC response after virus infection but failed to recall the memory responses following secondary challenge, further supporting the contribution of the BCR complex during post-GC memory responses (Fehr et al. 1998).

During the maintenance phase, memory B cells are found in circulation and distributed in the secondary lymphoid organs and bone marrow. In lymph nodes with no persisting GCs, memory B cells are found in a subcapsular niche where draining antigens, as well as subcapsular macrophages and memory Tfh cells, exist (Moran et al. 2018; Suan et al. 2015). Memory B cells are also in the periphery where, in infectious diseases, the antigen invades and immune responses take place. Following influenza infection, memory B cells are maintained not only in the draining lymph node and in the spleen, but also the lung tissue, as tissue-resident cells guarding against the re-infection (Allie et al. 2019; Onodera et al. 2012). Lung-resident memory B cells highly express CD69 and CXCR3, which are also expressed in lung-resident memory T cells for regulating prolonged T-cell retention in the peripheral tissue and T-cell commitment to effector fate, respectively (Allie et al. 2019; Kohlmeier et al. 2011; Kurachi et al. 2011; Mackay et al. 2015; Onodera et al. 2012). How tissue-resident memory B cells are recruited and retained in the cellular niches of the lung tissues remains to be important questions.

5.4 Reactivation of Memory B Cells

Reactivation of the memory B cells occurs in the lymphoid tissue and the periphery; they are maintained in both sites as discussed above and/or recruited from circulation. Upon reactivation via antigen recognition, memory B cells rapidly differentiate into terminally differentiated plasma cells or reenter the GC to undergo further affinity maturation. In this section, we focus on the mechanism of memory B-cell reactivation and their niche.

Memory B-cell reactivation following antigen exposure occurs with and without the help of T cells (Figs. 5.2 and 5.3). Upon exposure to a cognate antigen, together with TLR ligands provided by virus particles, memory B cells can differentiate into plasma cells and produce antibodies without T cell help (Hebeis et al. 2004; Onodera et al. 2016). T-cell-independent reactivation depends on the TLRs expressed in memory B cells and occurs before the onset of T-cell-dependent recall response, which leads to rapid terminal differentiation and higher-affinity antibody production (Onodera et al. 2016).

If T-cell-independent recall is restricted, then helper T cells are a key factor to guide memory B-cell reactivation. Following the primary infection, helper T cells are maintained as memory cells in the secondary lymphoid tissue, blood, and peripheral tissue and help memory B-cell reactivation rapidly after antigen re-exposure (Crotty 2019). Of note, the reactivation of memory Tfh cells is induced by cognate interaction with memory B cells rather than the interaction with dendritic cells, contributing to rapid memory responses (Ise et al. 2014).

The rapidness of T-cell-dependent memory B-cell activation, compared to naïve B cells, depends on the abundance of antigen-specific B cells and helper T cells, as well as the distinct cellular properties in the memory B cells themselves. One hypothesis is that the cytoplasmic tail of membrane IgG1 accounts for their rapid differentiation into plasma cells compared to IgM^+ B cells (Martin and Goodnow 2002). More recently, a study using nuclear-transferred antigen-specific BCR transgenic mice, with class-switched but naïve $IgG1^+$ B cells, showed that $IgG1^+$ memory B cells are more prone to differentiate into plasma cells than $IgG1^+$ naïve B cells, which differentiate into GC cells (Kometani et al. 2013). This suggests that BCR-independent memory phenotype is required for prompt differentiation into plasma cells. Mechanistically, lower Bach 2 expression in $IgG1^+$ memory B

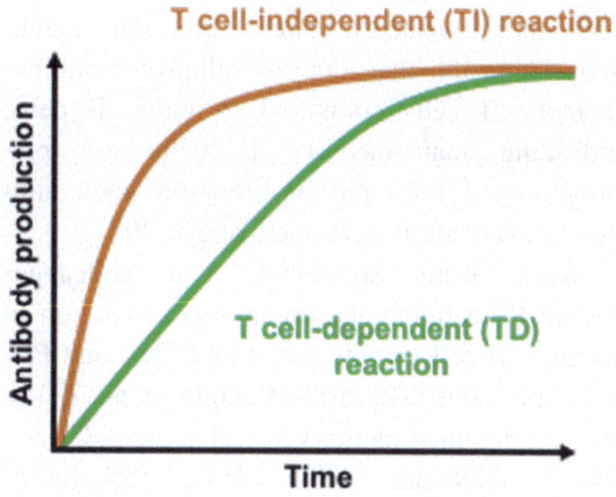

Fig. 5.2 T cell-dependent and -independent humoral responses. At secondary infection, especially in influenza A virus infection, two waves of memory B-cell differentiation occurs. In the early phase of reinfection, some memory B cells differentiate into plasma cells without T cell help (T cell-independent, TI, response). The remaining memory B cells respond through interaction with T cells (T cell-dependent, TD, response), catching up to the first wave response at later time points

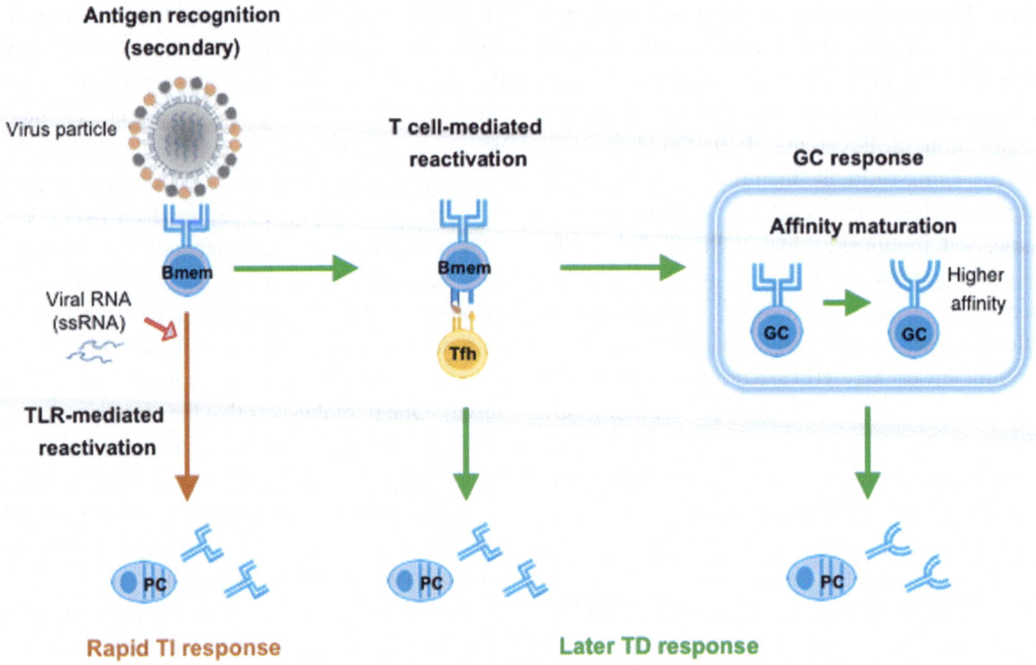

Fig. 5.3 Reactivation of memory B cells after antigen re-exposure. After antigen re-exposure, some memory B cells are activated without help from T cells but through TLR-mediated signals, leading to rapid antibody production (TI response). Following Tfh cell reactivation from the memory compartment, memory B cells are further activated with help from Tfh cells and rapidly differentiate into plasma cells (TD response). Some memory B cells differentiate into GC B cells for further affinity maturation. Bmem, memory B; Tfh, follicular helper T; GC, germinal center; PC, plasma cell; ssRNA, single-stranded RNA; TI, T cell-independent; TD, T cell-dependent

cells enhances plasma cell differentiation. A human study revealed a lower expression of transcription factors that suppress cell proliferation in memory B cells compared to naïve B cells, indicating that memory B cells are pre-programmed for rapid proliferation upon antigen re-exposure (Good and Tangye 2007).

Work from Shlomchik and colleagues revealed the functional compartmentalization of memory B-cell subsets based on CD80 and PD-L2 expression (Zuccarino-Catania et al. 2014). Among the three memory B-cell subsets, $CD80^-$ $PD\text{-}L2^-$ (DN) and $CD80^-$ $PD\text{-}L2^+$ (SP) $IgG1^-$ memory B cells are prone to differentiate into GC B cells, but $CD80^+$ $PD\text{-}L2^+$ (DP) $IgG1^-$ memory B cells are more likely to differentiate into IgG1-producing plasma cells at an earlier time point after re-challenge. Majority of class-switched memory B cells are DP cells, and $IgG1^-$ memory B cells are SP and DN cells. DP $IgG1^+$ and DP $IgG1^-$ memory B cells similarly produced $IgG1^+$ plasma cells, suggesting that the functional heterogeneity of memory B cells is governed independently of BCR-isotype. Lung class-switched memory B cells express CD80 and PD-L2 more frequently than their counterparts in secondary lymphoid organs, suggesting they are more prone to plasma cell differentiation.

IgE is an important immunoglobulin isotype involved in therapeutical and pathological responses such as anti-helminth immunity, allergy, and anaphylaxis. IgE can be rapidly produced upon antigen re-exposure. However, mouse studies using IgE-reporter mice show that IgE class-switched B cells differentiate into short-lived plasma cells, but not into memory B cells (Phan and Tangye 2017; Yang et al. 2014). This leads to the hypothesis that IgE is produced by plasma cells that undergo class-switching from IgM^+ or IgG^+ memory B cells upon antigen re-exposure. Indeed, a transfer study shows that $IgG1^+$ memory B cells undergo sequential class-switching and differentiate into IgE^+ plasma cells (He et al. 2017).

Memory B-cell reactivation takes place in the secondary lymphoid organs and the peripheral tissue by tissue-resident memory B cells or by memory B cells recruited from circulation. In the lymph nodes, an imaging study showed that memory B cells in the subcapsular niche rapidly respond to re-invading antigens (Moran et al. 2018). In the periphery, virus reinfection initiates tissue-resident memory B-cell reactivation in lungs, which contributes to the prompt supply of protective antibodies in situ (Allie et al. 2019; Onodera et al. 2012).

5.5 Conclusion

Human and mouse memory B cells are heterogeneous in their phenotypes, tissue residence, and responsiveness to re-challenged antigens. This heterogeneity may be the result of adaptation to protect the host from a variety of life-threatening pathogens. Tissue residence is a key property of memory B cells that is induced by an infection, and that is closely associated with the protective functions. In addition to an anatomical advantage to rapidly respond to re-infecting pathogens, tissue-resident memory B cells possess unique properties to counteract the pathogens, one of which is an increased breadth of antigen specificity that is essential for protection against mutating pathogens. Thus, future analyses of tissue-resident memory B cells at the front line of infections are likely to provide new and protective aspects of memory B cells that have, to this point, remained unaddressed by model antigen studies.

Acknowledgements The laboratory is funded by the Ministry of Education, Culture, Sports, Science, and Technology in Japan under JP19K17656 (to YA) and the Japan Agency for Medical Research and Development under JP19fk0108051, 19fk0108035, and 19fk0310120 (all to YT).

References

Adachi Y, Onodera T, Yamada Y, Daio R, Tsuiji M, Inoue T, Kobayashi K, Kurosaki T, Ato M, Takahashi Y (2015) Distinct germinal center selection at local sites shapes memory B cell response to viral escape. J Exp Med 212:1709–1723

Adachi Y, Tonouchi K, Nithichanon A, Kuraoka M, Watanabe A, Shinnakasu R, Asanuma H, Ainai A, Ohmi Y, Yamamoto T, Ishii KJ, Hasegawa H, Takeyama H, Lertmemongkolchai G, Kurosaki T, Ato M, Kelsoe G, Takahashi Y (2019) Exposure of an occluded hemagglutinin epitope drives selection of a class of cross-protective influenza antibodies. Nat Commun 10:3883

Allie SR, Bradley JE, Mudunuru U, Schultz MD, Graf BA, Lund FE, Randall TD (2019) The establishment of resident memory B cells in the lung requires local antigen encounter. Nat Immunol 20:97–108

Barrington RA, Pozdnyakova O, Zafari MR, Benjamin CD, Carroll MC (2002) B lymphocyte memory: role of stromal cell complement and FcgammaRIIB receptors. J Exp Med 196:1189–1199

Crotty S (2019) T follicular helper cell biology: a decade of discovery and diseases. Immunity 50:1132–1148

Denton AE, Innocentin S, Carr EJ, Bradford BM, Lafouresse F, Mabbott NA, Morbe U, Ludewig B, Groom JR, Good-Jacobson KL, Linterman MA (2019) Type I interferon induces CXCL13 to support ectopic germinal center formation. J Exp Med 216:621–637

Ehrhardt GR, Hsu JT, Gartland L, Leu CM, Zhang S, Davis RS, Cooper MD (2005) Expression of the immunoregulatory molecule FcRH4 defines a distinctive tissue-based population of memory B cells. J Exp Med 202:783–791

Fehr T, Rickert RC, Odermatt B, Roes J, Rajewsky K, Hengartner H, Zinkernagel RM (1998) Antiviral protection and germinal center formation, but impaired B cell memory in the absence of CD19. J Exp Med 188:145–155

Good KL, Tangye SG (2007) Decreased expression of Kruppel-like factors in memory B cells induces the rapid response typical of secondary antibody responses. Proc Natl Acad Sci U S A 104:13420–13425

He JS, Subramaniam S, Narang V, Srinivasan K, Saunders SP, Carbajo D, Wen-Shan T, Hidayah Hamadee N, Lum J, Lee A, Chen J, Poidinger M, Zolezzi F, Lafaille JJ, Curotto de Lafaille MA (2017) IgG1 memory B cells keep the memory of IgE responses. Nat Commun 8:641

Hebeis BJ, Klenovsek K, Rohwer P, Ritter U, Schneider A, Mach M, Winkler TH (2004) Activation of virus-specific memory B cells in the absence of T cell help. J Exp Med 199:593–602

Hikida M, Casola S, Takahashi N, Kaji T, Takemori T, Rajewsky K, Kurosaki T (2009) PLC-gamma2 is essential for formation and maintenance of memory B cells. J Exp Med 206:681–689

Ise W, Inoue T, McLachlan JB, Kometani K, Kubo M, Okada T, Kurosaki T (2014) Memory B cells contribute to rapid Bcl6 expression by memory follicular helper T cells. Proc Natl Acad Sci U S A 111:11792–11797

Kaji T, Ishige A, Hikida M, Taka J, Hijikata A, Kubo M, Nagashima T, Takahashi Y, Kurosaki T, Okada M, Ohara O, Rajewsky K, Takemori T (2012) Distinct cellular pathways select germline-encoded and somatically mutated antibodies into immunological memory. J Exp Med 209:2079–2097

Kohlmeier JE, Reiley WW, Perona-Wright G, Freeman ML, Yager EJ, Connor LM, Brincks EL, Cookenham T, Roberts AD, Burkum CE, Sell S, Winslow GM, Blackman MA, Mohrs M, Woodland DL (2011) Inflammatory chemokine receptors regulate CD8(+) T cell contraction and memory generation following infection. J Exp Med 208:1621–1634

Kometani K, Nakagawa R, Shinnakasu R, Kaji T, Rybouchkin A, Moriyama S, Furukawa K, Koseki H, Takemori T, Kurosaki T (2013) Repression of the transcription factor Bach2 contributes to predisposition of IgG1 memory B cells toward plasma cell differentiation. Immunity 39:136–147

Kurachi M, Kurachi J, Suenaga F, Tsukui T, Abe J, Ueha S, Tomura M, Sugihara K, Takamura S, Kakimi K, Matsushima K (2011) Chemokine receptor CXCR3 facilitates CD8(+) T cell differentiation into short-lived effector cells leading to memory degeneration. J Exp Med 208:1605–1620

Kuraoka M, Schmidt AG, Nojima T, Feng F, Watanabe A, Kitamura D, Harrison SC, Kepler TB, Kelsoe G (2016) Complex antigens drive permissive clonal selection in germinal centers. Immunity 44:542–552

Mackay LK, Braun A, Macleod BL, Collins N, Tebartz C, Bedoui S, Carbone FR, Gebhardt T (2015) Cutting edge: CD69 interference with sphingosine-1-phosphate receptor function regulates peripheral T cell retention. J Immunol 194:2059–2063

Martin SW, Goodnow CC (2002) Burst-enhancing role of the IgG membrane tail as a molecular determinant of memory. Nat Immunol 3:182–188

Maruyama M, Lam KP, Rajewsky K (2000) Memory B-cell persistence is independent of persisting immunizing antigen. Nature 407:636–642

Moran I, Nguyen A, Khoo WH, Butt D, Bourne K, Young C, Hermes JR, Biro M, Gracie G, Ma CS, Munier CML, Luciani F, Zaunders J, Parker A, Kelleher AD, Tangye SG, Croucher PI, Brink R, Read MN, Phan TG (2018) Memory B cells are reactivated in subcapsular proliferative foci of lymph nodes. Nat Commun 9:3372

Okada T, Miller MJ, Parker I, Krummel MF, Neighbors M, Hartley SB, O'Garra A, Cahalan MD, Cyster JG (2005) Antigen-engaged B cells undergo chemotaxis toward the T zone and form motile conjugates with helper T cells. PLoS Biol 3:e150

Onodera T, Hosono A, Odagiri T, Tashiro M, Kaminogawa S, Okuno Y, Kurosaki T, Ato M, Kobayashi K, Takahashi Y (2016) Whole-virion influenza vaccine recalls an early burst of high-affinity memory B cell response through TLR signaling. J Immunol 196:4172–4184

Onodera T, Takahashi Y, Yokoi Y, Ato M, Kodama Y, Hachimura S, Kurosaki T, Kobayashi K (2012) Memory B cells in the lung participate in protective humoral immune responses to pulmonary influenza virus reinfection. Proc Natl Acad Sci U S A 109:2485–2490

Phan TG, Tangye SG (2017) Memory B cells: total recall. Curr Opin Immunol 45:132–140

Portugal S, Obeng-Adjei N, Moir S, Crompton PD, Pierce SK (2017) Atypical memory B cells in human chronic infectious diseases: an interim report. Cell Immunol 321:18–25

Randall TD (2010) Bronchus-associated lymphoid tissue (BALT) structure and function. Adv Immunol 107:187–241

Shinnakasu R, Inoue T, Kometani K, Moriyama S, Adachi Y, Nakayama M, Takahashi Y, Fukuyama H, Okada T, Kurosaki T (2016) Regulated selection of germinal-center cells into the memory B cell compartment. Nat Immunol 17:861–869

Suan D, Nguyen A, Moran I, Bourne K, Hermes JR, Arshi M, Hampton HR, Tomura M, Miwa Y, Kelleher AD, Kaplan W, Deenick EK, Tangye SG, Brink R, Chtanova T, Phan TG (2015) T follicular helper cells have distinct modes of migration and molecular signatures in naive and memory immune responses. Immunity 42:704–718

Tas JM, Mesin L, Pasqual G, Targ S, Jacobsen JT, Mano YM, Chen CS, Weill JC, Reynaud CA, Browne EP, Meyer-Hermann M, Victora GD (2016) Visualizing antibody affinity maturation in germinal centers. Science 351:1048–1054

Taylor JJ, Pape KA, Jenkins MK (2012) A germinal center-independent pathway generates unswitched memory B cells early in the primary response. J Exp Med 209:597–606

Toyama H, Okada S, Hatano M, Takahashi Y, Takeda N, Ichii H, Takemori T, Kuroda Y, Tokuhisa T (2002) Memory B cells without somatic hypermutation are generated from Bcl6-deficient B cells. Immunity 17:329–339

Victora GD, Nussenzweig MC (2012) Germinal centers. Annu Rev Immunol 30:429–457

Weisel F, Shlomchik M (2017) Memory B cells of mice and humans. Annu Rev Immunol 35:255–284

Wirths S, Lanzavecchia A (2005) ABCB1 transporter discriminates human resting naive B cells from cycling transitional and memory B cells. Eur J Immunol 35:3433–3441

Yang Z, Robinson MJ, Allen CD (2014) Regulatory constraints in the generation and differentiation of IgE-expressing B cells. Curr Opin Immunol 28:64–70

Zuccarino-Catania GV, Sadanand S, Weisel FJ, Tomayko MM, Meng H, Kleinstein SH, Good-Jacobson KL, Shlomchik MJ (2014) CD80 and PD-L2 define functionally distinct memory B cell subsets that are independent of antibody isotype. Nat Immunol 15:631–637

Regulation of Plasma Cell Differentiation

6

W. Ise and T. Kurosaki

Abstract

Humoral immunity provides protection from pathogen infection, and this is mediated by antibodies that are produced by plasma cells. Plasma cells are terminally differentiated from activated B cells and are specialized for secreting antibodies. Plasma cells are generated during extrafollicular or germinal center (GC) responses, but GC-derived plasma cells are thought to be the major precursors of long-lived plasma cells, which confer long-term protection. Here, we review recent progress in our understanding of the cellular and molecular basis for plasma cell differentiation from GC B cells.

Keywords

Plasma cell · Antibody · B cell · Transcription factor · Germinal center

W. Ise (✉) · T. Kurosaki
Laboratory of Lymphocyte Differentiation,
WPI Immunology Frontier Research Center,
Osaka University, Osaka 565-0871, Japan
e-mail: wise@ifrec.osaka-u.ac.jp

T. Kurosaki
e-mail: kurosaki@ifrec.osaka-u.ac.jp

T. Kurosaki
Laboratory for Lymphocyte Differentiation,
RIKEN Center for Integrative Medical Sciences
(IMS), Yokohama, Kanagawa 230-0045, Japan

6.1 Introduction

Antibodies are effector proteins produced by terminally differentiated B cells termed plasma cells (Nutt et al. 2015) and play pivotal roles for both immediate and long-lasting host protection against viral, bacterial, and parasitic infections. Generation of antibodies with potent neutralizing and cross-reactive capacity against invading pathogens is one of the goals of our immune system and of most current vaccines.

The current paradigm proposes that there are two types of plasma cells, short- or long-lived plasma cells (Chang et al. 2018; Kometani and Kurosaki 2015). Most of the plasma cells that are generated immediately after antigen encounter die within a few days but confer initial and rapid protection to pathogens. In contrast, some of the plasma cells survive in specialized niches in the bone marrow or gut-associated lymphoid tissues for many years and contribute to long-term protection. Majority of such long-lived plasma cells are derived from the germinal center (GC), a transient structure formed in secondary lymphoid tissues (Victora and Nussenzweig 2012) and produce high affinity antibodies that effectively neutralize pathogens. Thus, the efficient induction of long-lived plasma cells is the key for successful vaccination. Here, we will review the basis of plasma cell generation from activated B cells and especially focus on the recent

J.-Y. Wang (ed.), *B Cells in Immunity and Tolerance*, Advances in Experimental Medicine and Biology 1254, https://doi.org/10.1007/978-981-15-3532-1_6

advances in our understanding of the mechanisms underlying plasma cell generation from GC B cells.

6.2 Initiation of Plasma Cell Differentiation

Upon challenge with T-dependent antigens, the cognate interaction between antigen-specific B cells and CD4+ T cells occurs at the border of the T and B zones, and the activated B cells migrate toward the outer region of the follicles. Then, those B cells proliferate extensively, form extracellular foci, and differentiate into antibody-secreting plasma cells (MacLennan et al. 2003). Most of these plasma cells are short-lived and die in situ within a few days (Jacob et al. 1991). During the extrafollicular B cell response, somatic hypermutation (SHM) is induced at very low levels (Di Niro et al. 2015; William et al. 2002), and thus, the variable regions of antibodies produced by the extrafollicular, short-lived plasma cells are usually unmutated (Jacob et al. 1991; McHeyzer-Williams et al. 1993). Majority of antibodies produced at this stage are IgM isotype. However, extrafollicular antibody response plays an important role by providing rapid protection against pathogens as a first defense by acquired immunity.

In addition to plasma cells, naïve B cells can differentiate into memory B cells or germinal center B cells (Kurosaki et al. 2015). One of the important factors that influence B cell fate decision is BCR affinity. Using BCR transgenic mice, it has elegantly been demonstrated that B cell fate toward effector cells is primarily determined by the strength of BCR interaction with antigen (Paus et al. 2006). Decreasing initial BCR affinity selectively abrogates the differentiation into extrafollicular plasma cells but does not impact GC B cell development. Besides the strength of BCR signaling, BCR affinity also influences the strength of T cell help that a B cell can receive. By internalizing more antigens, B cells expressing higher affinity BCR present more antigenic peptides to cognate T cells, thus receiving more T cell help.

6.3 Transcriptional and Epigenetic Regulation of Plasma Cell Differentiation

The differentiation into plasma cells is a terminal differentiation and lineage switch from B cells, which should be accompanied by dramatic changes in gene expression. Indeed, a remarkably distinct gene expression profile has been found during transition from activated B cells to plasma cells (Shi et al. 2015). However, only a few transcription factors facilitate the global changes in gene expression during this lineage switch. The transcription factors which direct the lineage switch from B cells to plasma cells are Blimp1, XBP-1, and IRF4. These factors basically extinguish B cell identity and initiate transcriptional program into plasma cells (Nutt et al. 2011). Blimp1 has been recognized as a "master regulator" for plasma cell development (Lin et al. 2002; Shaffer et al. 2002). Blimp1 functions primarily as a transcriptional repressor and inhibits B cell genes, such as Pax5 or Bcl6. However, recent work has revealed the multifunctional aspect of Blimp1. Blimp1 has functions to activate IRF4 expression, immunoglobulin transcription, and many components of the unfolded protein response (UPR), including XBP-1 (Minnich et al. 2016; Tellier et al. 2016). IRF4 is required to induce Blimp1 expression (Ochiai et al. 2013; Sciammas et al. 2006). A recent study has revealed that IRF4 is essential for plasma cell survival, as the acute inactivation of Irf4 from plasma cells results in complete loss of plasma cells (Tellier et al. 2016). In contrast, Blimp1 is dispensable for plasma cell survival (Tellier et al. 2016).

It has been demonstrated that epigenetic programs are also critical for the lineage transition from B cells to plasma cells. Recent work has revealed that plasma cell differentiation from B cells is associated with targeted hypomethylation of DNA (Barwick et al. 2016). DNA hypomethylation occurs after multiple cell divisions, which is associated with high expression of IRF4 or Blimp1. Indeed, inhibition of DNA methylation facilitates plasma cell differentiation. Likewise, deletion of de novo DNA methyltransferases from B cells results in a significant increase in plasma cell differentiation (Barwick et al. 2018), suggesting the role of DNA methylation in establishing the plasma cell program.

6.4 B Cell Selection in Germinal Center

After interaction with cognate T cells at the T-B border, some of the activated B cells return to the follicle, proliferate extensively, and form GCs. GCs are composed of two anatomically distinct compartments, the light zone (LZ) and dark zone (DZ), and B cells constantly cycle between LZ and DZ (Victora and Nussenzweig 2012). In the DZ, antigen-specific B cells expand vigorously. The proliferation of B cells in DZ is accompanied by BCR diversification through SHM. Unless silent mutation, the mutations that B cells receive in V region of BCR can result in change in BCR affinity for the antigen. Once exiting the cell cycle, B cells migrate to the LZ, where affinity selection takes place. In the LZ, the B cells first contact with follicular dendritic cells (FDCs) that display antigens on their surface as immune complexes. The B cells then internalize, process the antigens, and present them as peptide-MHC II complexes to cognate T follicular helper (Tfh) cells. BCR affinity has been believed to determine the amount of antigen that B cells internalize and present on their surface. Therefore, BCR affinity is directly linked to the amount of help that B cells would receive from the Tfh cells. LZ B cells expressing BCRs with an appropriate window of affinity receive signals for survival or differentiation. The "affinity-matured" GC B cells recycle back to DZ for a further round of SHM. Alternatively, those GC B cells exit the GC either as memory B cells or plasma cells.

6.5 GC-Derived Plasma Cells

The current paradigm that plasma cells generated during GC response migrate to BM and survive for many years is originally derived from the observation by Smith et al. (1997). By analyzing NP hapten-specific B cell response, it was first demonstrated that all NP-specific plasma cells in bone marrow had the affinity-enhancing mutation and produced high affinity antibodies, whereas a substantial fraction of memory B cells was of low affinity. This suggests that high affinity GC B cells are selected to differentiate into the precursors of long-lived plasma cells in bone marrow.

The following studies with genetically modified animals have confirmed that affinity-based selection of plasma cells actually operates in GCs. By tracing the SHM and affinity of anti-HEL transgenic BCR, Phan et al. have demonstrated that post-GC plasma cells already posses high affinity mutation, even at a time point when most of GC cells do not yet acquire such mutation (Phan et al. 2006). We have developed a system in which GC B cells and their progeny can be inducibly and irreversibly marked (Shinnakasu et al. 2016). As previously reported (Tomayko et al. 2010), GC-derived memory B cells exhibit extensive SHM in Ig genes but are composed of lower affinity cells, whereas post-GC plasma cells are uniformly of high affinity (Ise et al. 2018; Shinnakasu et al. 2016). Thus, BCR affinity tightly regulates the fate of GC B cells, and the high affinity clones are likely to be selected as plasma cells. Since majority of long-lived plasma cells in BM are GC-derived, this mechanism would help to ensure the quality of long-term antibody response.

6.6 Plasma Cell Precursors in the GC

Commitment to the plasma cell lineage has been thought to begin already during the GC response (Suan et al. 2017; Victora and Nussenzweig 2012). Previous immunohistochemical analyses of GCs have identified IRF4$^+$, Bcl6$^-$, or Blimp-1$^+$ cells within GCs (De Silva et al. 2016), suggesting that plasma cell-like cells can be already generated in the GC. However, it was unclear whether those cells were still GC B cells or already differentiated, early plasma cells. In LZ, 10–20% of B cells express c-Myc, a regulator of cell cycle progression (Calado et al. 2012; Dominguez-Sola et al. 2012). Because c-Myc expression is induced by Tfh cell help, and in B cells with high affinity BCRs, c-Myc$^+$ cells are likely to be positively selected cells, some of which should enter GC recycling. However, it was not unclear whether plasma cell precursors are in c-Myc$^+$ or distinct population.

Our recent study identified two populations of LZ GC B cells; Bcl6^{lo}CD69^{hi} and Bcl6^{hi}CD69^{hi} cells (Ise et al. 2018). Bcl6^{lo}CD69^{hi} cells, which constitute only 1–3% of LZ GC cells, are enriched for higher affinity BCRs (Ise et al. 2018). The cells express high levels of c-Myc and IRF4 and are biased to the plasma cell fate rather than to GC recycling. In contrast, 10–20% of LZ cells are Bcl6^{hi}CD69^{hi} cells with relatively lower affinity BCRs. The Bcl6^{hi}CD69^{hi} cells express c-Myc but not IRF4 and favor the GC recycling fate. Compared to Bcl6^{hi}CD69^{hi} cells, the Bcl6^{lo}CD69^{hi} cells require more Tfh cell help for their development. A transcriptome analysis showed that Bcl6^{lo}CD69^{hi} cells have down-regulated many of GC-signature genes, such as Bcl6, Bach2, S1pr2, and Efnb1. On the other hand, they have up-regulated an exit receptor Gpr183 (EBI2) and some of plasma cell signature genes. Hence, the c-Myc$^+$Bcl6^{lo}IRF4$^+$ cells are thought to be plasma cell precursors that are losing GC B cell identity but turning plasma cell program on, whereas the c-Myc$^+$Bcl6^{hi}IRF4$^-$ cells are likely to be the precursors to recycle back to DZ for further cell division and SHM (Fig. 6.1).

Given that the Bcl6^{lo}IRF4$^+$CD69^{hi} LZ GC cells do not express the plasma cell markers CD138 or Blimp-1 (Ise et al. 2018), these cells presumably represent the emerging, earliest plasma cell precursors. Bcl6^{lo} cells with higher expression of IRF4 or Blimp-1$^+$ are found among DZ GC B cells (Ise et al. 2018; Krautler et al. 2017), suggesting that plasma cell precursors in the LZ migrate to the DZ and this accompanies their maturation toward plasma cells. During this process, epigenetic modifications such as DNA hypomethylation (Barwick et al. 2016), which facilitates expression of Blimp-1 and stabilizes the plasma cell phenotype, might take place (Minnich et al. 2016). Finally, these early plasma cells would exit from the GC through the DZ, as predicted by computational modeling and imaging analysis (Fooksman et al. 2010; Meyer-Hermann et al. 2012).

6.7 Signals That Induce Plasma Cell Differentiation in GC

Positive selection of LZ GC B cells is initiated by binding of BCR to antigen displayed on FDCs. Recognition of antigen by higher affinity BCRs should give rise to stronger signals than that by lower affinity BCRs. Importantly, BCR affinity influences not only the strength of BCR signaling but the extent of signals provided by Tfh cells since B cells function as antigen-presenting cells for cognate Tfh cells, as mentioned earlier. Thus, B cells with high affinity would receive stronger T cell help. Generation of plasma cells from GC B cells requires both signals delivered through BCR and provided by Tfh cells (Krautler et al. 2017). Indeed, transcriptome analysis showed that the plasma cell precursors in the LZ are more strongly imprinted with the signatures

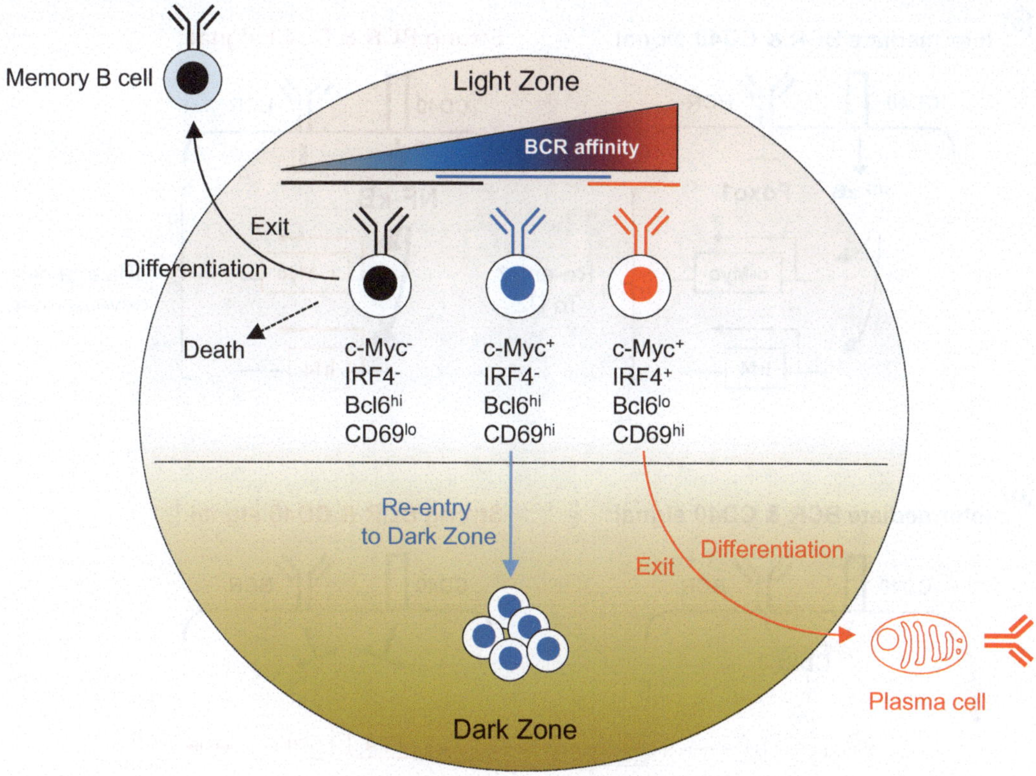

Fig. 6.1 Committed precursors for memory B cells, recycling, or plasma cells in GC LZ. c-Myc$^+$IRF4$^+$Bcl6^{lo}CD69^{hi} B cells are plasma cell precursors that express the highest affinity for Ags and exit the GC through DZ as early plasma cells. c-Myc$^+$IRF4$^-$Bcl6^{hi}CD69^{hi} B cells express BCRs with intermediate affinity and recycle back to the DZ for further somatic hypermutation. c-Myc$^-$IRF4$^-$Bcl6^{hi}CD69^{lo} B cells express lower affinity BCRs and differentiate into memory B cells or die by apoptosis

of both BCR- and CD40-activation than are other GC B cells (Ise et al. 2018). Thus, the question arises of how these strong BCR and/or Tfh help signals facilitate generation of plasma cells from LZ GC B cells.

Since BCR signaling in GC B cells is generally attenuated and is hard to be detected, the role of BCR signaling for plasma cell generation from GC B cells has been ambiguous. However, Luo et al. have recently demonstrated that crosslinking of BCR results in selective activation of Syk-PI3K-AKT pathway and inactivation of Foxo1 (Luo et al. 2018). Given that Foxo1 is a transcription factor that is required for GC B cell proliferation and the DZ phenotype (Dominguez-Sola et al. 2015; Inoue et al. 2017; Sander et al. 2015), the extent of BCR ligation might regulate Foxo1 activity and fate of GC B cells; strong PI3K-AKT signaling inactivates Foxo1, promoting exit from GC reaction, whereas weaker signaling maintains active Foxo1, facilitating cell cycle reentry.

Luo et al. have also demonstrated that ligation of CD40 on GC B cells promotes the translocation of RelA and cRel into the nucleus and results in the up-regulation of IRF4 (Luo et al. 2018). cRel is critical for GC maintenance, and RelA, as well as IRF4, is important for plasma cell differentiation (Heise et al. 2014). Furthermore, they observed that BCR and CD40 signals synergistically induce high-level expression of c-Myc (Luo et al. 2018), a critical driver of GC B cell survival and proliferation (Calado et al. 2012; Dominguez-Sola et al. 2012).

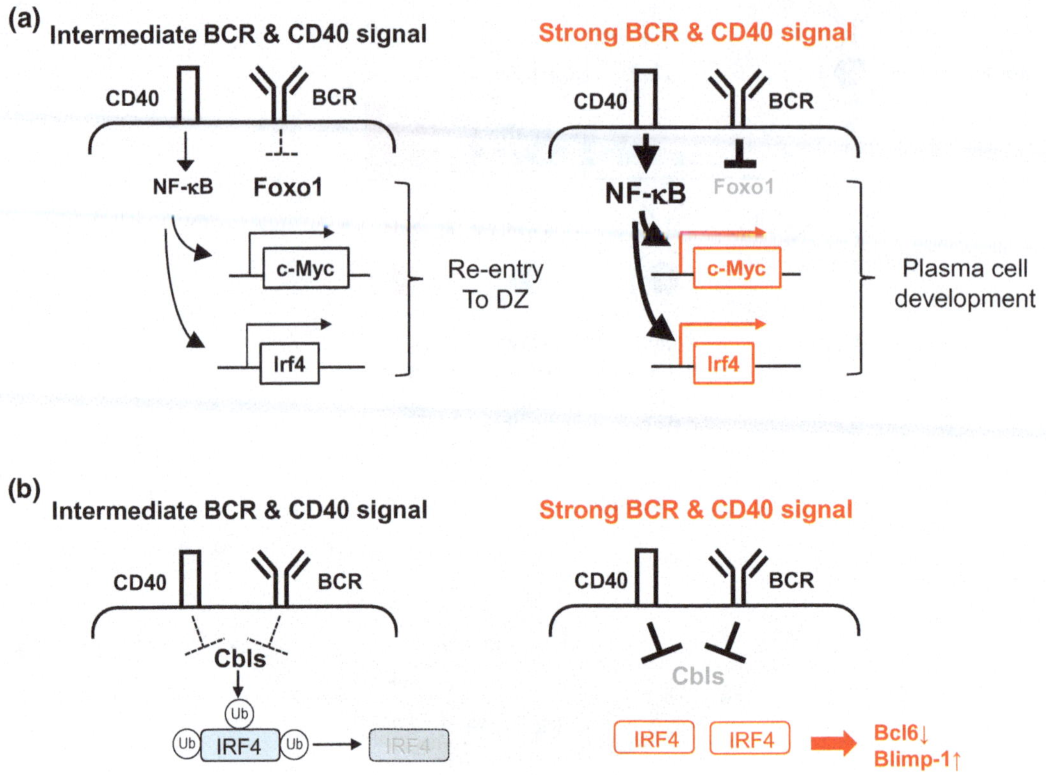

Fig. 6.2 Role of BCR and CD40 signals in the generation of plasma cells from GC B cells. **a** In GC B cells, CD40 signals activate NF-κB pathways and induce c-Myc or Irf4 expression, whereas strong BCR signals inactivate Foxo1, which is required for reentry into the DZ. In B cells receiving intermediate levels of CD40 and BCR stimulation, Foxo1 is not inactivated, and c-Myc or Irf4 is weakly induced, allowing the cells to recycle into the DZ. In contrast, when B cells are strongly activated through the BCR and CD40, Foxo1 is inactivated, and NF-κB activation leads to high expression of c-Myc or Irf4. High levels of IRF4 down-regulate Bcl6 and induce Blimp-1 expression, which promotes GC B cells to exit as plasma cells. **b** Cbl ubiquitin ligases are expressed in LZ B cells and prevent premature GC exit by promoting IRF4 degradation. Strong CD40 and BCR signals trigger degradation of Cbls in LZ B cells, resulting in high IRF4 expression, which promotes plasma cell development

The extent of BCR and/or CD40 signaling appears to generate heterogenous expression of fate-determining transcription factors within positively selected GC B cell population. Microscopic analysis has shown that c-Myc^{+} LZ B cell population consists of Foxo1^{+} or Foxo1^{-} cells (Sander et al. 2015). Likewise, GC B cells with high levels of IRF4 lack Pax5 and nuclear Foxo1, whereas those with lower IRF4 expression maintain Pax5 expression and nuclear Foxo1 localization (Lin et al. 2015). It is likely that a moderate level of BCR/CD40 signaling maintains Pax5 and active form of Foxo1 in c-Myc^{+} cells, which allows the cells to re-cycle to DZ, whereas strong BCR/CD40 ligation induces IRF4 in c-Myc^{+} cells, but down-regulates Pax5 and inactivates Foxo1, which facilitates to exit the GC program and differentiate into plasma cells (Fig. 6.2a).

Li et al. have reported a novel mechanism by which BCR/CD40 signaling regulates plasma cell generation by controlling IRF4 expression in GC B cells (Li et al. 2018). Cbl ubiquitin ligases, which are abundantly expressed in LZ B cells, down-regulate IRF4 protein expression through ubiquitin-dependent degradation. Importantly, strong BCR/CD40 stimulation somehow leads to the degradation of Cbl itself, allowing high expression of IRF4 protein. In Cbl-deficient mice, affinity maturation is impaired, and $Bcl6^{lo}IRF4^{hi}$ plasma cell precursors are significantly expanded, suggesting that Cbls prevent the development of plasma cells from premature GC B cells. The findings suggest a model, in which expression of Cbls determines GC B cell fate. In high affinity B cells, strong BCR signal and Tfh cell help extinguish Cbl expression, which allows high expression of IRF4 and plasma cell differentiation, while in lower affinity B cells, abundant Cbl expression prevents IRF4 expression (Fig. 6.2b).

6.8 GC B Cell-Tfh Cell Interactions for Plasma Cell Generation

Recent several works have emphasized the importance of strength of interaction between GC B cells and Tfh cells, which is mediated by several surface molecules, for efficient generation of plasma cells (Fig. 6.3). A crucial role for inducible T-cell co-stimulatory ligand (ICOSL) in GC B cell response has been demonstrated by Liu et al. (2015). Ligation of ICOSL with ICOS promotes entangled interaction between GC B cells and Tfh cells, which then results in increased CD40L expression by Tfh cells. Enhanced CD40L-CD40 interaction further up-regulates ICOSL on GC B cells. Generation of plasma cells, but not of memory B cells, is impaired by ICOSL-deficient GC B cells, demonstrating that intercellular positive feedback, which is initiated by ICOSL ligation, facilitates GC B cell activation and plasma cell differentiation. $ICOSL^{high}$ GC B cells express higher affinity BCRs, consistent with our recent observation that $Bcl6^{lo}CD69^{hi}$ plasma cell precursors with higher affinity BCRs express higher levels of CD40 than other LZ B cells (Ise et al. 2018). The plasma cell precursors also express higher levels of adhesion molecules, such as SLAM or ICAM-1 which supports long-lasting cognate Tfh-B cell interaction (Zaretsky et al. 2017). Indeed, our data suggest that stable conjugate formation with Tfh cells is prerequisite for IRF4 expression by LZ GC B cells. An imaging analysis has previously characterized how GC B cells interact with cognate Tfh cells in vivo (Allen et al. 2007). Most of GC B cells contact with Tfh cells for short duration (<2 min), but a few percent of the GC B-Tfh cells form much more stable conjugates (5–60 min) (Allen et al. 2007). It could be possible that GC B cells forming long-lasting conjugate with Tfh cells are plasma cell precursors. Taken together, stable contact with Tfh cells, which is facilitated by the bidirectional ICOS-ICOSL, CD40-Cd40L signaling, and by adhesion molecules, would provide strong T cell help to LZ B cells, resulting in initiation of genetic programs toward plasma cell differentiation (Fig. 6.3a, b).

Besides CD40L or ICOS, other surface molecules on Tfh cells are also involved in plasma cell development from GCs. The immunoinhibitory receptor PD-1, highly expressed on Tfh cells, is one of them. PD-1 ligands, PD-L1 or PD-L2, are up-regulated in GC B cells. In PD-1- or PD-L2-deficient mice, initial antibody response, including GC responses against immunized antigens, appears to be normal. However, later on, the number of GC-derived plasma cells become fewer (Good-Jacobson et al. 2010), suggesting that these molecules play some roles in the selection of plasma cells from GCs. Mechanistically, PD-1-PD-L1/L2 axis appears to regulate Tfh cell activity. First, PD-1 controls IL-21 production by Tfh cells (Fig. 6.3c) (Li et al. 2018; Liu et al. 2015). PD-1-deficient Tfh cells produce less IL-21, which results in decreased plasma cell generation (Good-Jacobson et al. 2010). Second, PD-1 controls the positioning of Tfh cells (Fig. 6.3a) (Shi et al. 2018). PD-1-deficient Tfh cells show impaired migration from B cell follicles into GCs. Thus, PD-1-PD-L1/L2 axis is involved in plasma cell development from GCs by regulating the quantity and quality of Tfh help.

Plexin B2-Semaphorin 4C (Sema 4C) aix regulates interaction between Tfh cells and GC B cells and is involved in plasma cell generation (Yan et al. 2017). Plexin B2 is highly expressed by GC B cells and its ligand, and Sema4C is

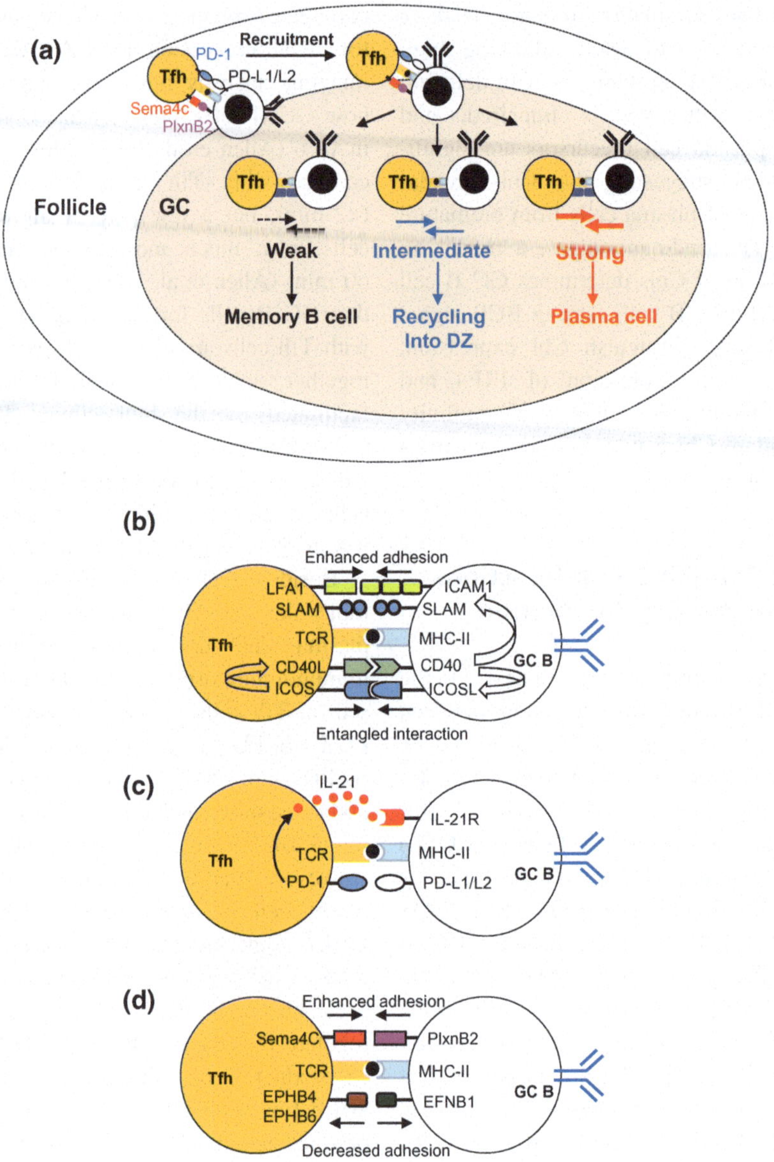

Fig. 6.3 GC B-Tfh cell interactions for plasma cell generation. **a** Plexin B2 expressed by GC B cells binds to Semaphorin 4C (Sema 4C) expressed on Tfh cells. The Plxn B2–Sema4C interaction promotes T-B adhesion and facilitates Tfh cell access to the GC. The interaction between PD-1 on Tfh cells and PD-L1/L2 on GC B cells also helps to recruit Tfh cells from follicles to the GC. Once positioned at the GC border, Tfh cells gain easier access into the center of the GC. In the GC, B cells with lower affinity BCRs receive weak T cell help, which favors differentiation into memory B cells. GC B cells with intermediate BCR affinity recycle into the DZ after transient contact with cognate T cells and receiving intermediate help. GC B cells with higher affinity BCRs receive stronger T cell help as a result of sustained T-B contacts, which favors plasma cell differentiation. **b** ICOSL signals delivered by GC B cells support sustained interactions with Tfh cells. ICOS stimulation increases CD40L expression by Tfh cells, which in turn activates CD40, and this leads to further up-regulation of ICOSL. CD40 activation in GC B cells also results in up-regulation of ICAM-1 or SLAM, which promotes stronger Tfh cell-GC B cell adhesion. **c** Ligation of PD-1 with PD-L1/L2 promotes IL-21 production by Tfh cells, and the IL-21 signal helps GC B cells for their proliferation or differentiation into plasma cells. **d** The interaction between Semaphorin 4C (Sema4C) in Tfh cells and Plexin B2 (PlxnB2) in GC B cells promotes Tfh-GC B cell adhesion. On the other hand, ligation of Ephrin-B1 (EFNB1) in GC B cells with Ephrin type-B receptor 4 (EPHB4) and EPHB6 in Tfh cells suppresses this adhesion

expressed on Tfh cells. The Plexin B2–Sema4C interaction promotes not only adhesion between these two cell types but migration of Tfh cells into the center of GC (Fig. 6.3a, d). In Plexin B2-deficient mice, Tfh cells localize at the GC border but not in GCs. Importantly, although GC formation is intact, plasma cell generation and affinity maturation are impaired. Thus, the Sema 4C–Plexin B2 axis helps plasma cell generation by efficiently recruiting Tfh cells into GCs.

The Ephrin family receptors and their ligands also regulate Tfh cell–GC B cell interaction. Ephrin type-B receptors EPHB4 and EPHB6 are expressed on Tfh cells (Lu et al. 2017). One of their ligands is Ephrin-B1 (EFNB1), which is highly expressed by GC B cells and acts as a repulsive guidance cue (Laidlaw et al. 2017; Lu et al. 2017). EFNB1 inhibits Th cell-GC B cell adhesion (Fig. 6.3d), and EFNB1-deficient B cells more efficiently interact with Tfh cells and generate more plasma cells (Lu et al. 2017). Intriguingly, EFNB1 is down-regulated in $Bcl6^{lo}CD69^{hi}$ LZ cells (Ise et al. 2018) but is expressed in a subset of LZ B cells, presumably memory B cells precursors in the GC (Laidlaw et al. 2017). Therefore, it could be possible that the extent of Ephrin interaction determines the fate of GC B cells into either memory B cells or plasma cells, by controlling Tfh-GC B cell adhesion.

6.9 Regulation of Plasma Cell Generation by Heterogenous Tfh Cells

The heterogeneity in Tfh cell population, in terms of cytokine profile, has recently been revealed. Thus, the quality of Tfh cell help could contribute to the GC output. Upon N. brasiliensis infection, it has been suggested that Tfh cells acquire distinct effector functions during the GC response, which critically influence the GC B cell response (Weinstein et al. 2016). Tfh cells secreted IL-21 at early phase of GC. However, at a later phase, Tfh cells produced IL-4 rather than IL-21 and showed robust expression of CD40L. Importantly, $IL\text{-}21^{+}IL\text{-}4^{+}$ Tfh cells or $IL\text{-}21^{-}IL\text{-}4^{+}$ Tfh cells were more potent to induce the differentiation of plasma cells than $IL\text{-}21^{+}IL\text{-}4^{-}$ Tfh cells (Weinstein et al. 2016). This might be correlated with a temporal switch in the GC reaction; the output from GCs switches from generation of memory B cells at earlier stage to generation of plasma cells at a later phase of GC response (Weisel et al. 2016).

More recently, IL-9 has been shown to be produced by only $\sim$2% of Tfh cells and to be required for the development of memory B cells from GCs (Wang et al. 2017). Furthermore, a rare population of IL-13-producing Tfh cells has also been discovered. $IL\text{-}13^{+}$Tfh cells showed a unique cytokine profile ($IL\text{-}13^{hi}$ $IL\text{-}4^{hi}$ $IL\text{-}5^{hi}$) and co-expressed transcription factors Bcl6 and GATA-3 (Gowthaman et al. 2019). $IL\text{-}13^{+}$Tfh cells elicited high affinity IgE production and allergen-induced anaphylaxis. Whether $IL\text{-}9^{+}$ or $IL\text{-}13^{+}$ Tfh cells emerge at early or late GC response has not been examined yet. Together, it could be possible that the relative abundance of functionally distinct Tfh cells affects the generation of memory B cells versus plasma cells or the isotype of antibodies produced.

6.10 Regulation of Plasma Cell Generation by T Follicular Regulatory Cells

Recent studies have discovered that an effector type of regulatory T (Treg) cells, called the T follicular regulatory (Tfr) cells, is involved in regulation of GC responses (Sage and Sharpe 2016). $CXCR5^{+}Foxp3^{+}Bcl6^{+}$ Tfr cells were discovered as a T cell subpopulation that phenotypically and functionally shares characteristics of Tfh cells and conventional Treg cells (Chung et al. 2011; Linterman et al. 2011; Wollenberg et al. 2011). Tfhr cells develop from thymus-derived $Foxp3^{+}$ Treg cells but not from Tfh cells (Chung et al. 2011; Linterman et al. 2011; Wollenberg et al. 2011; Wing et al. 2017).

Indeed, TCR repertoire of Tfr cells is distinct from that of Tfh cells and is skewed toward self-antigens (Maceiras et al. 2017). Consistent with this, earlier studies have clearly demonstrated an important role of Tfr cells in humoral autoimmunity. Deletion of Bcl6 in Foxp3+ Treg cells resulted in Tfr deficiency and led to late-onset spontaneous autoimmune diseases (Fu et al. 2018). In an experimental Sjogren's syndrome model, the ablation of Tfr greatly enhanced disease development (Fu et al. 2018). Regulation of humoral autoimmunity by Tfr was also confirmed in viral infection. Tfr cells were not detected at the early phase after influenza infection but were generated from Treg cells after the immune response resolved (Botta et al. 2017). Importantly, the ablation of Tfr cells induced the generation of self-reactive plasma cells, while influenza-specific GC B cell or plasma cell response remained relatively intact (Botta et al. 2017). A more recent work has demonstrated that Tfr cells control not only humoral autoimmunity but also antigen-specific allergic immunity. The ablation of Tfr cells resulted in increased self-reactive IgG and IgE (Clement et al. 2019). Interestingly, in house dust mite models, the absence of Tfr greatly increased house dust mite-specific IgE and lung inflammation (Clement et al. 2019). Importantly, Tfr cells inhibited Tfh13 cell-induced IgE response. Together, Tfr cells control the generation of plasma cells in response to vaccines, infections, allergens, and self-antigens.

6.11 Concluding Remarks

The concept of "affinity-based" selection of plasma cells during GC reaction has been established by the studies in late 90s. Recent work has proved it and demonstrated its cellular and molecular basis in great detail. BCR affinity is not the sole determinant but apparently a critical factor for fate decision of GC B cells, by influencing strength of BCR signaling or help from Tfh cells. The extent of interaction with Tfh cells, cytokine profile of Tfh cells, and involvement of Tfr control plasma cell generation from GC B cells. Targeting the key pathways or molecules that control plasma cell differentiation will help to promote efficient generation of high affinity antibodies for protection from invading pathogens or to limit humoral autoimmunity or allergic immunity.

References

Allen CD, Okada T, Tang HL, Cyster JG (2007) Imaging of germinal center selection events during affinity maturation. Science 315:528–531

Barwick BG, Scharer CD, Bally APR, Boss JM (2016) Plasma cell differentiation is coupled to division-dependent DNA hypomethylation and gene regulation. Nat Immunol 17:1216–1225

Barwick BG, Scharer CD, Martinez RJ, Price MJ, Wein AN, Haines RR, Bally APR, Kohlmeier JE, Boss JM (2018) B cell activation and plasma cell differentiation are inhibited by de novo DNA methylation. Nat Commun 9:1900

Botta D, Fuller MJ, Marquez-Lago TT, Bachus H, Bradley JE, Weinmann AS, Zajac AJ, Randall TD, Lund FE, Leon B, Ballesteros-Tato A (2017) Dynamic regulation of T follicular regulatory cell responses by interleukin 2 during influenza infection. Nat Immunol 18:1249–1260

Calado DP, Sasaki Y, Godinho SA, Pellerin A, Kochert K, Sleckman BP, de Alboran IM, Janz M, Rodig S, Rajewsky K (2012) The cell-cycle regulator c-Myc is essential for the formation and maintenance of germinal centers. Nat Immunol 13:1092–1100

Chang HD, Tokoyoda K, Radbruch A (2018) Immunological memories of the bone marrow. Immunol Rev 283:86–98

Chung Y, Tanaka S, Chu F, Nurieva RI, Martinez GJ, Rawal S, Wang YH, Lim H, Reynolds JM, Zhou XH, Fan HM, Liu ZM, Neelapu SS, Dong C (2011) Follicular regulatory T cells expressing Foxp3 and Bcl-6 suppress germinal center reactions. Nat Med 17:983–988

Clement RL, Daccache J, Mohammed MT, Diallo A, Blazar BR, Kuchroo VK, Lovitch SB, Sharpe AH, Sage PT (2019) Follicular regulatory T cells control humoral and allergic immunity by restraining early B cell responses. Nat Immunol 20:1360–1371

De Silva NS, Anderson MM, Carette A, Silva K, Heise N, Bhagat G, Klein U (2016) Transcription factors of the alternative NF-kappaB pathway are required for germinal center B-cell development. Proc Natl Acad Sci USA 113:9063–9068

Di Niro R, Lee SJ, Vander Heiden JA, Elsner RA, Trivedi N, Bannock JM, Gupta NT, Kleinstein SH, Vigneault F, Gilbert TJ, Meffre E, McSorley SJ, Shlomchik MJ (2015) Salmonella infection drives promiscuous B cell activation followed by extrafollicular affinity maturation. Immunity 43:120–131

Dominguez-Sola D, Kung J, Holmes AB, Wells VA, Mo T, Basso K, Dalla-Favera R (2015) The FOXO1 transcription factor instructs the germinal center dark zone program. Immunity 43:1064–1074

Dominguez-Sola D, Victora GD, Ying CY, Phan RT, Saito M, Nussenzweig MC, Dalla-Favera R (2012) The proto-oncogene MYC is required for selection in the germinal center and cyclic reentry. Nat Immunol 13:1083–1091

Fooksman DR, Schwickert TA, Victora GD, Dustin ML, Nussenzweig MC, Skokos D (2010) Development and migration of plasma cells in the mouse lymph node. Immunity 33:118–127

Fu W, Liu X, Lin X, Feng H, Sun L, Li S, Chen H, Tang H, Lu L, Jin W, Dong C (2018) Deficiency in T follicular regulatory cells promotes autoimmunity. J Exp Med 215:815–825

Good-Jacobson KL, Szumilas CG, Chen L, Sharpe AH, Tomayko MM, Shlomchik MJ (2010) PD-1 regulates germinal center B cell survival and the formation and affinity of long-lived plasma cells. Nat Immunol 11:535–542

Gowthaman U, Chen JS, Zhang B, Flynn WF, Lu Y, Song W, Joseph J, Gertie JA, Xu L, Collet MA, Grassmann JDS, Simoneau T, Chiang D, Berin MC, Craft JE, Weinstein JS, Williams A, Eisenbarth SC (2019) Identification of a T follicular helper cell subset that drives anaphylactic IgE. Science 365

Heise N, De Silva NS, Silva K, Carette A, Simonetti G, Pasparakis M, Klein U (2014) Germinal center B cell maintenance and differentiation are controlled by distinct NF-kappaB transcription factor subunits. J Exp Med 211:2103–2118

Inoue T, Shinnakasu R, Ise W, Kawai C, Egawa T, Kurosaki T (2017) The transcription factor Foxo1 controls germinal center B cell proliferation in response to T cell help. J Exp Med 214:1181–1198

Ise W, Fujii K, Shiroguchi K, Ito A, Kometani K, Takeda K, Kawakami E, Yamashita K, Suzuki K, Okada T, Kurosaki T (2018) T follicular helper cell-germinal center B cell interaction strength regulates entry into plasma cell or recycling germinal center cell fate. Immunity 48(702–715):e704

Jacob J, Kassir R, Kelsoe G (1991) In situ studies of the primary immune response to (4-hydroxy-3-nitrophenyl)acetyl. I. The architecture and dynamics of responding cell populations. J Exp Med 173: 1165–1175

Kometani K, Kurosaki T (2015) Differentiation and maintenance of long-lived plasma cells. Curr Opin Immunol 33:64–69

Krautler NJ, Suan D, Butt D, Bourne K, Hermes JR, Chan TD, Sundling C, Kaplan W, Schofield P, Jackson J, Basten A, Christ D, Brink R (2017) Differentiation of germinal center B cells into plasma cells is initiated by high-affinity antigen and completed by Tfh cells. J Exp Med 214:1259–1267

Kurosaki T, Kometani K, Ise W (2015) Memory B cells. Nat Rev Immunol 15:149–159

Laidlaw BJ, Schmidt TH, Green JA, Allen CD, Okada T, Cyster JG (2017) The Eph-related tyrosine kinase ligand Ephrin-B1 marks germinal center and memory precursor B cells. J Exp Med 214:639–649

Li X, Gadzinsky A, Gong L, Tong H, Calderon V, Li Y, Kitamura D, Klein U, Langdon WY, Hou F, Zou YR, Gu H (2018) Cbl ubiquitin ligases control B cell exit from the germinal-center reaction. Immunity 48(530–541):e536

Lin KI, Angelin-Duclos C, Kuo TC, Calame K (2002) Blimp-1-dependent repression of Pax-5 is required for differentiation of B cells to immunoglobulin M-secreting plasma cells. Mol Cell Biol 22:4771–4780

Lin WH, Adams WC, Nish SA, Chen YH, Yen B, Rothman NJ, Kratchmarov R, Okada T, Klein U, Reiner SL (2015) Asymmetric PI3K signaling driving developmental and regenerative cell fate bifurcation. Cell Rep 13:2203–2218

Linterman MA, Pierson W, Lee SK, Kallies A, Kawamoto S, Rayner TF, Srivastava M, Divekar DP, Beaton L, Hogan JJ, Fagarasan S, Liston A, Smith KG, Vinuesa CG (2011) Foxp3+ follicular regulatory T cells control the germinal center response. Nat Med 17:975–982

Liu D, Xu H, Shih C, Wan Z, Ma X, Ma W, Luo D, Qi H (2015) T-B-cell entanglement and ICOSL-driven feed-forward regulation of germinal centre reaction. Nature 517:214–218

Lu P, Shih C, Qi H (2017) Ephrin B1-mediated repulsion and signaling control germinal center T cell territoriality and function. Science 356

Luo W, Weisel F, Shlomchik MJ (2018) B cell receptor and CD40 signaling are rewired for synergistic induction of the c-Myc transcription factor in germinal center B cells. Immunity 48(313–326):e315

Maceiras AR, Almeida SCP, Mariotti-Ferrandiz E, Chaara W, Jebbawi F, Six A, Hori S, Klatzmann D, Faro J, Graca L (2017) T follicular helper and T follicular regulatory cells have different TCR specificity. Nat Commun 8:15067

MacLennan IC, Toellner KM, Cunningham AF, Serre K, Sze DM, Zuniga E, Cook MC, Vinuesa CG (2003) Extrafollicular antibody responses. Immunol Rev 194:8–18

McHeyzer-Williams MG, McLean MJ, Lalor PA, Nossal GJ (1993) Antigen-driven B cell differentiation in vivo. J Exp Med 178:295–307

Meyer-Hermann M, Mohr E, Pelletier N, Zhang Y, Victora GD, Toellner KM (2012) A theory of germinal center B cell selection, division, and exit. Cell Rep 2:162–174

Minnich M, Tagoh H, Bonelt P, Axelsson E, Fischer M, Cebolla B, Tarakhovsky A, Nutt SL, Jaritz M, Busslinger M (2016) Multifunctional role of the transcription factor Blimp-1 in coordinating plasma cell differentiation. Nat Immunol 17:331–343

Nutt SL, Hodgkin PD, Tarlinton DM, Corcoran LM (2015) The generation of antibody-secreting plasma cells. Nat Rev Immunol 15:160–171

Nutt SL, Taubenheim N, Hasbold J, Corcoran LM, Hodgkin PD (2011) The genetic network controlling plasma cell differentiation. Semin Immunol 23:341–349

Ochiai K, Maienschein-Cline M, Simonetti G, Chen J, Rosenthal R, Brink R, Chong AS, Klein U, Dinner AR, Singh H, Sciammas R (2013) Transcriptional regulation of germinal center B and plasma cell fates by dynamical control of IRF4. Immunity 38:918–929

Paus D, Phan TG, Chan TD, Gardam S, Basten A, Brink R (2006) Antigen recognition strength regulates the choice between extrafollicular plasma cell and germinal center B cell differentiation. J Exp Med 203:1081–1091

Phan TG, Paus D, Chan TD, Turner ML, Nutt SL, Basten A, Brink R (2006) High affinity germinal center B cells are actively selected into the plasma cell compartment. J Exp Med 203:2419–2424

Sage PT, Sharpe AH (2016) T follicular regulatory cells. Immunol Rev 271:246–259

Sander S, Chu VT, Yasuda T, Franklin A, Graf R, Calado DP, Li S, Imami K, Selbach M, Di Virgilio M, Bullinger L, Rajewsky K (2015) PI3 kinase and FOXO1 transcription factor activity differentially control B cells in the germinal center light and dark zones. Immunity 43:1075–1086

Sciammas R, Shaffer AL, Schatz JH, Zhao H, Staudt LM, Singh H (2006) Graded expression of interferon regulatory factor-4 coordinates isotype switching with plasma cell differentiation. Immunity 25:225–236

Shaffer AL, Lin KI, Kuo TC, Yu X, Hurt EM, Rosenwald A, Giltnane JM, Yang L, Zhao H, Calame K, Staudt LM (2002) Blimp-1 orchestrates plasma cell differentiation by extinguishing the mature B cell gene expression program. Immunity 17:51–62

Shi J, Hou S, Fang Q, Liu X, Liu X, Qi H (2018) PD-1 controls follicular T helper cell positioning and function. Immunity 49(264–274):e264

Shi W, Liao Y, Willis SN, Taubenheim N, Inouye M, Tarlinton DM, Smyth GK, Hodgkin PD, Nutt SL, Corcoran LM (2015) Transcriptional profiling of mouse B cell terminal differentiation defines a signature for antibody-secreting plasma cells. Nat Immunol 16:663–673

Shinnakasu R, Inoue T, Kometani K, Moriyama S, Adachi Y, Nakayama M, Takahashi Y, Fukuyama H, Okada T, Kurosaki T (2016) Regulated selection of germinal-center cells into the memory B cell compartment. Nat Immunol 17:861–869

Smith KG, Light A, Nossal GJ, Tarlinton DM (1997) The extent of affinity maturation differs between the memory and antibody-forming cell compartments in the primary immune response. EMBO J 16:2996–3006

Suan D, Krautler NJ, Maag JLV, Butt D, Bourne K, Hermes JR, Avery DT, Young C, Statham A, Elliott M, Dinger ME, Basten A, Tangye SG, Brink R (2017) CCR6 defines memory B cell precursors in mouse and human germinal centers, revealing light-zone location and predominant low antigen affinity. Immunity 47(1142–1153):e1144

Tellier J, Shi W, Minnich M, Liao Y, Crawford S, Smyth GK, Kallies A, Busslinger M, Nutt SL (2016) Blimp-1 controls plasma cell function through the regulation of immunoglobulin secretion and the unfolded protein response. Nat Immunol 17:323–330

Tomayko MM, Steinel NC, Anderson SM, Shlomchik MJ (2010) Cutting edge: hierarchy of maturity of murine memory B cell subsets. J Immunol 185:7146–7150

Victora GD, Nussenzweig MC (2012) Germinal centers. Annu Rev Immunol 30:429–457

Wang Y, Shi J, Yan J, Xiao Z, Hou X, Lu P, Hou S, Mao T, Liu W, Ma Y, Zhang L, Yang X, Qi H (2017) Germinal-center development of memory B cells driven by IL-9 from follicular helper T cells. Nat Immunol 18:921–930

Weinstein JS, Herman EI, Lainez B, Licona-Limon P, Esplugues E, Flavell R, Craft J (2016) TFH cells progressively differentiate to regulate the germinal center response. Nat Immunol 17:1197–1205

Weisel FJ, Zuccarino-Catania GV, Chikina M, Shlomchik MJ (2016) A temporal switch in the germinal center determines differential output of memory B and plasma cells. Immunity 44:116–130

William J, Euler C, Christensen S, Shlomchik MJ (2002) Evolution of autoantibody responses via somatic hypermutation outside of germinal centers. Science 297:2066–2070

Wing JB, Kitagawa Y, Locci M, Hume H, Tay C, Morita T, Kidani Y, Matsuda K, Inoue T, Kurosaki T, Crotty S, Coban C, Ohkura N, Sakaguchi S (2017) A distinct subpopulation of CD25(-) T-follicular regulatory cells localizes in the germinal centers. Proc Natl Acad Sci USA 114:E6400–E6409

Wollenberg I, Agua-Doce A, Hernandez A, Almeida C, Oliveira VG, Faro J, Graca L (2011) Regulation of the germinal center reaction by Foxp3+ follicular regulatory T cells. J Immunol 187:4553–4560

Yan H, Wu L, Shih C, Hou S, Shi J, Mao T, Chen W, Melvin B, Rigby RJ, Chen Y, Jiang H, Friedel RH, Vinuesa CG, Qi H (2017) Plexin B2 and Semaphorin 4C guide T cell recruitment and function in the germinal center. Cell Rep 19:995–1007

Zaretsky I, Atrakchi O, Mazor RD, Stoler-Barak L, Biram A, Feigelson SW, Gitlin AD, Engelhardt B, Shulman Z (2017) ICAMs support B cell interactions with T follicular helper cells and promote clonal selection. J Exp Med 214:3435–3448

Regulation of Humoral Immune Responses and B Cell Tolerance by the IgM Fc Receptor (FcμR)

7

Jun Liu, Ying Wang, Qing Min, Ermeng Xiong, Birgitta Heyman, and Ji-Yang Wang

Abstract

Immunoglobulin (Ig) M is the first antibody isotype produced during an immune response and is critical for host defense against infections. Recent studies have revealed that IgM also plays an important role in immune regulation and immunological tolerance. Mice lacking secretory IgM not only exhibit impaired production of antigen-specific IgG and are more susceptible to bacterial and viral infections, but also produce autoantibodies and are prone to develop autoimmune diseases. For many years, IgM has been thought to function predominantly by binding to antigen and activating complement (C′) system. It is now clear that IgM can also elicit its function through the IgM Fc receptor (FcμR). In this chapter, we will review the role of FcμR in B cell development, maturation, survival and activation, antibody production, host defense against bacterial and viral infections, and B cell tolerance. We will also discuss the relative contribution of IgM-C′ and IgM-FcμR pathways in humoral immune responses. Finally, we will discuss the possible involvement of FcμR in human chronic lymphocytic leukemia.

Keywords

IgM · FcμR · B cell receptor signaling · Humoral immune response · Complement

J. Liu · Y. Wang · Q. Min · E. Xiong · J.-Y. Wang (✉)
Department of Immunology, School of Basic Medical Sciences, Fudan University, Shanghai, China
e-mail: wang@fudan.edu.cn

B. Heyman
Department of Medical Biochemistry and Microbiology, Uppsala University, Uppsala, Sweden

7.1 Introduction

Antibodies (Ab) bind to the antigen (Ag) through their variable F(ab) region and elicit their function through the constant Fc portion. Cellular receptors for the Ab Fc portion (Fc receptor) mediate varieties of functions, including phagocytosis of Ab-opsonized pathogens, Ab-dependent cellular cytotoxicity, and regulation of immune cell activation (Fig. 7.1). Three Fc receptors for IgM have been identified, including Fcα/μ receptor (Fcα/μR), polymeric immunoglobulin receptor (pIgR), and the Fcμ receptor (FcμR) (Fig. 7.1). Fcα/μR is expressed by B cells and macrophages (Shibuya et al. 2000; Shibuya and Honda 2006) and was reported to play a role in pro-inflammatory functions of marginal zone B (MZB) cells in sepsis (Honda et al. 2016). pIgR is expressed in the mucosal epithelium (Stadtmueller et al. 2016; Schneeman et al. 2005) but

J.-Y. Wang (ed.), *B Cells in Immunity and Tolerance*, Advances in Experimental Medicine and Biology 1254, https://doi.org/10.1007/978-981-15-3532-1_7

	FcγRI (CD64) 70-kDa	FcγRII-A (CD32) 40-kDa	FcγRII-B (CD32) 40-kDa	FcγRIII (CD16)	FcεR1	FcαRI (CD89)	Fcα/μR	Poly-IgR	FcμR
Structure	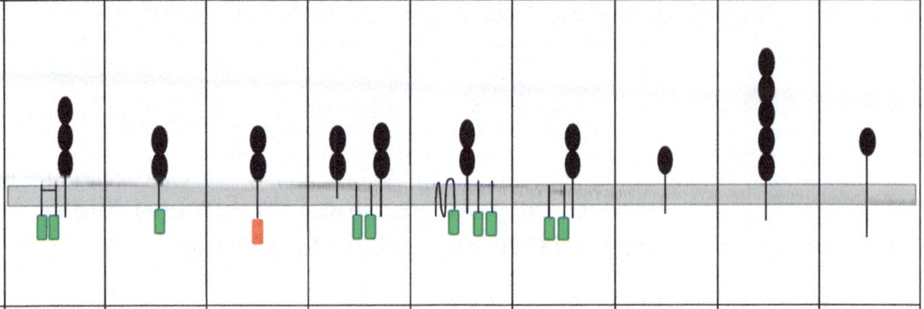								
Binding affinity	IgG1>3>4>2	IgG3>1>2>4	IgG3>1>4>2	IgG1,3>2,4	IgE	IgA1=IgA2	IgM>IgA	IgA, IgM	IgM
Expression	Mφ Neutrophils Eosinophils DC	Mφ Neutrophils Eosinophils Platelets LC	II-B1: B cells Mast cells II-B2: Mast cells Mφ Neutrophils Eosinophils Basophils DC LC	NK cells Mφ Neutrophils Eosinophils Mast cells DC LC	Mast cells Eosinophils Basophils	Mφ Neutrophils Eosinophils	Mφ B cells	Epithelium Liver Small intestine Lung	B cells (mice) B, T, NK cells (human)
Function	Uptake Stimulation of Activation Induction of killing	Uptake Granule release	II-B1: No uptake Inhibition of activation II-B2: Uptake Inhibition of activation	Induction of NK cell killing activity	Degranulation	Uptake Induction of killing	Uptake	Transcytosis	Regulation of humoral immunity and B cell tolerance

Green, ITAM; Red, ITIM

Fig. 7.1 Structure and function of human Fc receptors. ITAM and ITIM motifs are indicated by green and red rectangles, respectively. Mφ, macrophage; DC, dendritic cell; LC, langerhans cell; NK, natural killer cell

not in hematopoietic cells (Mostov 1994) and mediates the epithelial transport of J chain-containing dimeric IgA and polymeric IgM from the lamina propria (Kaetzel et al. 1991). FcμR is predominantly expressed by B cells in mice. Here, we review the role of FcμR in humoral immune responses and immunological tolerance.

7.2 Molecular Characteristics of FcμR

The existence of a receptor for IgM was reported since more than 40 years ago (Moretta et al. 1975; Lamon et al. 1976; Ferrarini et al. 1977; Pichler and Knapp 1977; Burns et al. 1979; Kikutani et al. 1986; Ikuta et al. 1987; Ludin et al. 1987; Kinet 1989). Molecular cloning of *FCMR*, the gene encoding human FcμR, revealed that it is a type I transmembrane protein (Kubagawa et al. 2009). *FCMR* is located on chromosome 1q32.2, adjacent to the polymeric Ig receptor (*PIGR*) and FcR for IgA and IgM (*FCAMR*) genes. Human FcμR is composed of a 234 amino acids (aa) extracellular domain, a 21-aa transmembrane segment, and a 118-aa cytoplasmic tail (Kubagawa et al. 2009; 2014a, b). Unlike Fc receptors for IgG, IgE, or IgA, FcμR, as well as Fcα/μR and pIgR, has no immunoreceptor tyrosine-based activation (ITAM) or inhibitory (ITIM) motifs in the cytoplasmic tail (Fig. 7.1). Instead, FcμR contains several conserved serine and tyrosine residues, which are similar to the Ig-tail tyrosine (ITT) motif (Engels et al. 2009; Engels and Wienands 2011). Stimulation of human FcμR with preformed IgM immune complexes induced the phosphorylation of these serine and tyrosine residues in BW5147 T cells stably expressing FcμR (Kubagawa et al. 2009), suggesting that FcμR could potentially transmit a signal upon ligand binding. Human FcμR is predominantly expressed by B, T, and NK cells but barely expressed by myeloid cells (Kubagawa et al. 2009). A recent study revealed that the binding of human FcμR to the Fc portion of IgM is more stable if the IgM simultaneously binds to surface proteins (Honjo et al. 2015).

The mouse FcμR gene (*Fcmr*) is also located adjacent to *Pigr* and *Fcamr* genes on chromosome 1 (Shima et al. 2010). Mouse and human FcμR are both type I transmembrane proteins with similar structure but share only 54% identity at the aa level. Like human FcμR, mouse FcμR also specifically binds to IgM (Shima et al. 2010; Kubagawa et al. 2017). Unlike human FcμR, mouse FcμR appears to be predominantly expressed in B lymphocytes, as revealed by our in-house microarray of a panel of immune cell types (Fig. 7.2a), BioGPS database (Fig. 7.2b) and FACS analyses (Fig. 7.2c) (Shima et al. 2010; Ouchida et al. 2012a; Liu et al. 2018). FcμR is most highly expressed in MZB cells (Liu et al. 2018). However, others have reported that myeloid cells also express FcμR (Lang et al. 2013; Brenner et al. 2014). The expression levels of mouse FcμR are variable among different B cell subsets (Choi et al. 2013; Liu et al. 2018). FcμR expression level in the germinal center (GC) B cells is much lower than that in naïve B cells (Ouchida et al. 2012a). One possibility is that FcμR may be down-modulated during GC reaction. FcμR is also expressed by IgG^{+} or IgA^{+} B cells (Honjo et al. 2012a).

Genes encoding FcμR, Fcα/μR, and pIgR are located in the same chromosomal region (Kubagawa et al. 2009; Shima et al. 2010), suggesting that they might have evolved from the same ancestor gene. However, while FcμR only binds to IgM, Fcα/μR binds to both IgM and IgA (Shibuya and Honda 2015; Honda et al. 2016; Shibuya et al. 2017). Moreover, pIgR binds to J chain-containing IgM and IgA and mediates their transcytosis to the gut (Turula and Wobus 2018). Although FcμR was originally designated as Fas apoptotic inhibitory molecule 3 or TOSO (Hitoshi et al. 1998), subsequent studies revealed that FcμR deficiency did not affect Fas-mediated apoptosis of either T or B cells (Honjo et al. 2012b; Ouchida et al. 2013).

7.3 FcμR in B Cell Development and Maturation

Several groups generated *Fcmr*-deficient and B cell-specific deletion of *Fcmr* (BKO) mouse strains. Studies from our and two other groups indicated that FcμR deficiency did not affect B cell development in the bone marrow (BM) but altered the numbers of different B cell subsets in the periphery (Ouchida et al. 2012a; Honjo et al. 2012a; Nguyen et al. 2017a). We and Honjo et al. found that MZB was severely reduced in $Fcmr^{-/-}$ mice (Ouchida et al. 2012a; Honjo et al. 2012a). We also found reduced tonic BCR signaling in $Fcmr^{-/-}$ MZB, which we think led to their decreased proportion and absolute numbers (Liu et al. 2018). In contrast, Honjo et al. proposed that MZB in $Fcmr^{-/-}$ mice rapidly differentiated into plasma cells, leading to their reduced proportion and numbers (Honjo et al. 2014). It was also reported that the splenic B-1 cells were increased (Honjo et al. 2012a; Nguyen et al, 2017a), and B cell numbers were decreased in the spleen and lymph nodes (Nguyen et al. 2011) in $Fcmr^{-/-}$ mice. Choi et al. reported increased B-1a but decreased B-2 population in the peritoneal cavity and reduced follicular B cells (FOB) in the spleen (Choi et al. 2013), which were similar to the phenotypes found in $S\mu^{-/-}$ mice that lack secreted IgM (Notley et al. 2010; Baker and Ehrenstein 2002). Collectively, FcμR deficiency did not significantly affect B cell development but affected B cell maturation and differentiation into various B cell subsets.

7.4 FcμR in B Cell Survival and Activation

We and others found that $Fcmr^{-/-}$ B cells showed reduced survival and proliferation in response to anti-IgM but not LPS stimulation (Ouchida et al.

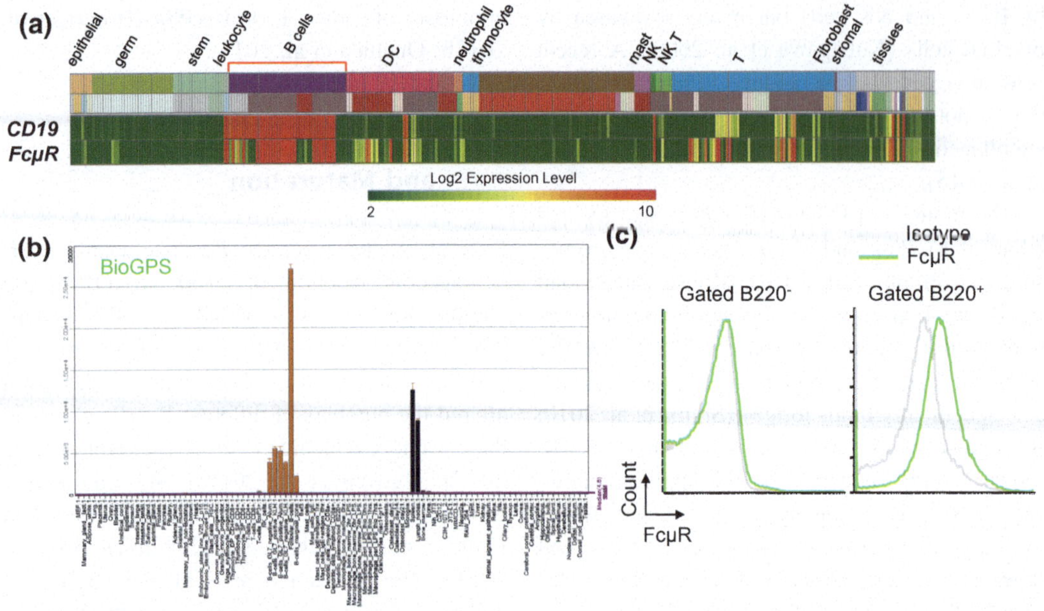

Fig. 7.2 FcμR is preferentially expressed by B cells. **a** Microarray analysis of different immune cell types and tissues of mice. Red and green indicate high and low expression, respectively. For comparison, the expression profile of B-cell-specific *CD19* gene is also shown. **b** FcμR expression in different mouse tissues and immune cells (adopted from BioGPS: http://biogps.org/#goto=genereport&id=69169). FcμR is preferentially expressed by both $GL7^-$ and $GL7^+$ B cells isolated from mice immunized with KLH (keyhole limpet hemocyanin) or alum (aluminum sulfate) and follicular B and marginal zone B cells (orange columns) and by the spleen and lymph node (black columns), but not expressed in other immune cells and tissues. **c** FACS analysis for FcμR cell surface expression. FcμR was expressed by $B220^+$ B cells but barely detectable in $B220^-$ cells (adopted from Ouchida et al. 2012a)

2012a; Choi et al. 2013). Conversely, crosslinking FcμR with an agonistic Ab, 4B5, specifically enhanced anti-IgM-induced survival and proliferation of WT B cells (Ouchida et al. 2012a, 2015), suggesting that FcμR is able to transmit a signal that can cooperate with BCR-derived signal to promote B cell activation. Consistent with this notion, we found that FcμR and BCR physically interact with each other on the plasma membrane of primary B cells by immunofluorescence and co-immunoprecipitation (Ouchida et al. 2015). FcμR deficiency did not affect early BCR signaling including Ca^{2+} influx but impaired the late response such as B cell survival (Ouchida et al. 2015). Biochemical analysis revealed that FcμR did not affect BCR-triggered IκB phosphorylation but promoted the activation of the non-canonical NF-κB pathway and the induction of BCL-xL (Ouchida et al. 2012, 2015). These results suggest that FcμR and BCR cooperate to regulate the late phase, rather than the early phase, of BCR signaling and enhance B cell survival. FcμR does not contain typical ITAM motifs but instead contains an ITT-like motif in its cytoplasmic tail (Kubagawa et al. 2014a, b, 2017; Wang et al. 2016). It is unclear how FcμR specifically affects the late phase, but not the early phase, of BCR signaling and whether the ITT motif is involved. Nguyen et al. reported a role for FcμR in limiting the tonic BCR signaling in immature B cells by attenuating the cell surface expression of IgM BCR (Nguyen et al. 2017a).

As described above, FcμR functions to promote BCR-mediated B cell survival and activation. It is well known that B cells express FcγRIIB, which inhibits B cell activation upon IgG-Ag immune complex-mediated coligation of FcγRIIB and BCR. Therefore, B cells express two types of Fc receptors with

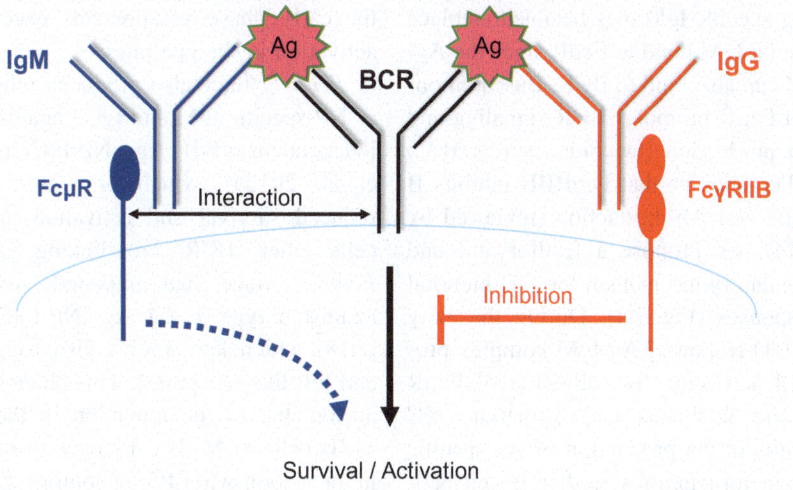

Fig. 7.3 B cells express two types of Fc receptors of opposing functions. We have shown that FcμR promotes B cell activation via interacting with the BCR and potentiating BCR signaling (Ouchida et al. 2015). B cells also express FcγRIIB, which inhibits B cell activation upon Ag-IgG complex-mediated co-engagement of FcγRIIB and BCR. B cells thus express two types of Fc receptors of opposing functions (adopted from Liu et al. 2019)

opposing functions (Fig. 7.3). We will discuss in the next section how FcμR and FcγRIIB might participate in the regulation of humoral immune responses in vivo.

7.5 Role of FcμR in Humoral Immune Responses

Analysis of serum Abs in *Fcmr*$^{-/-}$ mice revealed that basal serum IgM levels were elevated in the mutant mice, which inversely correlated with the cell surface levels of FcμR on B cells (Ouchida et al. 2012a). This observation suggests that some portion of the serum IgM in WT and heterozygous mice binds to the FcμR on B cells whereupon it is sequestered. Supporting this possibility, exogenously administered 4-hydroxy-3-nitrophenylacetyl (NP)-specific monoclonal IgM had a similar half-life in WT and *Fcmr*$^{-/-}$ mice, implicating that FcμR in WT mice was already occupied by IgM in vivo and thus unable to bind the exogenously administered IgM (Ouchida et al. 2012a). Nguyen et al. also found increased levels of serum IgM but attributed such an increase to the elevated numbers and hyper-activation of B-1 cells in the spleen (Nguyen et al. 2017a). In addition, Honjo et al. found increased levels of IgM and to a less extent, IgG3 in *Fcmr*$^{-/-}$ mice (Honjo et al. 2012a). These results collectively implicate a role for FcμR in maintaining optimal IgM levels and B cell homeostasis in vivo.

Fcmr$^{-/-}$ mice produced reduced amount of NP-specific IgG1 during both primary and secondary responses against a T-dependent (T-D) Ag, NP-chicken γ globulin (Ouchida et al. 2012a). The decreased Ab production was associated with decreased sizes and numbers of GCs and reduced numbers of memory and plasma cells. Honjo et al. reported impaired production of primary IgG1 and secondary IgM anti-CGG Ab but normal Ab affinity maturation (Honjo et al. 2012a). Choi et al. found decreased production of NP-specific IgG2b against NP-conjugated keyhole limpet hemocyanin (Choi et al. 2013). These results collectively suggest a role for FcμR in enhancing T-D responses. During a typical T-D humoral immune response, Ag-specific IgM is first produced, followed by the production of Ag-specific IgG. While FcμR appears to be occupied by IgM in vivo and cannot be replaced by exogenously administered NP-specific IgM (Ouchida et al. 2012a), we think that during an immune response, locally produced Ag-specific IgM may be able to replace the non-specific IgM bond to FcμR since the Ag-specific IgM can also bind to BCR. Based on our findings that FcμR promotes BCR signaling and efficient Ab production (Ouchida et al. 2012a) and the earlier findings that FcγRIIB inhibits B cell activation and Ab production (reviewed by Daëron 2014), we propose a feedforward and feedback regulatory mechanism for T-D humoral immune responses (Fig. 7.4). During the early phase of a T-D response, Ag-IgM complex promotes B cell activation by coligation of FcμR and BCR and facilitates GC formation. GC reaction results in the production of Ag-specific IgG, which in turn inhibits further B cell activation via FcγRIIB-mediated inhibitory signals (Fig. 7.4). We propose that B cell activation status is affected by the relative amount of Ag-specific IgM and IgG present in the local environment. We think that the sequential production of Ag-specific IgM and IgG during a T-D response allows sufficient B cell activation in the early phase yet prevents excessive B cell activation in the late phase.

Fcmr$^{-/-}$ mice also produced reduced amount of NP-specific IgM and IgG3 against a type 2 T-independent (T-I) Ag, NP-FICOLL (Ouchida et al. 2012a), which is consistent with the reduced survival and activation in *Fcmr*$^{-/-}$ B cells after BCR crosslinking. Additionally, *Fcmr*$^{-/-}$ mice had impaired Ab production against a type 1 T-I Ag, NP-LPS (Liu et al. 2018), which activates B cells through both BCR and toll-like receptor 4. This phenotype is likely attributable to the reduction in the number of MZB cells as MZB cells play an important role in the response to LPS. In contrast, Choi et al. did not find decreased Ab production against type 1 and 2 T-I Ag (Choi et al. 2013). The reason for the discrepancies between our and their results is unclear but could be due to the differences in the amount of the Ag used for immunization, the time point when the serum Ab was analyzed or age of the mice. Collectively, these results

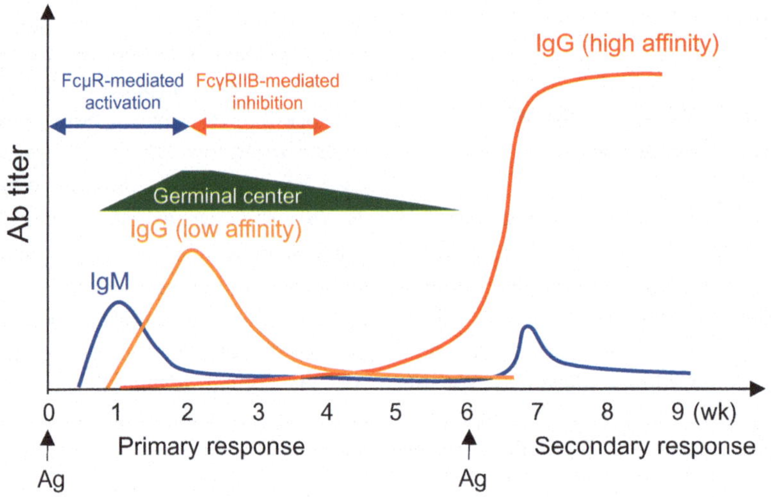

Fig. 7.4 Feedforward and feedback regulation of humoral immune responses by FcμR and FcγRIIB. During a typical T-D humoral immune response, Ag-specific IgM is produced first, followed by the production of Ag-specific IgG. Based on the findings that FcμR promotes while FcγRIIB inhibits B cell activation, we propose an autoregulatory mechanism for T-D humoral immune responses. During the early phase of the response, Ag-IgM complex coligates FcμR and BCR and enhances B cell survival and activation (see also Fig. 7.3). However, at a later phase of the response, Ag-IgG complex coligates FcγRIIB and BCR and suppresses further B cell activation. We think that this mechanism allows sufficient B cell activation during the early phase of an immune response yet prevents excessive B cell activation at a later phase (adopted from Liu et al. 2019)

suggest that FcμR regulates humoral immune responses to both T-D and T-I Ag.

7.6 FcμR in Infectious Immunity

Fcmr$^{-/-}$ mice produced increased levels of phosphorylcholine-specific Ab but decreased levels of protein-specific Ab than did WT mice upon infection with a low dose of live nonencapsulated strain of *Streptococcus pneumoniae* (R36A) (Honjo et al. 2012a). Our recent study revealed that FcμR was important in protecting mice from sepsis induced by a gram-negative bacterium *Citrobacter rodentium* (Liu et al. 2018). Consistently, Lang et al. reported that *Fcmr*$^{-/-}$ mice produced limited amount of cytokines after infection with a gram-positive bacterium *Listeria monocytogenes* and had increased mortality compared with WT mice (Lang et al. 2013). They also reported that FcμR was involved in the control of persistence-prone virus infection in a lymphocytic choriomeningitis virus model system (Lang et al. 2015). Yu et al. reported that conditional deletion of FcμR in B cells resulted in impaired pro-inflammatory T cell responses, which was associated with increased numbers of IL-10 producing B cells (Yu et al. 2018). Nguyen et al. reported that IgM-FcμR interactions regulated early B cell activation and plasma cell differentiation after influenza virus infection (Nguyen et al. 2017b). These results collectively suggest that FcμR plays an important role in protecting the mice against infection.

7.7 FcμR in B Cell Tolerance

Autoreactive B cells are eliminated by at least two distinct mechanisms. B cell central tolerance functions in the BM and eliminates autoreactive immature B cells by inducing their apoptosis, anergy or receptor editing, whereas peripheral tolerance functions to delete autoreactive B cells that escaped the central tolerance or that were generated during GC reaction by Ig gene somatic hypermutation. We and others found that *Fcmr*$^{-/-}$ mice produced autoreactive antibodies including anti-dsDNA, rheumatoid factor, and anti-nuclear antibodies (Ouchida et al. 2012a; Honjo et al. 2012a; Nguyen et al. 2017a; Honjo et al. 2014; Yu et al. 2018). Honjo et al. found that *Fcmr*$^{-/-}$ B6 *Fas*$^{lpr/lpr}$ mice had accelerated development of autoreactive Ab including anti-dsDNA and anti-Sm Ab. They also found enhanced formation of Mott cells and aberrant plasma cells in *Fcmr*$^{-/-}$ mice. Nevertheless, *Fcmr*$^{-/-}$ mice with autoimmune-prone background had normal kidney function and equal mortality compared to control group (Honjo et al. 2014). Brenner et al. reported that FcμR regulated the function of dendritic cells and regulatory T cells and that *Fcmr*$^{-/-}$ mice were more resistant to the experimental autoimmune encephalomyelitis (EAE), a mouse model of human multiple sclerosis (Brenner et al. 2014). We have shown that FcμR physically interacts with BCR and promotes foreign Ag-triggered survival and activation signals in mature B cells (Fig. 7.5, left panel). By analogy, we think that FcμR might also promote self Ag-triggered apoptosis or anergy in immature B cells in the BM and contribute to B cell central tolerance (Fig. 7.5, right panel). It remains to be explored whether autoantibody production in *Fcmr*$^{-/-}$ mice is due to the breakdown of B cell central tolerance, peripheral tolerance, or both.

7.8 Functional Relationship Between IgM-C′ and IgM-FcμR Pathways

IgM is the only isotype produced by all species of jawed vertebrates (Fellah et al. 1992; Boyden 1966; Ehrenstein and Notley 2010). It is also the first Ab to appear during evolution and the first isotype produced during a T-D immune response and usually the only isotype produced in T-I immune responses (Dorner and Radbruch 2007).

IgM is not only an effector molecule important for the early protection against infection but also regulates humoral immune responses (Sörman and Heyman 2017). When IgM is passively administered together with large antigens, the

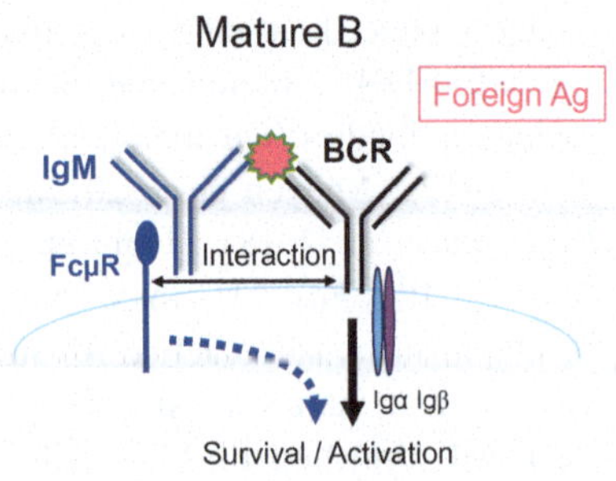

Fig. 7.5 Hypothetical model for a role of FcμR in immunity and tolerance. FcμR physically interacts with the BCR and potentiates foreign Ag-triggered survival and activation signals in mature B cells (left panel). By analogy, FcμR might also promote self Ag-triggered apoptosis or anergy of immature B cells and contribute to B cell central tolerance in the BM (right panel). Although FcμR and BCR are co-engaged by IgM-Ag complex in both mature and immature B cells in the illustration, given the fact that FcμR and BCR physically interact with each other (Ouchida et al. 2015), IgM alone in the absence of Ag may also be able to promote BCR signaling in both mature and immature B cells (modified from Liu et al. 2019)

resulting antibody response is enhanced as compared to the response to the antigen alone. This effect is dependent on the ability of IgM to activate C′ (Heyman et al. 1988; Ding et al. 2013). Moreover, classical C′ components C1, C2, C4, and C3 as well as C′ receptors 1 (CD35) and 2 (CD21) are required for the generation of normal antibody responses to many antigens (Carroll 2008). A puzzling finding is that primary antibody responses require classical C′ components because in naïve animals there would be very little specific antibodies available to activate the classical pathway. One hypothesis has been that natural IgM, which is available already during a first immunization in a naïve animal, would bind to the antigen and activate the classical pathway. This idea was tested in mutant mice (Cμ13) expressing mutant IgM unable to activate C′. However, these mice had a normal antibody response thus demonstrating that IgM-mediated C′ activation cannot explain why animals lacking classical C′ components have extremely low antibody responses (Rutemark et al. 2011). This observation suggests that in addition to C′ activation, there are alternative pathways by which IgM elicits its function. As discussed above, *Fcmr*$^{-/-}$ mice had reduced production of antigen-specific IgG, implicating that IgM can also function through FcμR. Therefore, it appears that both IgM-C′ and IgM-FcμR pathways are involved in the regulation of B cell survival and activation (Fig. 7.6). Currently, it is unclear whether these two pathways function independently or competitively. A detailed comparison of the immunological phenotypes of *Sμ*$^{-/-}$, *Fcmr*$^{-/-}$, Cμ13, and *Fcmr*$^{-/-}$Cμ13 mice should provide useful information

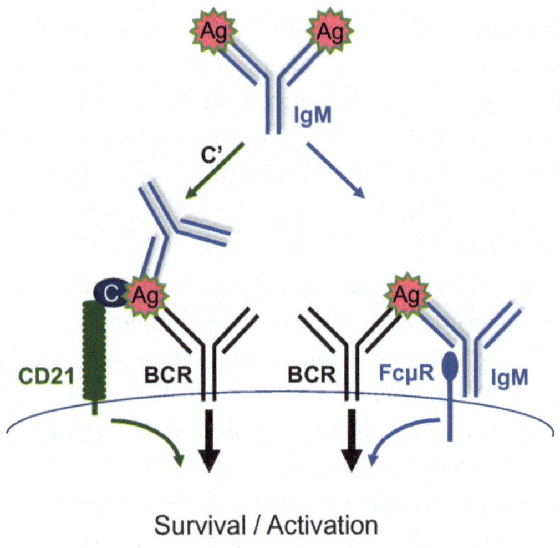

Fig. 7.6 IgM promotes B cell survival and activation through C′ receptor and FcμR. (1) IgM-Ag-C′ complex can activate Ag-specific B cells by coligation of BCR and C′ receptor (CD21) on B cells (green arrow). (2) IgM-Ag complex can also activate B cells by coligation of BCR and FcμR on B cells (blue arrow). The relative contribution of these two pathways in B cell activation remains to be elucidated (modified from Ouchida et al. 2012b) (author summary)

and allow the elucidation of the relationship between IgM-C′ and IgM-FcμR pathways.

7.9 FcμR in Human Diseases

Several groups reported that human FcμR was overexpressed in chronic lymphocytic leukemia (CLL) (Yi et al. 2011; Vire et al. 2011). CLL is a malignancy of mature IgM^+ B cells that exhibit features of polyreactive, partially anergized B cells related to memory B cells (Vire et al. 2011). *FCMR* expression in CLL was significantly higher than that in healthy controls and other B cell lymphoproliferative diseases (Yi et al. 2011; Hancer et al. 2012; Proto-Siqueira et al. 2008; Pallasch et al. 2008). In addition, CLL patients also had higher serum titers of FcμR, a 40-kDa soluble form of the receptor generated by alternative splicing, compared with healthy donors and high expression of *FCMR* was an independent indicator for shorter treatment-free survival in CLL (Li et al. 2011). Therefore, FcμR appears to be associated with the disease progression and patient survival and may serve as a prognostic factor. The elevated expression of FcμR in CLL also made it an ideal target for a more selective treatment of CLL by chimeric antigen receptor T cells (CAR-T). Indeed, initial studies implicated that anti-FcμR CAR-T cells selectively eliminated CLL cells without attacking healthy B cells and had superior therapeutic effect compared with the currently used therapies (Faitschuk et al. 2016).

The reason for the elevated FcμR expression in CLL remains unclear. FcμR expression was found to be decreased with age (Yi et al. 2011). Overexpression of FCMR was reported to promote the chromosomal abnormalities, implicating that FcμR may be related to the degree of genomic activity (Hancer et al. 2012). FcμR expression in CLL is upregulated by BCR stimulation, which suggested that autoreactive BCR signaling might cause its elevated expression (Pallasch et al. 2008). In contrast, CD40 ligation or stimulation of TLRs could downregulate FcμR expression (Vire et al. 2011). FcμR is highly expressed on CLL cells, internalized upon IgM binding and shuttled to lysosomes (Vire et al. 2011). FcμR thus may serve as a receptor for the delivery of IgM–drug conjugates into CLL cells (Vire et al. 2011). Additional studies suggested that human FcμR may have some roles in TNFα-mediated liver damage (Nguyen et al. 2011), malaria vaccine promotion (Lapke et al. 2015), and the function of pancreatic islets (Dharmadhikari et al. 2012).

7.10 Conclusion

Accumulating evidence, in particular the results of $S\mu^{-/-}$ mice, indicates that IgM has two major functions: (1) Enhancing humoral immune responses against foreign antigens and (2) Suppressing autoantibody production. With its pentameric structure, IgM can bind to Ag with high avidity and can efficiently activate the C′ cascade and elicit its function. As reviewed in this chapter, IgM can also function through FcμR. Analyses of conventional and B cell-specific $Fcmr^{-/-}$ mice by different groups have revealed the following common abnormal phenotypes: (1) altered B cell maturation and/or B cell subset differentiation; (2) impaired humoral immune responses against particular antigens and infections; (3) autoantibody production. Yet still many questions remain to be answered. Does FcμR play a role in the survival and activation of memory B cells? As the natural ligand for FcμR, is there any functional difference between innate IgM produced by B-1 cells and Ag-specific IgM produced by B-2 cells? Since IgM can elicit its function through both C′ activation and FcμR, it remains to be elucidated to what extent each of these two pathways contributes to IgM-mediated immunity against foreign antigens and tolerance against autoantigens.

Acknowledgements We thank Lumin Zhang for secretarial assistance and the members in Wang lab for helpful suggestions. This work was supported by the Major Research Plan of the National Natural Science Foundation of China (91942302 to J.Y.W.), the National Key R & D Plan of the Ministry of Science and Technology

(SQ2019YFE0100600 to J.Y.W.), the National Natural Science Foundation of China (81571529 and 31870898 to J.Y.W), Projects of International Cooperation and Exchanges NSFC (81811540035 to J.Y.W.), a grant-in-aid for scientific research (C) from Japan Society for the Promotion of Science (17K08878 to J.Y.W), China Postdoctoral Science Foundation Grant (2018M641929 to J.L.), and National Natural Science Foundation for Young Scholar (81901594 to J.L.).

References

Baker N, Ehrenstein MR (2002) Cutting edge: selection of B lymphocyte subsets is regulated by natural IgM. J Immunol 169(12):6686–6690

Boyden SV (1966) Natural antibodies and the immune response. Adv Immunol 5:1–28

Brenner D, Brustle A, Lin GH, Lang PA, Duncan GS, Knobbe-Thomsen CB et al (2014) Toso controls encephalitogenic immune responses by dendritic cells and regulatory T cells. Proc Natl Acad Sci USA 111 (3):1060–1065. https://doi.org/10.1073/pnas.1323166111

Burns GF, Cawley JC, Barker CR (1979) Characterization of the receptor for IgM present on human B lymphocytes. Immunology 36(3):569–577

Carroll MC (2008) Complement and humoral immunity. Vaccine 26 Suppl 8:I28–I33. https://doi.org/10.1016/j.vaccine.2008.11.022

Choi SC, Wang H, Tian L, Murakami Y, Shin DM, Borrego F et al (2013) Mouse IgM Fc receptor, FCMR, promotes B cell development and modulates antigen-driven immune responses. J Immunol 190(3):987–996. https://doi.org/10.4049/jimmunol.1202227

Daëron M (2014) Fc receptors as adaptive immunoreceptors. Curr Top Microbiol Immunol 382:131–164. https://doi.org/10.1007/978-3-319-07911-0_7

Dharmadhikari G, Muhle M, Schulthess FT, Laue S, Oberholzer J, Pattou F et al (2012) TOSO promotes beta-cell proliferation and protects from apoptosis. Mol Metab 1(1-2):70–78. https://doi.org/10.1016/j.molmet.2012.08.006

Ding Z, Bergman A, Rutemark C, Ouchida R, Ohno H, Wang JY et al (2013) Complement-activating IgM enhances the humoral but not the T cell immune response in mice. PLoS One 8(11):e81299. https://doi.org/10.1371/journal.pone.0081299

Dorner T, Radbruch A (2007) Antibodies and B cell memory in viral immunity. Immunity 27(3):384–392. https://doi.org/10.1016/j.immuni.2007.09.002

Ehrenstein MR, Notley CA (2010) The importance of natural IgM: scavenger, protector and regulator. Nat Rev Immunol 10(11):778–786. https://doi.org/10.1038/nri2849

Engels N, Konig LM, Heemann C, Lutz J, Tsubata T, Griep S et al (2009) Recruitment of the cytoplasmic adaptor Grb2 to surface IgG and IgE provides antigen receptor-intrinsic costimulation to class-switched B cells. Nat Immunol 10(9):1018–1025. https://doi.org/10.1038/ni.1764

Engels N, Wienands J (2011) The signaling tool box for tyrosine-based costimulation of lymphocytes. Curr Opin Immunol 23(3):324–329. https://doi.org/10.1016/j.coi.2011.01.005

Faitschuk E, Hombach AA, Frenzel LP, Wendtner CM, Abken H (2016) Chimeric antigen receptor T cells targeting Fc mu receptor selectively eliminate CLL cells while sparing healthy B cells. Blood 128 (13):1711–1722. https://doi.org/10.1182/blood-2016-01-692046

Fellah JS, Wiles MV, Charlemagne J, Schwager J (1992) Evolution of vertebrate IgM: complete amino acid sequence of the constant region of Ambystoma mexicanum mu chain deduced from cDNA sequence. Eur J Immunol 22(10):2595–2601. https://doi.org/10.1002/eji.1830221019

Ferrarini M, Hoffman T, Fu SM, Winchester R, Kunkel HG (1977) Receptors for IgM on certain human B lymphocytes. J Immunol 119(4):1525–1529

Hancer VS, Diz-Kucukkaya R, Aktan M (2012) Overexpression of Fc mu receptor (FCMR, TOSO) gene in chronic lymphocytic leukemia patients. Med Oncol 29 (2):1068–1072. https://doi.org/10.1007/s12032-011-9821-3

Heyman B, Pilström L, Shulman MJ (1988) Complement activation is required for IgM-mediated enhancement of the antibody response. J Exp Med 167(6):1999–2004. https://doi.org/10.1084/jem.167.6.1999

Hitoshi Y, Lorens J, Kitada SI, Fisher J, LaBarge M, Ring HZ et al (1998) Toso, a cell surface, specific regulator of Fas-induced apoptosis in T cells. Immunity 8(4):461–471

Honda S, Sato K, Totsuka N, Fujiyama S, Fujimoto M, Miyake K et al (2016) Marginal zone B cells exacerbate endotoxic shock via interleukin-6 secretion induced by Fcalpha/muR-coupled TLR4 signalling. Nat Commun 7:11498. https://doi.org/10.1038/ncomms11498

Honjo K, Kubagawa Y, Jones DM, Dizon B, Zhu Z, Ohno H et al (2012a) Altered Ig levels and antibody responses in mice deficient for the Fc receptor for IgM (FcmuR). Proc Natl Acad Sci USA 109(39):15882–15887. https://doi.org/10.1073/pnas.1206567109

Honjo K, Kubagawa Y, Kubagawa H (2012b) Is Toso an antiapoptotic protein or an Fc receptor for IgM? Blood 119(7):1789–1790. https://doi.org/10.1182/blood-2011-09-380782

Honjo K, Kubagawa Y, Kearney JF, Kubagawa H (2015) Unique ligand-binding property of the human IgM Fc receptor. J Immunol 194(4):1975–1982. https://doi.org/10.4049/jimmunol.1401866

Honjo K, Kubagawa Y, Suzuki Y, Takagi M, Ohno H, Bucy RP et al (2014) Enhanced auto-antibody production and Mott cell formation in FcmuR-deficient autoimmune mice. Int Immunol 26 (12):659–672. https://doi.org/10.1093/intimm/dxu070

Ikuta K, Takami M, Kim CW, Honjo T, Miyoshi T, Tagaya Y et al (1987) Human lymphocyte Fc receptor for IgE: sequence homology of its cloned cDNA with animal lectins. Proc Natl Acad Sci USA 84(3):819–823

Kaetzel CS, Robinson JK, Chintalacharuvu KR, Vaerman JP, Lamm ME (1991) The polymeric immunoglobulin receptor (secretory component) mediates transport of immune complexes across epithelial cells: a local defense function for IgA. Proc Natl Acad Sci USA 88(19):8796–8800

Kikutani H, Inui S, Sato R, Barsumian EL, Owaki H, Yamasaki K et al (1986) Molecular structure of human lymphocyte receptor for immunoglobulin E. Cell 47(5):657–665

Kinet JP (1989) Antibody-cell interactions: Fc receptors. Cell 57(3):351–354

Kubagawa H, Kubagawa Y, Jones D, Nasti TH, Walter MR, Honjo K (2014a) The old but new IgM Fc receptor (FcmuR). Curr Top Microbiol Immunol 382:3–28. https://doi.org/10.1007/978-3-319-07911-0_1

Kubagawa H, Oka S, Kubagawa Y, Torii I, Takayama E, Kang DW et al (2014b) The long elusive IgM Fc receptor, FcmuR. J Clin Immunol 34(Suppl 1):S35–S45. https://doi.org/10.1007/s10875-014-0022-7

Kubagawa H, Oka S, Kubagawa Y, Torii I, Takayama E, Kang DW et al (2009) Identity of the elusive IgM Fc receptor (FcmuR) in humans. J Exp Med 206(12):2779–2793. https://doi.org/10.1084/jem.20091107

Kubagawa H, Skopnik CM, Zimmermann J, Durek P, Chang HD, Yoo E et al (2017) Authentic IgM Fc Receptor (FcmuR). Curr Top Microbiol Immunol 408:25–45. https://doi.org/10.1007/82_2017_23

Lamon EW, Andersson B, Whitten HD, Hurst MM, Ghanta V (1976) IgM complex receptors on subpopulations of murine lymphocytes. J Immunol 116(5):1199–1203

Lang KS, Lang PA, Meryk A, Pandyra AA, Boucher LM, Pozdeev VI et al (2013) Involvement of Toso in activation of monocytes, macrophages, and granulocytes. Proc Natl Acad Sci USA 110(7):2593–2598. https://doi.org/10.1073/pnas.1222264110

Lang PA, Meryk A, Pandyra AA, Brenner D, Brustle A, Xu HC et al (2015) Toso regulates differentiation and activation of inflammatory dendritic cells during persistence-prone virus infection. Cell Death Differ 22(1):164–173. https://doi.org/10.1038/cdd.2014.138

Lapke N, Tartz S, Lee KH, Jacobs T (2015) The application of anti-Toso antibody enhances CD8(+) T cell responses in experimental malaria vaccination and disease. Vaccine 33(48):6763–6770. https://doi.org/10.1016/j.vaccine.2015.10.065

Li FJ, Kubagawa Y, McCollum MK, Wilson L, Motohashi T, Bertoli LF et al (2011) Enhanced levels of both the membrane-bound and soluble forms of IgM Fc receptor (FcmuR) in patients with chronic lymphocytic leukemia. Blood 118(18):4902–4909. https://doi.org/10.1182/blood-2011-04-350793

Liu J, Zhu H, Qian J, Xiong E, Zhang L, Wang YQ et al (2018) Fcmicro receptor promotes the survival and activation of marginal zone B cells and protects mice against bacterial sepsis. Front Immunol 9:160. https://doi.org/10.3389/fimmu.2018.00160

Liu J, Wang Y, Xiong E, Hong R, Lu Q, Ohno H et al (2019) Role of the IgM Fc receptor in immunity and tolerance. Front Immunol 10:529. https://doi.org/10.3389/fimmu.2019.00529

Ludin C, Hofstetter H, Sarfati M, Levy CA, Suter U, Alaimo D et al (1987) Cloning and expression of the cDNA coding for a human lymphocyte IgE receptor. EMBO J 6(1):109–114

Moretta L, Ferrarini M, Durante ML, Mingari MC (1975) Expression of a receptor for IgM by human T cells in vitro. Eur J Immunol 5(8):565–569. https://doi.org/10.1002/eji.1830050812

Mostov KE (1994) Transepithelial transport of immunoglobulins. Annu Rev Immunol 12:63–84. https://doi.org/10.1146/annurev.iy.12.040194.000431

Nguyen TT, Klasener K, Zurn C, Castillo PA, Brust-Mascher I, Imai DM et al (2017a) The IgM receptor FcmuR limits tonic BCR signaling by regulating expression of the IgM BCR. Nat Immunol 18(3):321–333. https://doi.org/10.1038/ni.3677

Nguyen TTT, Graf BA, Randall TD, Baumgarth N (2017b) sIgM-FcmuR interactions regulate early B cell activation and plasma cell development after influenza virus infection. J Immunol 199(5):1635–1646. https://doi.org/10.4049/jimmunol.1700560

Nguyen XH, Lang PA, Lang KS, Adam D, Fattakhova G, Foger N et al (2011) Toso regulates the balance between apoptotic and nonapoptotic death receptor signaling by facilitating RIP1 ubiquitination. Blood 118(3):598–608. https://doi.org/10.1182/blood-2010-10-313643

Notley CA, Baker N, Ehrenstein MR (2010) Secreted IgM enhances B cell receptor signaling and promotes splenic but impairs peritoneal B cell survival. J Immunol 184(7):3386–3393. https://doi.org/10.4049/jimmunol.0902640

Ouchida R, Lu Q, Liu J, Li Y, Chu Y, Tsubata T et al (2015) FcmuR interacts and cooperates with the B cell receptor to promote B cell survival. J Immunol 194(7):3096–3101. https://doi.org/10.4049/jimmunol.1402352

Ouchida R, Mori H, Hase K, Takatsu H, Kurosaki T, Tokuhisa T et al (2012a) Critical role of the IgM Fc receptor in IgM homeostasis, B-cell survival, and humoral immune responses. Proc Natl Acad Sci USA 109(40):E2699–E2706. https://doi.org/10.1073/pnas.1210706109

Ouchida R, Mori H, Hase K, Takatsu H, Kurosaki T, Tokuhisa T, Ohno H, Wang J-Y (2012b) Critical role of the IgM Fc receptor in IgM homeostasis, B cell survival and humoral immune responses. Proc Natl Acad Sci USA 109:15989–15990 (Author Summary)

Ouchida R, Mori H, Ohno H, Wang JY (2013) FcmuR (Toso/Faim3) is not an inhibitor of Fas-mediated cell death in mouse T and B cells. Blood 121(12):2368–2370. https://doi.org/10.1182/blood-2012-12-470906

Pallasch CP, Schulz A, Kutsch N, Schwamb J, Hagist S, Kashkar H et al (2008) Overexpression of TOSO in CLL is triggered by B-cell receptor signaling and associated with progressive disease. Blood 112 (10):4213–4219. https://doi.org/10.1182/blood-2008-05-157255

Pichler WJ, Knapp W (1977) Receptors for IgM-coated erythrocytes on chronic lymphatic leukemia cells. J Immunol 118(3):1010–1015

Proto-Siqueira R, Panepucci RA, Careta FP, Lee A, Clear A, Morris K et al (2008) SAGE analysis demonstrates increased expression of TOSO contributing to Fas-mediated resistance in CLL. Blood 112(2):394–397. https://doi.org/10.1182/blood-2007-11-124065

Rutemark C, Alicot E, Bergman A, Ma M, Getahun A, Ellmerich S et al (2011) Requirement for complement in antibody responses is not explained by the classic pathway activator IgM. Proc Natl Acad Sci USA 108 (43):E934–E942. https://doi.org/10.1073/pnas.1109831108

Schneeman TA, Bruno ME, Schjerven H, Johansen FE, Chady L, Kaetzel CS (2005) Regulation of the polymeric Ig receptor by signaling through TLRs 3 and 4: linking innate and adaptive immune responses. J Immunol 175(1):376–384

Shibuya A, Honda S (2006) Molecular and functional characteristics of the Fcalpha/muR, a novel Fc receptor for IgM and IgA. Springer Semin Immunopathol 28 (4):377–382. https://doi.org/10.1007/s00281-006-0050-3

Shibuya A, Honda S (2015) Immune regulation by Fcalpha/mu receptor (CD351) on marginal zone B cells and follicular dendritic cells. Immunol Rev 268 (1):288–295. https://doi.org/10.1111/imr.12345

Shibuya A, Honda SI, Shibuya K (2017) A pro-inflammatory role of Fcalpha/muR on marginal zone B cells in sepsis. Int Immunol 29(11):519–524. https://doi.org/10.1093/intimm/dxx059

Shibuya A, Sakamoto N, Shimizu Y, Shibuya K, Osawa M, Hiroyama T et al (2000) Fc alpha/mu receptor mediates endocytosis of IgM-coated microbes. Nat Immunol 1(5):441–446. https://doi.org/10.1038/80886

Shima H, Takatsu H, Fukuda S, Ohmae M, Hase K, Kubagawa H et al (2010) Identification of TOSO/FAIM3 as an Fc receptor for IgM. Int Immunol 22(3):149–156. https://doi.org/10.1093/intimm/dxp121

Sörman A, Heyman B (2017) Specific IgM and regulation of antibody responses. Curr Top Microbiol Immunol 408:67–87. https://doi.org/10.1007/82_2017_24

Stadtmueller BM, Huey-Tubman KE, Lopez CJ, Yang Z, Hubbell WL, Bjorkman PJ (2016) The structure and dynamics of secretory component and its interactions with polymeric immunoglobulins. Elife 5. https://doi.org/10.7554/eLife.10640

Turula H, Wobus CE (2018) The role of the polymeric immunoglobulin receptor and secretory immunoglobulins during mucosal infection and immunity. Viruses 10(5). https://doi.org/10.3390/v10050237

Vire B, David A, Wiestner A (2011) TOSO, the Fcmicro receptor, is highly expressed on chronic lymphocytic leukemia B cells, internalizes upon IgM binding, shuttles to the lysosome, and is downregulated in response to TLR activation. J Immunol 187(8):4040–4050. https://doi.org/10.4049/jimmunol.1100532

Wang H, Coligan JE, Morse HC 3rd (2016) Emerging functions of natural IgM and its Fc receptor FCMR in immune homeostasis. Front Immunol 7:99. https://doi.org/10.3389/fimmu.2016.00099

Yi S, Yu Z, Zhou K, Wang Y, An G, Li Z et al (2011) TOSO is overexpressed and correlated with disease progression in Chinese patients with chronic lymphocytic leukemia. Leuk Lymphoma 52(1):72–78. https://doi.org/10.3109/10428194.2010.531411

Yu J, Duong VHH, Westphal K, Westphal A, Suwandi A, Grassl GA et al (2018) Surface receptor Toso controls B cell-mediated regulation of T cell immunity. J Clin Invest 128(5):1820–1836. https://doi.org/10.1172/jci97280

Regulatory B Cells

8

Luman Wang, Ying Fu and Yiwei Chu

Abstract

B cells are typically characterized by their ability to produce antibodies, function as secondary antigen-present cells, and produce various immunoregulatory cytokines. The regulatory B (Breg)-cell population is now widely accepted as an important modulatory component of the immune system that suppresses inflammation. Recent studies indicate that Breg-cell populations are small under physiological conditions but expand substantially in both human patients and murine models of chronic inflammatory diseases, autoimmune diseases, infection, transplantation, and cancer. Almost all B-cell subsets can be induced to form Breg cells. In addition, there are unique Breg-cell subsets such as B10 and Tim-1^{+} B cells. Immunoregulatory function may be mediated by production of cytokines such as IL-10 and TGF-β and ensuing suppression of T cells, by direct cell–cell interactions, and (or) by altering the immune microenvironment. In this chapter, we describe in detail the discovery of Breg cells, their phenotypes, differentiation, function, contributions to disease, and therapeutic potential.

Keywords

Regulatory B cells · IL-10 · Diseases

8.1 Introduction

Morris et al. were the first to identify antibodies (Abs) with both pro- and anti-inflammatory activities in mice (Morris and Moller 1968). Subsequently, several groups described the ability of splenic B cells to suppress delayed-type hypersensitivity (DTH) responses in guinea pigs (Katz et al. 1974; Neta and Salvin 1974). Kennedy et al. also demonstrated that memory B cells can act as suppressors–inducers of feedback control (Kennedy and Thomas 1983). These and subsequent studies demonstrated that B cells could exert immunosuppressive effects, at least in part by regulating T-cell function. However, it has taken several decades to definitively identify regulatory B (Breg) cells and their immunosuppressive mechanisms. In the 1990s, Janeway and colleagues first reported the existence of an immunoregulatory B-cell subset that when transplanted induced complete recovery of acute experimental autoimmune encephalomyelitis

L. Wang · Y. Fu · Y. Chu (✉)
Department of Immunology, School of Basic Medical Sciences, and Institutes of Biomedical Sciences, Fudan University, No. 138, Yi Xue Yuan Rd, 226, Shanghai 200032, China
e-mail: yiweichu@fudan.edu.cn

J.-Y. Wang (ed.), *B Cells in Immunity and Tolerance*, Advances in Experimental Medicine and Biology 1254, https://doi.org/10.1007/978-981-15-3532-1_8

(EAE) in mice (Wolf et al. 1996). Mizoguchi and Bhan then demonstrated that B-cell-deficient mice with experimental inflammatory bowel disease (IBD) had more severe colitis symptoms, again suggesting that some B-cell populations have suppressive activity in immunological diseases. These authors also first coined the term "regulatory B cells" to designate B cells with immunoregulatory properties (Mizoguchi et al. 1997).

Since these initial discoveries, it has been established that B cells can contribute to the maintenance of immune tolerance and the suppression of inflammatory responses (Mizoguchi et al. 2002). However, there is still no consensus phenotypic definition of Breg cells. Immunomodulatory B cells have been ascribed various phenotypes, ranging from immature B2-lineage cells such as transitional-2 marginal zone precursor (T2-MZP) cells to mature B1-lineage B cells (Evans et al. 2007; Lenert et al. 2005; Lundy and Boros 2002). In 2008, the Tedder group identified a unique $CD19^{+}CD5^{+}CD1d^{hi}$ B-cell subset that produced IL-10 and functioned as a suppresser of diseases (Yanaba et al. 2008). In the following decade, several distinct Breg-cell subtypes and functions were identified in various disease models, including models of IBD, EAE, and cancer. Breg cells regulate disease development through multiple mechanisms, such as by producing IL-10, IL-35, and IL-21 (Shen et al. 2014; Tedder and Leonard 2014; Wang et al. 2014). Several research groups have examined Breg-cell function by treating isolated cells with exogenous factors followed by adoptive transfer into disease model mice to test for therapeutic effects. For instance, granulocyte—macrophage colony-stimulating factor and interleukin-15 fusokine (GIFT-15) converted naïve B cells into Breg cells that were subsequently shown to suppress EAE (Rafei et al. 2009). Human Breg cells with distinct phenotypes have also been identified (Blair et al. 2010; Bouaziz et al. 2010; Iwata et al. 2011). Tedder et al. defined human $CD19^{+}CD24^{+}CD27^{hi}$ B cells as Breg cells (Iwata et al. 2011), and Mauri et al. found that $CD19^{+}CD24^{hi}CD38^{hi}$ cells are immunosuppressive (Blair et al. 2010). Subsequently, a large number of studies confirmed the presence of Breg cells in the peripheral blood of patients with different diseases, suggesting broad clinical importance and potential therapeutic utility. Milestones and highlights in Breg-cell research are summarized in Table 8.1.

8.2 Breg-Cell Phenotype

Unlike Treg cells, there are no unique surface markers or released factors (i.e., specific cytokine profiles) that define Breg cells. Thus, the term Breg refers to B cells with regulatory functions. Nonetheless, multiple Breg-cell subsets with distinct phenotypes and effector functions have been described (summarized in Table 8.2).

8.2.1 Breg Cells in Mouse

8.2.1.1 Common Breg-Cell Subsets

Unlike natural Treg cells, there are a few if any "natural Breg cells." However, any B-cell subset can differentiate into Breg cells under the appropriate stimulus environment, such as the presence of toll-like receptor (TLR) ligands and anti-CD40 stimuli (Rosser and Mauri 2015). Bulk $CD19^{+}$ B cells can produce IL-10 upon lipopolysaccharide (LPS) stimulation (Matsushita and Tedder 2011). Innate B-cell subsets such as B-1, marginal zone (MZ), and transitional (T) B cells reportedly can be induced into Breg cells. For instance, stimulation of MZ B cells with TLR agonists facilitated production of IL-10, TGF-β, and IL-6, cytokines released by Breg cells (Tian et al. 2001). Further, these B-cell-derived populations have ameliorative effects in disease models. For example, CD40-stimulated T2 B cells suppressed lupus in MRL/lpr mice (Blair et al. 2009), while oral immunization with ovalbumin (OVA) enabled B-1 cells to negatively regulate intestinal immunity (De-Gennaro et al. 2009). Even follicular B (FOB) cells can express high levels of CD11b in response to TLR ligands plus IL-10, thus "acquiring" strong regulatory functions and suppressing autoimmune disease (Liu et al. 2015; Wang et al. 2018).

Table 8.1 Milestones and highlights in Breg-cell research

Year	Mouse	Human
1968	Inhibitory antibodies are exist (Morris and Moller 1968)	
1974	B cells suppress DTH (Katz et al. 1974; Neta and Salvin 1974)	
1983	Memory B cells are immunosuppressive (Kennedy and Thomas 1983)	
1996	B-cell-deficient mice develop more severe EAE (Wolf et al. 1996)	
1997	B-cell-deficient mouse develop more severe colitis (Mizoguchi et al. 1997)	
2002	The term "Breg" coined (Mizoguchi et al. 2002)	
2007	Transitional 2 B cells suppress arthritis (Evans et al. 2007)	
2008	Breg cells isolated with a unique $CD19^{+}CD1d^{hi}CD5^{+}$ phenotype (Yanaba et al. 2008)	
2010	Breg cells differentiate via TLR or CD40 stimulation (Neves et al. 2010; Zheng et al. 2010)	$CD19^{+}CD24^{hi}CD38^{hi}$ B cells exhibit regulatory capacity in human blood (Blair et al. 2010)
2011	Regulatory B cells identified in mice (Matsushita and Tedder 2011)	Identification of regulatory B cells in humans that resemble mouse-regulatory B cells (Iwata et al. 2011)
2012	IL-21 involved in Breg-cell development (Yoshizaki et al. 2012)	
2015	IL-35 involved in Breg-cell development (Wang et al. 2014) $CD11b^{+}$ Breg-cell-subset suppresses EAH (Liu et al. 2015)	
2018	LAG-3 expression identifies regulatory plasma cells (Lino et al. 2018)	

8.2.1.2 The Unique $CD5^{+}CD1d^{hi}$ Breg Cells

Currently, there are no known phenotypic or lineage markers that are unique to Breg cells; rather, Breg cells are more likely defined by their function and behavior. Tedder and colleagues found a specific Breg-cell subset, $CD5^{+}CD1d^{hi}$, present only in the mouse spleen and showing dramatic changes under disease conditions (Yanaba et al. 2008). Under physiological conditions, $CD5^{+}CD1d^{hi}$ Breg cells accounted for only 1–3% of the total B-cell population, but this proportion rose to 10–20% under various disease conditions (Yanaba et al. 2008). These $CD5^{+}CD1d^{hi}$ Breg cells highly expressed IL-10, and transferring these cells into mice with autoimmune diseases effectively alleviated disease symptoms (Kalampokis et al. 2013; Watanabe et al. 2010). Since the first report in 2008, many research groups have found this Breg subset and documented a regulatory role in various diseases. For example, Sheng et al. reported that $CD5^{+}CD1d^{hi}$ Breg cells regulate experimental autoimmune myasthenia gravis (MG) via IL-10 release (Sheng et al. 2015). In addition, B-cell activating factor (BAFF) induced IL-35 production by $CD5^{+}CD1d^{hi}$ Breg cell in lupus (Zhang et al. 2017). This $CD5^{+}CD1d^{hi}$ Breg-cell subset also appears indispensable for maintaining immune homeostasis (Xing et al. 2014). Further, $CD5^{+}CD1d^{hi}$

Table 8.2 Breg-cell phenotypes

Location	Subset	Phenotypes
Peritoneal cavity	B-1 cells	$CD19^+CD5^+IgM^{hi}CD23^-$ $CD21^-CD11b^+$ (Shimomura et al. 2008; Yanaba et al. 2008)
Spleen	$CD1d^{hi}CD5^+$ B cells	$CD19^{hi}CD1d^{hi}CD5^+IgM^{hi}CD24^{hi}B220^{hi}$ (Yanaba et al. 2008)
	MZ B cells	$CD19^+CD21^+CD1d^{+/-}CD5^+CD23^{low}$ (Bankoti et al. 2012)
	T2-MZP B cells	$CD19^+CD21^{hi}CD23^{hi}CD24^{hi}IgM^{hi}IgD^{hi}CD1d^{hi}$ (Evans et al. 2007; Moreau et al. 2015)
Intestine	IgA^+ plasmacytes	$CD19^+B220^+IgA^+PD\text{-}1^+$ (Liu et al. 2017)
"New"	$PD\text{-}1^+$	$CD19^+PD\text{-}1^+$ (Xiao et al. 2016)
	$CD73^+$ B cells	$CD19^+CD39^+CD73^+$ (Kaku et al. 2014)
	$TIM\text{-}1^+$ B cells	$CD19^+TIM^+$ (Ding et al. 2011)
	GrB^+ B cells	$CD19^+CD38^+CD1d^+IgM^+CD147^+$ (Lindner et al. 2013)
	$Foxp3^+$	$CD19^+$ $Foxp3^+$ (Guo et al. 2015; Vadasz and Toubi 2016)
	Killer B cells	$CD19^+Fas^+$ (Zhang et al. 2018)
	$CD11b^+$ B cells	$CD19^+CD11b^+$ (Liu et al. 2015)
Human blood	$CD27^+$ B cell	$CD19^+CD24^{hi}CD27^+$ (Iwata et al. 2011)
	$CD38^{hi}$ B cell	$CD19^+CD24^{hi}CD38^{hi}$ (Blair et al. 2010)

Breg cells have been found in humans where they likely exert inhibitory effects on various diseases (Chen et al. 2017).

8.2.1.3 Other New Breg-Cell Subsets

In addition to the $CD5^+CD1d^{hi}$ Breg-cell subset, several additional Breg-cell subsets have been reported in recent years, such as $Tim\text{-}1^+$, $CD11b^+$, $LAG\text{-}3^+$, $foxp3^+$, and $PD\text{-}1^+$ Breg cells. Ding et al. first reported Breg cells expressing TIM-1 and that TIM-1 ligation could promote Breg-cell expansion in mice (Ding et al. 2011). Kuchroo and colleagues confirmed that Tim-1 is essential for induction and maintenance of IL-10 expression by Breg cells and for their function in regulation of tissue inflammation (Xiao et al. 2012, 2015). Our group has been investigating a Breg-cell subset since 2015 (Liu et al. 2015; Qian et al. 2019; Wang et al. 2018) with high surface expression of CD11b under disease conditions. These $CD11b^+$ Breg cells have a crucial regulatory role in experimental autoimmune hepatitis (EAH) and are able to inhibit inflammation by disrupting T-cell receptor (TCR) signaling. In a colitis model, $CD11b^+$ B cells cooperate with Tregs in the maintenance of gut homeostasis. Using epigenomic detection, Lino et al. (2018) reported that LAG3 (CD223) identified another subset of regulatory plasma cell in vivo and in vitro. Other Breg cells express Treg-specific features such as $Foxp3^+$ expression (Noh et al. 2010; Vadasz and Toubi 2016). Finally, $PD\text{-}1^+$ B cells have been identified and functions in tumor immunity reported (Ren et al. 2016; Wang et al. 2019; Xiao et al. 2016).

8.2.2 Breg Cells in Human

Studies showing that Breg-cell populations expand under disease conditions in mice have led to numerous investigations on the presence and functions of Breg-cell subsets in humans, including various disease patients. However, the phenotypes of human Breg cells, their resemblances to mouse subsets, and relationships to specific diseases are controversial (Blair et al. 2010; Bouaziz et al. 2010; Iwata et al. 2011). Both $CD19^+CD24^{hi}CD27^+$ and $CD19^+CD24^{hi}CD38^{hi}$ Breg cells have been identified and shown to inhibit the proliferation and function of pro-inflammatory cells, but do not show consistent expression in disease. In the healthy population, $CD19^{+}CD24^{hi}CD27^{+}$ B cells account for about 25% of total B cells, but the proportion can either increase or decrease in specific diseases (de Masson et al. 2015; Yang et al. 2015, 2017; Zha et al. 2012). Further, immunosuppressive functions are only partially dependent on IL-10. In addition, $CD19^{+}CD24^{hi}CD38^{hi}$ B-cell function is actually impaired under disease conditions in contrast to most murine Breg-cell subsets (Blair et al. 2010; Hasan et al. 2019; Li et al. 2019b; Yu et al. 2017; Zhu et al. 2014).

8.2.3 Regulatory and Effector B Cells

With the discovery of Breg cells, B cells are now divided into effector (Beff) and regulatory subsets. Given that nearly every B-cell subset can "acquire" regulatory or effector functions, Breg and Beff cells are difficult to distinguish. Normally, cytokine expression is used to distinguish between these two groups since Breg-cell subsets predominantly produce IL-10, TGF-β, and IL-35, while Beff subsets produce IL-6, TNF-α, and IFN-γ (Matsushita 2019). The Tedder group demonstrated complex relationships between Breg and Beff cells in an EAE model (Matsushita et al. 2008). However, due to the lack of Breg-cell lineage commitment factors, it is difficult to distinguish these two B cell groups for further study of cell–cell interactions, a condition essential for future therapeutic applications.

8.3 Development and Differentiation of Breg Cells

Compared to Tregs, relatively little is known about Breg-cell biology as there are not known reliable surface markers or master transcription factors. Further, the Breg cell may be a transitional state rather than an independent stable B-cell lineage (Berthelot et al. 2013; Rosser and Mauri 2015), creating additional difficulties for studies on basic biology, particularly in vivo. Thus, it is believed that all Breg-cell subsets arise from a common progenitor by external stimulation and that all B cells can differentiate into Breg cells (Fig. 8.1). Immature B cells like T2-MZP B cells can develop into Breg cells after TLR ligand stimulation, and mature B cells and even

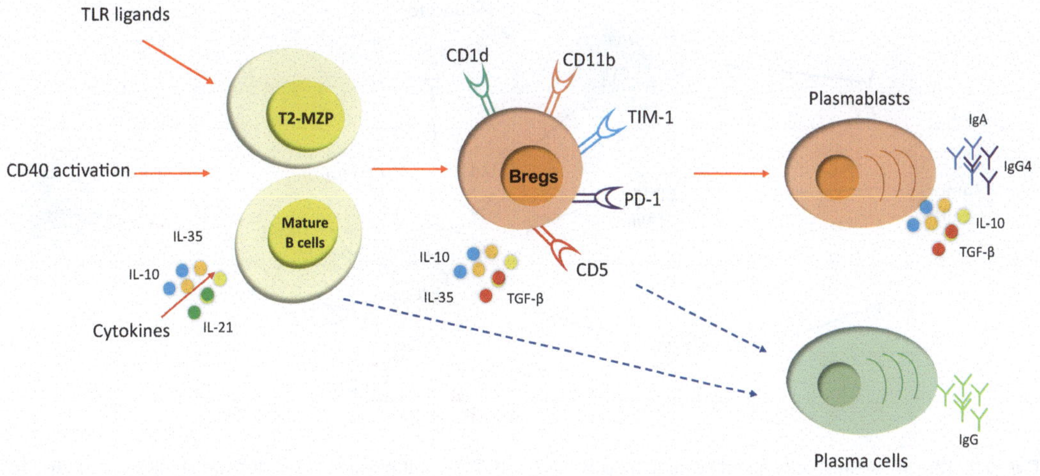

Fig. 8.1 Proposed development and differentiation pathways of Breg cells. Both T2-MZP B cells and mature B cells can differentiate into Breg cells under TLR ligand stimulation and CD40 activation by cytokines. Also, IL-10- and/or IL-35-producing plasmablasts can develop from mature B cells. All Breg-cell types can also differentiate into conventional plasma cells

plasma B cells can be transformed into Breg cells by appropriate stimuli. B cells transitioning into Breg cells are called B10 progenitor or B10pro cells. Functional Breg cells can be induced by CD40 ligand, LPS, or CpG oligonucleotides (Kalampokis et al. 2013). Tedder's group reported that mouse and human B10pro cells matured after in vitro stimulation by TLRs, disease-specific stimuli such as LPS in infection promote Breg-cell maturation. Myeloid differentiation primary response gene 88 (MyD88) signaling is required for IL-10 production in Breg cells but not for Breg-cell development. Thus, similar to Tregs, MyD88 is thought to be involved but not critical for Breg-cell development (Lino et al. 2018). Stromal interaction via stromal interaction molecules 1(STIM1) and 2(STIM2) is also necessary for IL-10 production by Breg cells (Matsumoto et al. 2011), while the cytokines IL-21 (Yoshizaki et al. 2012) and IL-35 (Shen et al. 2014) are essential for Breg-cell development. Lack of IL-21 or IL-35 decreases Breg-cell numbers both in vivo and in vitro. Furthermore, an earlier report suggested that splenic Breg cells eventually differentiate into antibody-producing plasmablasts after stimulation in vivo and in vitro (Maseda et al. 2012). Plasmablasts also have regulatory functions in autoimmune diseases and cancer (Liu et al. 2017; Matsumoto et al. 2014). Recent studies have suggested similarities in the in vivo development of Breg cells in mice and in humans.

8.4 The Mechanisms of Breg-Cell Regulation

Production of IL-10 is crucial for the immunosuppressive actions of Breg cells, although questions remain as to the intracellular pathways that induce IL-10 secretion. The target cells of Breg-cell immunomodulation and fundamental mechanisms are shown schematically in Fig. 8.2.

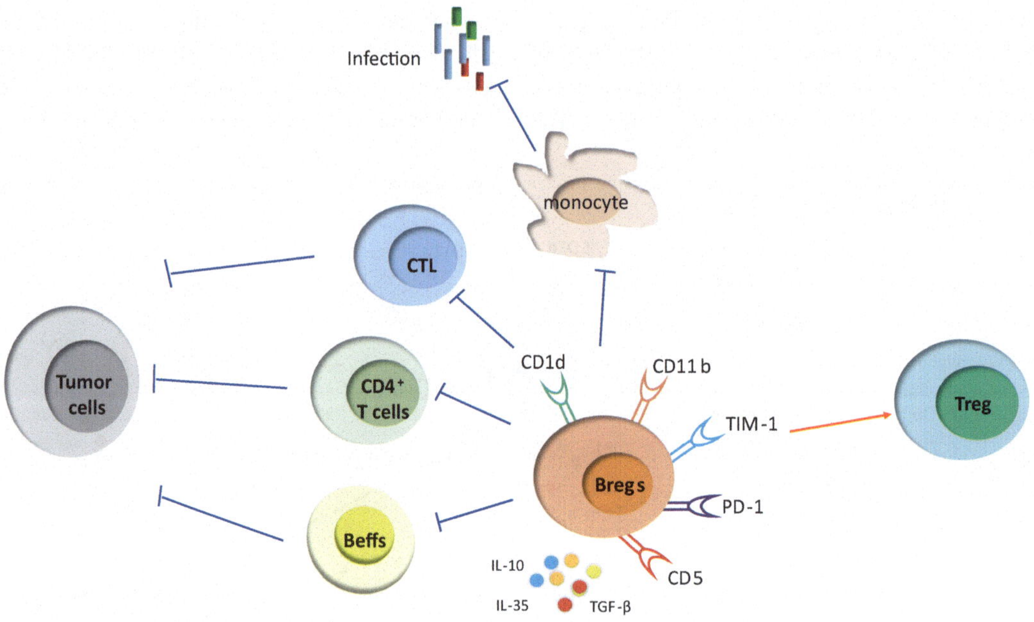

Fig. 8.2 Effects of Breg cells on other immune cells and tumor cells. Breg cells suppress the differentiation of monocytes, $CD4^+$ T cells, and cytotoxic T lymphocytes (CTLs), but promote Treg differentiation by secreting IL-10, IL-35, and TGF-β as well as through cell–cell contact, thereby inhibiting antitumor activity and inflammation

8.4.1 Cytokine-Producing Breg Cell

B cells release a variety of cytokines after stimulation (such as IL-4, IL-6, IL-10, IFN-γ, TNF-α, and TGF-β) and are classified into Breg or Beff subsets depending on cytokine release profile. Although the cellular origins of cytokine-producing B-cell subsets are still unclear and there are no definitive cell surface or transcription factor biomarkers for these cells, accumulating evidence indicates that B cells are critical for both innate and adaptive immune regulations (Bao and Cao 2014). Among them, B cells secreting IL-10, TGF-β, and IL-35 are defined as Breg cells.

It is now widely accepted that most primary Breg-cell functions are dependent on IL-10 expression and release. Indeed, several studies have used IL-10 expression as a marker for Breg cells, and the *il-10* reporter mouse has been used to study the phenotype and molecular mechanisms of immunomodulation by Breg cells. Fillatreau et al. first demonstrated that B cells regulate autoimmunity by IL-10 release. Subsequently, dozens of studies reported the role of IL-10 in B-cell regulation (Fillatreau et al. 2002). It has been reported that LAG-3, STIM1, and MYD88 are involved in mediating B-cell production of IL-10 (Kirkland et al. 2012; Lino et al. 2018; Matsumoto et al. 2011). However, other studies suggest IL-10-independent Breg-cell functions. Teichmann et al. performed lineage-specific deletion of *Il10* from B cells, and found that IL-10^{+} B cells were rare in vivo and that Breg-cell phenotypic subsets, such as CD1d^{hi}CD5^{+} and CD21^{hi}CD23^{lo}, were not enriched in *Il10* transcription (Teichmann et al. 2012), indicating that Breg-cell development does not rely on IL-10. These IL-10-independent mechanisms include promotion and maintenance of Tregs by production of TGF-β, IL-35, IgA, and adenosine as well as by surface expression of CD11b, Tim-1, PD-L1, and FasL (Ray et al. 2012, 2015; Wang et al. 2015; Zhao et al. 2019).

8.4.2 Regulatory Plasma Cells and Anti-Inflammatory Antibodies

Plasmablasts can also suppress inflammatory responses. Maseda et al. reported that splenic B10 cells differentiated into antibody-producing plasmablasts after stimulation in vivo and in vitro (Maseda et al. 2012). Mice deficient in B-cell *Irf4* and *Prdm1* expression exhibited defective plasma cell differentiation, and consequently developed exacerbated EAE (Matsumoto et al. 2014), again suggesting that some antibodies have anti-inflammatory functions. Moreover, IL-10- and IL-35-producing CD138^{+} plasma cells suppressed pro-inflammatory responses during EAE and Salmonella infection (Shen et al. 2014). Matsumoto et al. suggested that human CD19^{+}CD24^{hi}CD38^{hi} B cells are actually IL-10-producing plasmablasts (Matsumoto et al. 2014), and that CD19^{+}CD24^{hi}CD27^{+} Breg cells belong to memory B cells. Antibodies can also induce immunoregulation by B cells, one of the earliest Breg studies found that antibodies can have regulatory functions in vivo (Morris and Moller 1968). IgG4 has been repeatedly implicated in B-cell regulatory function, and IgG4-expressing B cells are confined to the IL-10^{+} B-cell subset in human subjects (Lin et al. 2014, 2017; van de Veen et al. 2013). Our group proposed a role for Breg-cell-derived IgA in maintaining mucosal immunity. In colitis, IgA-expressing B cells maintain intestinal homeostasis and suppress IBD (Wang et al. 2015). Alternatively, these cells may have deleterious effects in cancer by suppressing tumor inflammation, as IgA^{+} B cells promoted colorectal tumors by inhibiting CTLs (Liu et al. 2017).

8.5 Cellular Targets of Breg Cell-Mediated Suppression

8.5.1 Suppression of Effector T Cells

Several disease model studies have demonstrated that controlling the overactivation of $CD4^+$ T cells is one of the most important regulatory functions of B cells (Lund and Randall 2010; Rosser et al. 2014). Adoptive transfer of Breg cells suppresses inflammatory responses and $CD4^+$ T-cell activation. For instance, adoptive transfer of $CD11b^+$ B cells to EAH model mice suppressed $CD4^+$ T-cell proliferation and IFN-γ/TNF-α production, ameliorating the disease (Liu et al. 2015). Moreover, Tim-1^+ Breg cells isolated from mice receiving MHC-mismatched islet allografts prolonged islet graft survival in secondary graft recipients (Ding et al. 2011). The same study reported that $CD4^+$ T cells from graft recipients that received Tim-1^+ Breg cells produced lower levels of IFN-γ and $CD4^+$ T polarization was tend to a type 2 response compared to T cells from control mice (Ding et al. 2011). Similarly, transfer of generated Breg cells which induced by GIFT-15 in vitro, suppressed the function of Teffs and consequently alleviate EAE symptoms (Rafei et al. 2009). In addition, Breg cells can also suppress inflammatory responses by inducing T-cell death. Studies revealed that after LPS stimulation, B cells express Fas ligand (FasL) and TGF-β, induces apoptosis of both B and T cells in diabetic environment (Tian et al. 2001). In addition, studies have found that B1 cells express FasL and target $CD4^+$ T cells for apoptosis in schistosomiasis, preventing the development of schistosome granulomatous disease (Lundy and Boros 2002).

Breg-cell inhibition of $CD8^+$ T cells and suppression of inflammation have been studied extensively in infectious diseases and cancers. In μMT mice, B cells can limit $CD8^+$ T-cell-mediated immune surveillance, resulting in more frequent tumorigenesis (Schioppa et al. 2011). For instance, B-cell-deficient mice were resistant to the development of breast tumors in mouse. The B-cell-deficient mouse has an increased CTL response to breast-tumor antigen, leading to effective clearance of tumor cells (Qin et al. 1998). Similarly, Liu et al. reported that IgA^+ B cells effectively inhibited CTLs, leaded to poor prognosis of colorectal tumors (Liu et al. 2017).

8.5.2 Enhancing the Production of Tregs

Breg cells can also promote the production and activity of Tregs (Chien and Chiang 2018), Breg and Treg cells cooperate to control inflammation in infection (Jeong et al. 2012) and diseases such as EAE (Matsushita et al. 2010). Reichardt et al. found that B-cell-induced Tregs, termed "bTregs," secreted IL-10 and suppressed inflammation. Further, Shao et al. found that $Foxp3^-$IL-10^- bTregs suppress inflammation by expressing high levels of CTLA, GITR, ICOS, LAG3, and OX40, but not IL-10 (Shao et al. 2016). In addition to inducing naive T cells to differentiate into Tregs, B cells can also promote the proliferation of Tregs. In μMT mouse models of oral tolerance and arthritis, reconstitution of wild-type (WT) B cells restored $Foxp3^+$ Treg expansion (Carter et al. 2011; Sun et al. 2008). Moreover, B cells mitigate autoimmune diseases including IBD by promoting Treg proliferation through GITR ligand signaling (Ray et al. 2012; Shao et al. 2016; Wang et al. 2015). In mouse-tumor models, the absence of B lymphocytes reduced the number and function of Tregs, thus enhancing the antitumor response (Tadmor et al. 2011). The therapeutic effects of bTregs have been described in a variety of other mouse disease models, such as allergic asthma (Chu and Chiang 2012), rheumatoid arthritis (Chen et al. 2016), and breast cancer (Olkhanud et al. 2011). These functions in animal models of disease suggest that bTregs are a promising target for broad-based clinical treatments.

8.5.3 B Cells

In many Breg-cell-mediated immunosuppressive animal models, the production of pathogenic antibodies is reduced, which may be the indirect effect of inhibiting helper T cells but may also be the result of Breg-cell acting directly on the antibody-secreting B cells (Rosser et al. 2014). In the rat model of cardiac transplantation, Breg cells inhibited the production of B-cell antibodies. Antibody unable to class switch from IgM to IgG, thus the graft can survive for a long time (Le Texier et al. 2011). Furthermore, adoptive transfer of Breg cells into graft-recipient mice prevented cardiac allograft rejection, and the suppression was related to the decrease in total IgG levels and increase in Th2-related antibody isotype IgG1 (Le Texier et al. 2011). In other animal models of Breg-cell-mediated immunosuppression, the transfer of Breg cells also elicits a similar type 2 antibody response (Evans et al. 2007; Gray et al. 2007; Mauri et al. 2003; Miles et al. 2012). These studies suggest that Breg cells can alter B-cell effector functions directly or indirectly via helper T cells.

8.5.4 Other Cell Targets of Breg Cell-Mediated Suppression

Breg cells have been shown to suppress IL-12 production by dendritic cells (DCs). Lenert et al. reported that MZ B cells from lupus mice produced larger amounts of IL-10 than WT mice, and IL-10 suppressed IL-12 production by total splenocytes in vitro (Lenert et al. 2005). Further studies have shown that CpG-stimulated $CD5^+$ B cells inhibit the response of neonatal DCS to IL-12 in an IL-10-dependent manner, thereby activating Th1 cells. This interaction helps prevent neonatal death by suppressing excessive inflammation after infection (Sun et al. 2005; Zhang et al. 2007). In addition, leishmania infection induces a large number of IL-10-producing B cells in vitro, which reduce IL-12 secretion through DCs (Ronet et al. 2010). In contrast to T cells and DCs, Breg-cell effects on monocytes and macrophages are largely uninvestigated. However, $CD19^{-/-}$ mice lacking $CD1d^{h}iCD5^+$ B cells demonstrated promoted phagocytosis of *Listeria monocytogenes* by macrophages, possibly due to the lack of a Breg-cell response. In vitro, LPS-activated $CD1d^{hi}CD5^+$ B cells suppressed macrophage produced nitric oxide, TNF-α, and IFN-γ production (Horikawa et al. 2013), which may explain the enhanced phagocytosis and cytotoxicity in the absence of Breg cells. This aspect of Breg-cell function warrants more intensive investigation. In tumor and infection models, Breg cells are able to suppress immune responses by natural killer (NK) cells (Bankoti et al. 2012; Inoue et al. 2006). The interaction between B cells and CD40L on tumor cells induces IL-10 production, consequently suppresses NK cell produced IFN-γ (Inoue et al. 2006). Reconstitution of WT B cells into μMT mice restored breast-tumor growth, while inhibited NK cell activity (Inoue et al. 2006). B cells can also inhibit the infiltration of $CD49^+$ NK cells by interacting with Treg cells, thereby preventing the effective elimination of tumor cells in and out of the body (Zhang et al. 2013). Breg-cell-mediated IL-10-dependent suppression of neutrophil responses has also been demonstrated in murine infection models (Neves et al. 2010). Both B-$Myd88^{-/-}$and B-$TLR2^{-/-}$chimeric mice showed defects in the IL-10 response of B cells and increased activity of neutrophils, NK cells and T cells, resulting in more effective clearance of *salmonella typhimurium.* In this model, there were more neutrophils and a high production of TNF-α (Neves et al. 2010).

8.6 Breg Cells in Diseases

Among the most interesting aspects of Breg-cell behavior is expansion and functional activation in disease-associated microenvironments, suggesting contributions to disease pathogenesis or amelioration and underscoring Breg cells as promising targets from immunotherapy.

8.6.1 Breg Cell in Autoimmune Diseases

As described before, the existence of Breg cells was first posited in an autoimmune disease model and their functions have been most extensively studied in various autoimmune disease models and human patients (Rosser and Mauri 2015). B cells and plasma cells are considered the primary drivers of autoimmune diseases through the production of autoantibodies, so B-cell depletion and reduced autoantibody titers should theoretically be an effective treatment. However, such treatments have not demonstrated experimental or clinical success. In fact, Goetz et al. found that ulcerative colitis was exacerbated by depletion of peripheral B cells using rituximab (RTX) (Goetz et al. 2007), and Lehmann-Horn and colleagues found that B-cell depletion accentuated pro-inflammatory reactions in neuroimmunological disorders (Lehmann-Horn et al. 2011). These studies indicate that Breg cells are of vital importance for controlling autoimmune inflammation.

In terms of specific autoimmune diseases, Tedder and colleagues have examined the interactions of regulatory and pathogenic B cells in the EAE disease environment and how Treg and Breg cells contribute to disease progression (Matsushita et al. 2008, 2010). In IBD, the Breg subsets B-1 (Shimomura et al. 2008), $CD19^+CD5^+CD1d^{hi}$ (Yanaba et al. 2011), and CD11b (Wang et al. 2018) have strong inhibitory effects on autoimmune processes when transferred in vivo. Mauri and colleagues suggested that murine tissue-resident T2-MZP cells (Evans et al. 2007) and peripheral blood $CD19^+CD24^+CD38^+$ cells (Flores-Borja et al. 2013) are essential for arthritis remission (Mauri and Menon 2017). In addition, contributions of Breg cells to the amelioration of other autoimmune diseases such as autoimmune hepatitis (Liu et al. 2015) and thyroiditis (Zha et al. 2012) have been suggested.

8.6.2 Breg Cells in Cancer

In B-cell- or Breg-cell-deficient mice, enhanced antitumor immunity is associated with increased activity of CTLs (Liu et al. 2017) and NK cells (Terabe et al. 2005). The antitumor effects of immune cells are suppressed by IL-10 and TGF-β produced by B cells (Cai et al. 2019; Inoue et al. 2006; Liu et al. 2017). For instance, in ovarian cancer, Breg cells significantly suppressed IFN-γ production by CTLs via IL-10 release (Wei et al. 2016). Breg cells also promote the transformation of naïve T cells into Tregs through TGF-β release, which in turn inhibits the proliferation of CTLs and increases tumor metastasis (Olkhanud et al. 2011). In the mouse model of breast cancer, tumor-environment-induced Breg cells produced TGF-β and conversion of Teffs to Tregs, suppressing the proliferation of T cells and NK cells (Zhang et al. 2016). Similarly, PD-1 transforms B cells into Breg cells, resulting in the suppression of tumor-specific T cells and the promotion of human hepatoma growth (Ren et al. 2016). Also, tumor cells can convert normal B cells into Breg cells, inhibiting the antitumor immune process (Olkhanud et al. 2011). Nonmetastatic cancer cells express and utilize metabolites of the 5-lipoxygenase (5-LO) pathway to induce generation of Breg (Wejksza et al. 2013). Similarly, glioma cell-derived placenta growth factors (PlGFs) can induce Breg cells to suppress $CD8^+$ T-cell antitumor activities (Ye et al. 2014). Moreover, GrB^+ Breg cells are found in many tumor microenvironments, where they contribute to escape from the antitumor immune response (Lindner et al. 2013). Collectively, these results suggest that Breg cells suppress immune responses to murine and human tumors and thus may contribute to carcinogenesis, progression, and metastasis.

8.6.3 Breg Cell in Transplantation

Breg-cell transplantation is a potential strategy for enhancing graft tolerance (Chu et al. 2018; Li et al. 2019a; Mohib et al. 2018; Wortel and Heidt 2017). In two recent clinical studies, a few patients with stable graft function for years after immunosuppressive drug withdrawal demonstrated greater absolute numbers and proportions of peripheral B cells compared to recipients with graft rejection (Chesneau et al. 2013; Viklicky et al. 2013). In addition, B-cell depletion with RTX can promote transplant rejection. For example, B-cell depletion plus RTX treatment accelerated allograft rejection in a skin graft model (DiLillo et al. 2011; Marino et al. 2016). Alternatively, B cells reconstituted after depletion, differentiated into an immunosuppressive phenotype and promoted long-term survival of allogeneic islets in a nonhuman primate model (Liu et al. 2007). Moreover, the stimulated transitional B cells from graft-tolerant patients expressed higher levels of IL-10, suggesting that Breg cells may help prevent rejection following organ transplantation (Chesneau et al. 2013).

A number of experimental tolerogenic agents, including anti-TIM-1, anti-TIM-4, and anti-CD45, all require B cells for tolerance induction in mice (Ding et al. 2011, 2017; Lee et al. 2012). For instance, anti-TIM1 Ab induced transplant tolerance to allogeneic islets only when B cells were present in recipients (Lee et al. 2012). Furthermore, the synergistic effect of combining anti-CD45RB with anti-TIM1 mAbs for tolerance of allogeneic islets also depended on the presence of recipient B cells (Lee et al. 2012). Mice T2 B cells that tolerant to MHC-mismatched skin grafts expressed lower levels of CD86 and higher levels of TIM-1, and transfer of T2 B cells prolonged skin allograft survival by suppression T-cell activation (Moreau et al. 2015).

8.6.4 Breg Cell in Infection

Breg cells also modulate inflammatory responses to parasitic, viral, and bacterial infections. In *Babesia microti* infection, B cells produce more IL-10 and adoptive transfer of IL-10-producing B cells increases the susceptibility to infection (Jeong et al. 2012). The functions of Breg cells in bacterial infection have been investigated mainly using B-cell-deficient mouse models (lMT, JHD, or JHT). Breg cells can be either beneficial or deleterious for infection outcome due to functional diversity. For instance, Breg cells can either suppress anti-infective immunity and/or overactive cellular immunity (Fillatreau 2011). Virus such as HIV and HBV can induce the development of IL-10-producing B cells, which are able to inhibit effective anti-HIV-1 T-cell responses (Liu et al. 2014). Multiple subsets of Breg cell are induced by infection; for instance, peritoneal B-1 cells produce high levels of IL-10 upon stimulation by TLR ligands (Sindhava et al. 2010). Marginal zone B cells (MZBs) participate in the early immune response to several pathogens. Bankoti et al. (2012) reported that depletion of MZBs enhanced T-cell responses and led to insufficient resistance to parasitic infections.

8.6.5 Other Conditions

Pregnancy also influences the development and function of Breg cells. The pregnancy-associated hormones estradiol, progesterone, and human chorionic gonadotropin are known to suppress the capacity of both innate and adaptive immune cells (Guzman-Genuino and Diener 2017; Lima et al. 2016; Muzzio et al. 2014). In a murine model of pregnancy loss, Jensen et al. reported that $CD19^{+}CD5^{+}CD1d^{+}$ B cells were diminished in abortion-prone animals, while transfer of IL-10-producing Breg cells prevented fetal rejection (Jensen et al. 2013). This same group found that $CD19^{+}CD24^{hi}CD27^{+}$ Breg-cell number increased during the first trimester of human pregnancy, while cell numbers in spontaneous abortion patients remained as low as in non-pregnant women (Rolle et al. 2013). It is not yet clear why Breg-cell numbers change during pregnancy. B cells express receptors for hormones and are critical regulators of immune status during pregnancy. Further studies on the effects of pregnancy-associated hormones on regulatory B cells may facilitate novel preventative treatments for spontaneous abortion (Muzzio et al. 2014).

8.7 Breg Cell-Targeted Therapies

Studies on Breg cells in health and disease have provided compelling evidence for possible therapeutic applications. However, since the phenotype and transcription factors are not yet clear, there have been no clinical trials on Breg cell-based treatments. Several studies have shown that

RTX therapy induces repopulation of B10 cells. Sun et al. demonstrated that RTX therapy for MG delayed IL-10-producing cell repopulation (Sun et al. 2013). Targeting Breg cells may benefit multiple sclerosis and colitis (Goetz et al. 2007; Lehmann-Horn et al. 2013). Many studies in humans have shown significant changes in the number of Breg cells over the course of disease, suggesting that Breg cells are crucial to disease progression (Mauri and Blair 2014). Moreover, numerous studies in murine models clearly demonstrate that transferring B cells with induced regulatory function can effectively mitigate disease processes (Matsushita 2019; Zhao et al. 2019). Given this clinical potential, it is critical to identify biomarkers for more precise phenotypic analysis and purification of Breg cells.

8.8 Conclusions and Outstanding Questions

While Breg cells may have a myriad of clinical applications, clinical trials are hampered by the lack of reliable biomarkers and distinct phenotypes. In fact, Breg-cell subsets are most likely B-cell populations induced by specific inflammatory environments during disease. Therefore, there are many questions to be solved before such therapeutic applications can be considered, such as what biomarkers can be used for identification and purification, what transcription factors control differentiation, and the precise environmental conditions required for Breg-cell differentiation. Moreover, it must be determined if these processes are organ- and disease-specific. Also, the metabolic and epigenetic pathways involved in Breg-cell differentiation must be elucidated. Answers to these questions could facilitate the development of Breg-cell-based immunotherapies for a variety of diseases, including autoimmune disorders, other inflammatory disorders, and cancer.

References

Bankoti R, Gupta K, Levchenko A, Stager S (2012) Marginal zone B cells regulate antigen-specific T cell responses during infection. J Immunol 188:3961–3971

Bao Y, Cao X (2014) The immune potential and immunopathology of cytokine-producing B cell subsets: a comprehensive review. J Autoimmun 55:10–23

Berthelot JM, Jamin C, Amrouche K, Le Goff B, Maugars Y, Youinou P (2013) Regulatory B cells play a key role in immune system balance. Joint Bone Spine 80:18–22

Blair PA, Chavez-Rueda KA, Evans JG, Shlomchik MJ, Eddaoudi A, Isenberg DA, Ehrenstein MR, Mauri C (2009) Selective targeting of B cells with agonistic anti-CD40 is an efficacious strategy for the generation of induced regulatory T2-like B cells and for the suppression of lupus in MRL/lpr mice. J Immunol 182:3492–3502

Blair PA, Norena LY, Flores-Borja F, Rawlings DJ, Isenberg DA, Ehrenstein MR, Mauri C (2010) CD19 (+)CD24(hi)CD38(hi) B cells exhibit regulatory capacity in healthy individuals but are functionally impaired in systemic Lupus Erythematosus patients. Immunity 32:129–140

Bouaziz JD, Calbo S, Maho-Vaillant M, Saussine A, Bagot M, Bensussan A, Musette P (2010) IL-10 produced by activated human B cells regulates CD4 (+) T-cell activation in vitro. Eur J Immunol 40:2686–2691

Cai X, Zhang L, Wei W (2019) Regulatory B cells in inflammatory diseases and tumor. Int Immunopharmacol 67:281–286

Carter NA, Vasconcellos R, Rosser EC, Tulone C, Munoz-Suano A, Kamanaka M, Ehrenstein MR, Flavell RA, Mauri C (2011) Mice lacking endogenous IL-10-producing regulatory B cells develop exacerbated disease and present with an increased frequency of Th1/Th17 but a decrease in regulatory T cells. J Immunol 186:5569–5579

Chen SY, Hsu WT, Chen YL, Chien CH, Chiang BL (2016) Lymphocyte-activation gene 3(+) (LAG3(+)) forkhead box protein 3(-) (FOXP3(-)) regulatory T cells induced by B cells alleviates joint inflammation in collagen-induced arthritis. J Autoimmun 68:75–85

Chen Y, Li C, Lu Y, Zhuang H, Gu W, Liu B, Liu F, Sun J, Yan B, Weng D, Chen J (2017) IL-10-producing CD1d(hi)CD5(+) regulatory B cells may play a critical role in modulating immune homeostasis in silicosis patients. Front Immunol 8:110

Chesneau M, Michel L, Degauque N, Brouard S (2013) Regulatory B cells and tolerance in transplantation: from animal models to human. Front Immunol 4:497

Chien CH, Chiang BL (2018) Recent advances in regulatory T cells induced by B cells. Cell Mol Immunol 15:539–541

Chu KH, Chiang BL (2012) Regulatory T cells induced by mucosal B cells alleviate allergic airway hypersensitivity. Am J Respir Cell Mol Biol 46:651–659

Chu Z, Zou W, Xu Y, Sun Q, Zhao Y (2018) The regulatory roles of B cell subsets in transplantation. Expert Rev Clin Immunol 14:115–125

De-Gennaro LA, Popi AF, Almeida SR, Lopes JD, Mariano M (2009) B-1 cells modulate oral tolerance in mice. Immunol Lett 124:63–69

de Masson A, Bouaziz JD, Le Buanec H, Robin M, O'Meara A, Parquet N, Rybojad M, Hau E, Monfort JB, Branchtein M et al (2015) CD24(hi)CD27(+) and plasmablast-like regulatory B cells in human chronic graft-versus-host disease. Blood 125:1830–1839

DiLillo DJ, Griffiths R, Seshan SV, Magro CM, Ruiz P, Coffman TM, Tedder TF (2011) B lymphocytes differentially influence acute and chronic allograft rejection in mice. J Immunol 186:2643–2654

Ding Q, Mohib K, Kuchroo VK, Rothstein DM (2017) TIM-4 identifies IFN-gamma-expressing proinflammatory B effector 1 cells that promote tumor and allograft rejection. J Immunol 199:2585–2595

Ding Q, Yeung M, Camirand G, Zeng Q, Akiba H, Yagita H, Chalasani G, Sayegh MH, Najafian N, Rothstein DM (2011) Regulatory B cells are identified by expression of TIM-1 and can be induced through TIM-1 ligation to promote tolerance in mice. J Clin Invest 121:3645–3656

Evans JG, Chavez-Rueda KA, Eddaoudi A, Meyer-Bahlburg A, Rawlings DJ, Ehrenstein MR, Mauri C (2007) Novel suppressive function of transitional 2 B cells in experimental arthritis. J Immunol 178:7868–7878

Fillatreau S (2011) Novel regulatory functions for toll-like receptor-activated B cells during intracellular bacterial infection. Immunol Rev 240:52–71

Fillatreau S, Sweenie CH, McGeachy MJ, Gray D, Anderton SM (2002) B cells regulate autoimmunity by provision of IL-10. Nat Immunol 3:944–950

Flores-Borja F, Bosma A, Ng D, Reddy V, Ehrenstein MR, Isenberg DA, Mauri C (2013) CD19+CD24hiCD38hi B cells maintain regulatory T cells while limiting TH1 and TH17 differentiation. Sci Transl Med 5:173ra123

Goetz M, Atreya R, Ghalibafian M, Galle PR, Neurath MF (2007) Exacerbation of ulcerative colitis after rituximab salvage therapy. Inflamm Bowel Dis 13:1365–1368

Gray M, Miles K, Salter D, Gray D, Savill J (2007) Apoptotic cells protect mice from autoimmune inflammation by the induction of regulatory B cells. Proc Natl Acad Sci USA 104:14080–14085

Guo Y, Zhang X, Qin M, Wang X (2015) Changes in peripheral CD19(+)Foxp3(+) and CD19(+)TGFbeta(+) regulatory B cell populations in rheumatoid arthritis patients with interstitial lung disease. J Thorac Dis 7:471–477

Guzman-Genuino RM, Diener KR (2017) Regulatory B cells in pregnancy: lessons from autoimmunity, graft tolerance, and cancer. Front Immunol 8:172

Hasan MM, Thompson-Snipes L, Klintmalm G, Demetris AJ, O'Leary J, Oh S, Joo H (2019) CD24(hi)CD38(hi) and CD24(hi)CD27(+) human regulatory B cells display common and distinct functional characteristics. J Immunol 203:2110–2120

Horikawa M, Weimer ET, DiLillo DJ, Venturi GM, Spolski R, Leonard WJ, Heise MT, Tedder TF (2013) Regulatory B cell (B10 Cell) expansion during Listeria infection governs innate and cellular immune responses in mice. J Immunol 190:1158–1168

Inoue S, Leitner WW, Golding B, Scott D (2006) Inhibitory effects of B cells on antitumor immunity. Cancer Res 66:7741–7747

Iwata Y, Matsushita T, Horikawa M, Dilillo DJ, Yanaba K, Venturi GM, Szabolcs PM, Bernstein SH, Magro CM, Williams AD et al (2011) Characterization of a rare IL-10-competent B-cell subset in humans that parallels mouse regulatory B10 cells. Blood 117:530–541

Jensen F, Muzzio D, Soldati R, Fest S, Zenclussen AC (2013) Regulatory B10 cells restore pregnancy tolerance in a mouse model. Biol Reprod 89(4):90

Jeong YI, Hong SH, Cho SH, Lee WJ, Lee SE (2012) Induction of IL-10-producing CD1dhighCD5+ regulatory B cells following Babesia microti-infection. PLoS ONE 7:e46553

Kaku H, Cheng KF, Al-Abed Y, Rothstein TL (2014) A novel mechanism of B cell-mediated immune suppression through CD73 expression and adenosine production. J Immunol 193:5904–5913

Kalampokis I, Yoshizaki A, Tedder TF (2013) IL-10-producing regulatory B cells (B10 cells) in autoimmune disease. Arthritis Res Ther 15(Suppl 1):S1

Katz SI, Parker D, Turk JL (1974) B-cell suppression of delayed hypersensitivity reactions. Nature 251:550–551

Kennedy MW, Thomas DB (1983) A regulatory role for the memory B cell as suppressor-inducer of feedback control. J Exp Med 157:547–558

Kirkland D, Benson A, Mirpuri J, Pifer R, Hou B, DeFranco AL, Yarovinsky F (2012) B cell-intrinsic MyD88 signaling prevents the lethal dissemination of commensal bacteria during colonic damage. Immunity 36:228–238

Le Texier L, Thebault P, Lavault A, Usal C, Merieau E, Quillard T, Charreau B, Soulillou JP, Cuturi MC, Brouard S, Chiffoleau E (2011) Long-term allograft tolerance is characterized by the accumulation of B

cells exhibiting an inhibited profile. Am J Transplant 11:429–438
Lee KM, Kim JI, Stott R, Soohoo J, O'Connor MR, Yeh H, Zhao G, Eliades P, Fox C, Cheng N et al (2012) Anti-CD45RB/anti-TIM-1-induced tolerance requires regulatory B cells. Am J Transplant 12:2072–2078
Lehmann-Horn K, Kronsbein HC, Weber MS (2013) Targeting B cells in the treatment of multiple sclerosis: recent advances and remaining challenges. Ther Adv Neurol Disord 6:161–173
Lehmann-Horn K, Schleich E, Hertzenberg D, Hapfelmeier A, Kumpfel T, von Bubnoff N, Hohlfeld R, Berthele A, Hemmer B, Weber MS (2011) Anti-CD20 B-cell depletion enhances monocyte reactivity in neuroimmunological disorders. J Neuroinflammation 8:146
Lenert P, Brummel R, Field EH, Ashman RF (2005) TLR-9 activation of marginal zone B cells in lupus mice regulates immunity through increased IL-10 production. J Clin Immunol 25:29–40
Li J, Luo Y, Wang X, Feng G (2019a) Regulatory B cells and advances in transplantation. J Leukoc Biol 105:657–668
Li T, Yu Z, Qu Z, Zhang N, Crew R, Jiang Y (2019b) Decreased number of CD19(+)CD24(hi)CD38(hi) regulatory B cells in diabetic nephropathy. Mol Immunol 112:233–239
Lima J, Martins C, Leandro MJ, Nunes G, Sousa MJ, Branco JC, Borrego LM (2016) Characterization of B cells in healthy pregnant women from late pregnancy to post-partum: a prospective observational study. BMC Pregnancy Childbirth 16:139
Lin W, Jin L, Chen H, Wu Q, Fei Y, Zheng W, Wang Q, Li P, Li Y, Zhang W et al (2014) B cell subsets and dysfunction of regulatory B cells in IgG4-related diseases and primary Sjogren's syndrome: the similarities and differences. Arthritis Res Ther 16:R118
Lin W, Zhang P, Chen H, Chen Y, Yang H, Zheng W, Zhang X, Zhang F, Zhang W, Lipsky PE (2017) Circulating plasmablasts/plasma cells: a potential biomarker for IgG4-related disease. Arthritis Res Ther 19:25
Lindner S, Dahlke K, Sontheimer K, Hagn M, Kaltenmeier C, Barth TF, Beyer T, Reister F, Fabricius D, Lotfi R et al (2013) Interleukin 21-induced granzyme B-expressing B cells infiltrate tumors and regulate T cells. Cancer Res 73:2468–2479
Lino AC, Dang VD, Lampropoulou V, Welle A, Joedicke J, Pohar J, Simon Q, Thalmensi J, Baures A, Fluhler V et al (2018) LAG-3 inhibitory receptor expression identifies immunosuppressive natural regulatory plasma cells. Immunity 49(120–133):e129
Liu C, Noorchashm H, Sutter JA, Naji M, Prak EL, Boyer J, Green T, Rickels MR, Tomaszewski JE, Koeberlein B et al (2007) B lymphocyte-directed immunotherapy promotes long-term islet allograft survival in nonhuman primates. Nat Med 13:1295–1298
Liu J, Zhan W, Kim CJ, Clayton K, Zhao H, Lee E, Cao JC, Ziegler B, Gregor A, Yue FY et al (2014) IL-10-producing B cells are induced early in HIV-1 infection and suppress HIV-1-specific T cell responses. PLoS ONE 9:e89236
Liu R, Lu Z, Gu J, Liu J, Huang E, Liu X, Wang L, Yang J, Deng Y, Qian J et al (2017) MicroRNAs 15A and 16-1 activate signaling pathways that mediate chemotaxis of immune regulatory B cells to colorectal tumors. Gastroenterology 154:637–651
Liu X, Jiang X, Liu R, Wang L, Qian T, Zheng Y, Deng Y, Huang E, Xu F, Chu Y (2015). B cells expressing CD11b effectively inhibit CD4 T cell responses and ameliorate experimental autoimmune hepatitis. Hepatology 62:1563–1575
Lund FE, Randall TD (2010) Effector and regulatory B cells: modulators of CD4(+) T cell immunity. Nat Rev Immunol 10:236–247
Lundy SK, Boros DL (2002) Fas ligand-expressing B-1a lymphocytes mediate CD4(+)-T-cell apoptosis during schistosomal infection: induction by interleukin 4 (IL-4) and IL-10. Infect Immun 70:812–819
Marino J, Paster JT, Trowell A, Maxwell L, Briggs KH, Crosby Bertorini P, Benichou G (2016) B cell depletion with an anti-CD20 antibody enhances alloreactive memory T cell responses after transplantation. Am J Transplant 16:672–678
Maseda D, Smith SH, DiLillo DJ, Bryant JM, Candando KM, Weaver CT, Tedder TF (2012) Regulatory B10 cells differentiate into antibody-secreting cells after transient IL-10 production in vivo. J Immunol 188:1036–1048
Matsumoto M, Baba A, Yokota T, Nishikawa H, Ohkawa Y, Kayama H, Kallies A, Nutt SL, Sakaguchi S, Takeda K et al (2014) Interleukin-10-producing plasmablasts exert regulatory function in autoimmune inflammation. Immunity 41:1040–1051
Matsumoto M, Fujii Y, Baba A, Hikida M, Kurosaki T, Baba Y (2011) The calcium sensors STIM1 and STIM2 control B cell regulatory function through interleukin-10 production. Immunity 34:703–714
Matsushita T (2019) Regulatory and effector B cells: friends or foes? J Dermatol Sci 93:2–7
Matsushita T, Horikawa M, Iwata Y, Tedder TF (2010) Regulatory B cells (B10 cells) and regulatory T cells have independent roles in controlling experimental autoimmune encephalomyelitis initiation and late-phase immunopathogenesis. J Immunol 185:2240–2252
Matsushita T, Tedder TF (2011) Identifying regulatory B cells (B10 cells) that produce IL-10 in mice. Methods Mol Biol 677:99–111
Matsushita T, Yanaba K, Bouaziz JD, Fujimoto M, Tedder TF (2008) Regulatory B cells inhibit EAE initiation in mice while other B cells promote disease progression. J Clin Invest 118:3420–3430
Mauri C, Blair PA (2014) Editorial: regulatory B cells: are we really ready to manipulate them for the benefit of patients with autoimmune diseases? Arthritis Rheumatol 66:1982–1983

Mauri C, Gray D, Mushtaq N, Londei M (2003) Prevention of arthritis by interleukin 10-producing B cells. J Exp Med 197:489–501

Mauri C, Menon M (2017) Human regulatory B cells in health and disease: therapeutic potential. J Clin Invest 127:772–779

Miles K, Heaney J, Sibinska Z, Salter D, Savill J, Gray D, Gray M (2012) A tolerogenic role for toll-like receptor 9 is revealed by B-cell interaction with DNA complexes expressed on apoptotic cells. Proc Natl Acad Sci USA 109:887–892

Mizoguchi A, Mizoguchi E, Smith RN, Preffer FI, Bhan AK (1997) Suppressive role of B cells in chronic colitis of T cell receptor alpha mutant mice. J Exp Med 186:1749–1756

Mizoguchi A, Mizoguchi E, Takedatsu H, Blumberg RS, Bhan AK (2002) Chronic intestinal inflammatory condition generates IL-10-producing regulatory B cell subset characterized by CD1d upregulation. Immunity 16:219–230

Mohib K, Cherukuri A, Rothstein DM (2018) Regulatory B cells and transplantation: almost prime time? Curr Opin Organ Transplant 23:524–532

Moreau A, Blair PA, Chai JG, Ratnasothy K, Stolarczyk E, Alhabbab R, Rackham CL, Jones PM, Smyth L, Elgueta R et al (2015) Transitional-2 B cells acquire regulatory function during tolerance induction and contribute to allograft survival. Eur J Immunol 45:843–853

Morris A, Moller G (1968) Regulation of cellular antibody synthesis effect of adoptively transferred antibody-producing spleen cells on cellular antibody synthesis. J Immunol 101:439–445

Muzzio D, Zygmunt M, Jensen F (2014) The role of pregnancy-associated hormones in the development and function of regulatory B cells. Front Endocrinol 5:39

Neta R, Salvin SB (1974) Specific suppression of delayed hypersensitivity: the possible presence of a suppressor B cell in the regulation of delayed hypersensitivity. J Immunol 113:1716–1725

Neves P, Lampropoulou V, Calderon-Gomez E, Roch T, Stervbo U, Shen P, Kuhl AA, Loddenkemper C, Haury M, Nedospasov SA et al (2010) Signaling via the MyD88 adaptor protein in B cells suppresses protective immunity during Salmonella typhimurium infection. Immunity 33:777–790

Noh J, Choi WS, Noh G, Lee JH (2010) Presence of Foxp3-expressing CD19(+)CD5(+) B cells in human peripheral blood mononuclear cells: human CD19(+) CD5(+)Foxp3(+) regulatory B cell (Breg). Immune Netw 10:247–249

Olkhanud PB, Damdinsuren B, Bodogai M, Gress RE, Sen R, Wejksza K, Malchinkhuu E, Wersto RP, Biragyn A (2011) Tumor-evoked regulatory B cells promote breast cancer metastasis by converting resting CD4(+) T cells to T-regulatory cells. Cancer Res 71:3505–3515

Qian T, Hong J, Wang L, Wang Z, Lu Z, Li Y, Liu R, Chu Y (2019) Regulation of CD11b by HIF-1alpha and the STAT3 signaling pathway contributes to the immunosuppressive function of B cells in inflammatory bowel disease. Mol Immunol 111:162–171

Qin Z, Richter G, Schuler T, Ibe S, Cao X, Blankenstein T (1998) B cells inhibit induction of T cell-dependent tumor immunity. Nat Med 4:627–630

Rafei M, Hsieh J, Zehntner S, Li M, Forner K, Birman E, Boivin MN, Young YK, Perreault C, Galipeau J (2009) A granulocyte-macrophage colony-stimulating factor and interleukin-15 fusokine induces a regulatory B cell population with immune suppressive properties. Nat Med 15:1038–1045

Ray A, Basu S, Williams CB, Salzman NH, Dittel BN (2012) A novel IL-10-independent regulatory role for B cells in suppressing autoimmunity by maintenance of regulatory T cells via GITR ligand. J Immunol 188:3188–3198

Ray A, Wang L, Dittel BN (2015) IL-10-independent regulatory B-cell subsets and mechanisms of action. Int Immunol 27:531–536

Ren Z, Peng H, Fu YX (2016) PD-1 shapes B cells as evildoers in the tumor microenvironment. Cancer Discov 6:477–478

Rolle L, Memarzadeh Tehran M, Morell-Garcia A, Raeva Y, Schumacher A, Hartig R, Costa SD, Jensen F, Zenclussen AC (2013) Cutting edge: IL-10-producing regulatory B cells in early human pregnancy. Am J Reprod Immunol 70:448–453

Ronet C, Hauyon-La Torre Y, Revaz-Breton M, Mastelic B, Tacchini-Cottier F, Louis J, Launois P (2010) Regulatory B cells shape the development of Th2 immune responses in BALB/c mice infected with Leishmania major through IL-10 production. J Immunol 184:886–894

Rosser EC, Blair PA, Mauri C (2014) Cellular targets of regulatory B cell-mediated suppression. Mol Immunol 62:296–304

Rosser EC, Mauri C (2015) Regulatory B cells: origin, phenotype, and function. Immunity 42:607–612

Schioppa T, Moore R, Thompson RG, Rosser EC, Kulbe H, Nedospasov S, Mauri C, Coussens LM, Balkwill FR (2011) B regulatory cells and the tumor-promoting actions of TNF-alpha during squamous carcinogenesis. Proc Natl Acad Sci USA 108:10662–10667

Shao TY, Hsu LH, Chien CH, Chiang BL (2016) Novel Foxp3(-) IL-10(-) regulatory T-cells induced by B-cells alleviate intestinal inflammation in vivo. Sci Rep 6:32415

Shen P, Roch T, Lampropoulou V, O'Connor RA, Stervbo U, Hilgenberg E, Ries S, Dang VD, Jaimes Y, Daridon C et al (2014) IL-35-producing B cells are critical regulators of immunity during autoimmune and infectious diseases. Nature 507:366–370

Sheng JR, Quan S, Soliven B (2015) IL-10 derived from CD1d(hi)CD5(+) B cells regulates experimental autoimmune myasthenia gravis. J Neuroimmunol 289:130–138

Shimomura Y, Mizoguchi E, Sugimoto K, Kibe R, Benno Y, Mizoguchi A, Bhan AK (2008) Regulatory role of B-1 B cells in chronic colitis. Int Immunol 20:729–737

Sindhava V, Woodman ME, Stevenson B, Bondada S (2010) Interleukin-10 mediated autoregulation of murine B-1 B-cells and its role in Borrelia hermsii infection. PLoS ONE 5:e11445

Sun CM, Deriaud E, Leclerc C, Lo-Man R (2005) Upon TLR9 signaling, CD5+ B cells control the IL-12-dependent Th1-priming capacity of neonatal DCs. Immunity 22:467–477

Sun F, Ladha SS, Yang L, Liu Q, Shi SX, Su N, Bomprezzi R, Shi FD (2013) Interleukin-10 producing-B cells and their association with responsiveness to rituximab in myasthenia gravis. Muscle Nerve 49:487–494

Sun JB, Flach CF, Czerkinsky C, Holmgren J (2008) B lymphocytes promote expansion of regulatory T cells in oral tolerance: powerful induction by antigen coupled to cholera toxin B subunit. J Immunol 181:8278–8287

Tadmor T, Zhang Y, Cho HM, Podack ER, Rosenblatt JD (2011) The absence of B lymphocytes reduces the number and function of T-regulatory cells and enhances the anti-tumor response in a murine tumor model. Cancer Immunol Immunother 60:609–619

Tedder TF, Leonard WJ (2014) Autoimmunity: regulatory B cells–IL-35 and IL-21 regulate the regulators. Nat Rev Rheumatol 10:452–453

Teichmann LL, Kashgarian M, Weaver CT, Roers A, Muller W, Shlomchik MJ (2012) B cell-derived IL-10 does not regulate spontaneous systemic autoimmunity in MRL.Fas(lpr) mice. J Immunol 188:678–685

Terabe M, Swann J, Ambrosino E, Sinha P, Takaku S, Hayakawa Y, Godfrey DI, Ostrand-Rosenberg S, Smyth MJ, Berzofsky JA (2005) A nonclassical non-Valpha14Jalpha18 CD1d-restricted (type II) NKT cell is sufficient for down-regulation of tumor immunosurveillance. J Exp Med 202:1627–1633

Tian J, Zekzer D, Hanssen L, Lu Y, Olcott A, Kaufman DL (2001) Lipopolysaccharide-activated B cells down-regulate Th1 immunity and prevent autoimmune diabetes in nonobese diabetic mice. J Immunol 167:1081–1089

Vadasz Z, Toubi E (2016) FoxP3 expression in macrophages, cancer, and B cells-is it real? Clin Rev Allergy Immunol 52(3):364–372

van de Veen W, Stanic B, Yaman G, Wawrzyniak M, Sollner S, Akdis DG, Ruckert B, Akdis CA, Akdis M (2013) IgG4 production is confined to human IL-10-producing regulatory B cells that suppress antigen-specific immune responses. J Allergy Clin Immunol 131:1204–1212

Viklicky O, Krystufkova E, Brabcova I, Sekerkova A, Wohlfahrt P, Hribova P, Wohlfahrtova M, Sawitzki B, Slatinska J, Striz I et al (2013) B-cell-related biomarkers of tolerance are up-regulated in rejection-free kidney transplant recipients. Transplantation 95: 148–154

Wang L, Ray A, Jiang X, Wang JY, Basu S, Liu X, Qian T, He R, Dittel BN, Chu Y (2015) T regulatory cells and B cells cooperate to form a regulatory loop that maintains gut homeostasis and suppresses dextran sulfate sodium-induced colitis. Mucosal Immunol 8:1297–1312

Wang RX, Yu CR, Dambuza IM, Mahdi RM, Dolinska MB, Sergeev YV, Wingfield PT, Kim SH, Egwuagu CE (2014) Interleukin-35 induces regulatory B cells that suppress autoimmune disease. Nat Med 20:633–641

Wang X, Wang G, Wang Z, Liu B, Han N, Li J, Lu C, Liu X, Zhang Q, Yang Q, Wang G (2019) PD-1-expressing B cells suppress CD4(+) and CD8(+) T cells via PD-1/PD-L1-dependent pathway. Mol Immunol 109:20–26

Wang Z, Zhang H, Liu R, Qian T, Liu J, Huang E, Lu Z, Zhao C, Wang L, Chu Y (2018) Peyer's patches-derived CD11b(+) B cells recruit regulatory T cells through CXCL9 in DSS-induced colitis. Immunology 155:356–366

Watanabe R, Ishiura N, Nakashima H, Kuwano Y, Okochi H, Tamaki K, Sato S, Tedder TF, Fujimoto M (2010) Regulatory B cells (B10 cells) have a suppressive role in murine lupus: CD19 and B10 cell deficiency exacerbates systemic autoimmunity. J Immunol 184:4801–4809

Wei X, Jin Y, Tian Y, Zhang H, Wu J, Lu W, Lu X (2016) Regulatory B cells contribute to the impaired antitumor immunity in ovarian cancer patients. Tumour Biol: J Int Soc Oncodevelopmental Biol Med 37:6581–6588

Wejksza K, Lee-Chang C, Bodogai M, Bonzo J, Gonzalez FJ, Lehrmann E, Becker K, Biragyn A (2013) Cancer-produced metabolites of 5-lipoxygenase induce tumor-evoked regulatory B cells via peroxisome proliferator-activated receptor alpha. J Immunol 190:2575–2584

Wolf SD, Dittel BN, Hardardottir F, Janeway CA Jr (1996) Experimental autoimmune encephalomyelitis induction in genetically B cell-deficient mice. J Exp Med 184:2271–2278

Wortel CM, Heidt S (2017) Regulatory B cells: phenotype, function and role in transplantation. Transpl Immunol 41:1–9

Xiao S, Brooks CR, Sobel RA, Kuchroo VK (2015) Tim-1 is essential for induction and maintenance of IL-10 in regulatory B cells and their regulation of tissue inflammation. J Immunol 194:1602–1608

Xiao S, Brooks CR, Zhu C, Wu C, Sweere JM, Petecka S, Yeste A, Quintana FJ, Ichimura T, Sobel RA et al (2012) Defect in regulatory B-cell function and development of systemic autoimmunity in T-cell Ig mucin 1 (Tim-1) mucin domain-mutant mice. Proc Natl Acad Sci USA 109:12105–12110

Xiao X, Lao XM, Chen MM, Liu RX, Wei Y, Ouyang FZ, Chen DP, Zhao XY, Zhao Q, Li XF et al (2016) PD-1hi Identifies a novel regulatory B-cell population in human hepatoma that promotes disease progression. Cancer Discov 6:546–559

Xing C, Ma N, Xiao H, Wang X, Zheng M, Han G, Chen G, Hou C, Shen B, Li Y, Wang R (2014) Critical role for thymic CD19+CD5+CD1dhiIL-10+ regulatory B cells in immune homeostasis. J Leukoc Biol 97 (3):547–556

Yanaba K, Bouaziz JD, Haas KM, Poe JC, Fujimoto M, Tedder TF (2008) A regulatory B cell subset with a unique CD1dhiCD5+ phenotype controls T cell-dependent inflammatory responses. Immunity 28:639–650

Yanaba K, Yoshizaki A, Asano Y, Kadono T, Tedder TF, Sato S (2011) IL-10-producing regulatory B10 cells inhibit intestinal injury in a mouse model. Am J Pathol 178:735–743

Yang J, Li W, Luo F, Zhao N, Zhang W, Zhang D, Qian J, Yu Y, Zheng X, Wang Y et al (2015) Low percentage of CD24hiCD27(+)CD19(+) B cells decelerates gastric cancer progression in XELOX-treated patients. Int Immunopharmacol 26:322–327

Yang M, Du C, Wang Y, Liu J (2017) Increased CD19 +CD24+CD27+ B regulatory cells are associated with insulin resistance in patients with type I Hashimoto's thyroiditis. Mol Med Rep 15:4338–4345

Ye ZP, He HY, Wang H, Li WS, Luo L, Huang ZC, Guo Y (2014) Glioma-derived ADAM10 induces regulatory B cells to suppress CD8+ T Cells. PLoS ONE 9:e105350

Yoshizaki A, Miyagaki T, DiLillo DJ, Matsushita T, Horikawa M, Kountikov EI, Spolski R, Poe JC, Leonard WJ, Tedder TF (2012) Regulatory B cells control T-cell autoimmunity through IL-21-dependent cognate interactions. Nature 491:264–268

Yu S, Qi Y, Wang H, Jiang J, Sun L, Zhou Q (2017) Dysfunction of CD24+CD38+ B cells in patients with Hashimoto's thyroiditis is associated with a lack of interleukin 10. Int J Biochem Cell Biol 90:114–120

Zha B, Wang L, Liu X, Liu J, Chen Z, Xu J, Sheng L, Li Y, Chu Y (2012) Decrease in proportion of CD19 + CD24(hi) CD27+ B cells and impairment of their suppressive function in Graves' disease. PLoS ONE 7: e49835

Zhang H, Wang Z, Liu R, Qian T, Liu J, Wang L, Chu Y (2018) Reactive oxygen species stimulated pulmonary epithelial cells mediate the alveolar recruitment of FasL(+) killer B cells in LPS-induced acute lung injuries. J Leukoc Biol 104:1187–1198

Zhang X, Deriaud E, Jiao X, Braun D, Leclerc C, Lo-Man R (2007) Type I interferons protect neonates from acute inflammation through interleukin 10-producing B cells. J Exp Med 204:1107–1118

Zhang Y, Eliav Y, Shin SU, Schreiber TH, Podack ER, Tadmor T, Rosenblatt JD (2013) B lymphocyte inhibition of anti-tumor response depends on expansion of Treg but is independent of B-cell IL-10 secretion. Cancer Immunol Immunother 62:87–99

Zhang Y, Li J, Zhou N, Zhang Y, Wu M, Xu J, Shen C, An X, Shen G, Yang M et al (2017) The unknown aspect of BAFF: inducing IL-35 production by a CD5 (+)CD1d(hi)FcgammaRIIb(hi) regulatory B-cell subset in Lupus. J Invest Dermatol 137:2532–2543

Zhang Y, Morgan R, Chen C, Cai Y, Clark E, Khan WN, Shin SU, Cho HM, Bayati AA, Pimentel A, Rosenblatt JD (2016) Mammary tumor educated B cells acquire LAP/TGF- and PD-L1 expression and suppress anti-tumor immune response. Int Immunol 28:423–433

Zhao H, Feng R, Peng A, Li G, Zhou L (2019) The expanding family of noncanonical regulatory cell subsets. J Leukoc Biol 106:369–383

Zheng J, Liu Y, Lau YL, Tu W (2010) CD40-activated B cells are more potent than immature dendritic cells to induce and expand CD4(+) regulatory T cells. Cell Mol Immunol 7:44–50

Zhu HQ, Xu RC, Chen YY, Yuan HJ, Cao H, Zhao XQ, Zheng J, Wang Y, Pan M (2014) Impaired function of CD19 CD24 CD38 regulatory B cells in pemphigus patients. Br J Dermatol 172(1):101–110

Diversified IgA–Bacteria Interaction in Gut Homeostasis

9

Keiichiro Suzuki

Abstract

Immunoglobulin A (IgA) is the major immunoglobulin isotype produced by the gut immune system, and many studies revealed key roles of IgA in establishing host-bacteria mutualism. This chapter will review current understandings for the function of gut IgA in regulating commensal microbiota. IgA specifically recognizes bacterial species that strongly stimulate host's immune responses, and suppresses their overgrowth or reduces the expressions of bacterial pro-inflammatory genes. On the other hand, IgA coatings on symbiotic bacteria enhance bacteria–mucus and bacteria–bacteria interactions, which induce production of metabolites enforcing mucosal barrier functions. Such diversified effects suggest that multiple factors may be involved in the mechanisms of IgA–bacteria interactions, including IgA specificity to microbial epitopes, mode of cellular responses of IgA synthesis (T-dependent and T-independent) and post-translational modifications of IgA proteins, such as glycosylation.

Keywords

IgA · Gut · Commensal bacteria · Diversification

9.1 Introduction

Immunoglobulin A (IgA) forms a first-line defense to eliminate intestinal pathogens and toxins. The amount of IgA is extraordinarily abundant (40–60 mg/kg/day in humans) and mammalian species devote a huge energy to produce IgA on the mucosal surfaces. It has been estimated that about 80% of plasma cells in whole body are IgA^+ cells in the gut lamina propria (LP) (Brandtzaeg et al. 1999; Fagarasan and Honjo 2003). Importantly, IgA is generated upon the interaction with commensal microbiota at the steady state. The composition of gut commensal is disturbed with IgA deficiency in mice and humans, associated with recurrent infections, allergy, and autoimmunity (Fadlallah et al. 2018; Singh et al. 2014; Yel 2010). Recent studies with fluorescence-activated cell sorter (FACS) purification and 16S-based sequencing of IgA-coated bacteria allowed to identify the members of IgA-targeted bacteria (Bunker et al.

K. Suzuki (✉)
Laboratory for Mucosal Immunity, Center for Integrative Medical Sciences (IMS), RIKEN, 1-7-22 Suehiro-Cho, Tsurumi-Ku Yokohama, 230-0045 Kanagawa, Japan
e-mail: keiichiro.suzuki@riken.jp

J.-Y. Wang (ed.), *B Cells in Immunity and Tolerance*, Advances in Experimental Medicine and Biology 1254, https://doi.org/10.1007/978-981-15-3532-1_9

2017; Kau et al. 2015; Kawamoto et al. 2014; Palm et al. 2014; Planer et al. 2016). Some of these bacteria have strong stimuli to the immune system, and mono-colonization or overgrowth of the members of IgA-coated bacteria induce inflammation in gut and systemic immune compartment (Fagarasan et al. 2002; Palm et al. 2014; Planer et al. 2016; Suzuki et al. 2004; Wu et al. 2010). Other members of IgA-coated bacteria produce "protective" metabolites such as short-chain fatty acids. Affinity-selected and high-quality IgA are required to maintain the diversity of symbiotic bacteria in the gut lumen (Kawamoto et al. 2012). The disturbed selection of germinal centers (GCs) B cells results in the loss of selective IgA-coating on symbiotic taxa, and reduces the microbial diversity and expands the numbers of potentially pathogenic strains (Kawamoto et al. 2014). Furthermore, glycan-dependent and epitope-independent IgA–bacteria binding enhances the expression of mucus-associated bacterial genes, and modify the metabolic function of whole gut microbiota (Nakajima et al. 2018). Thus, IgA has the capacity to enhance retention, growth, and metabolic function of the symbiotic bacteria in the gut. This chapter will review the current knowledge about complex and diversified function of IgA in the interaction with gut microbiota, and briefly summarize the mechanisms of IgA induction in the gut.

9.2 Selective Bacteria Suppression by Gut IgA

IgA is critical to remove gut pathogens. Initial studies revealed that IgA inhibits pathogen adherence to epithelial cells by inducing bacterial agglutination and prevent their entry into deeper tissues (Stokes et al. 1975; Williams and Gibbons 1972). A recent study using *Salmonella typhymurium* showed that IgA induced cross-linking of dividing bacterial cells, and thus enchain the daughter cells to the mother cells (Moor et al. 2017) (Fig. 9.1). The cross-linking of the growing bacteria, called enchained growth, prevented the separation of daughter cells after the division. Enchained growth finally formed bacterial clumps and enhanced clearance of the pathogen from the gut lumen (Moor et al. 2017).

The mechanism of how IgA regulates commensal bacteria is less clear. The initial observation for the role of IgA in commensal regulation was made in activation-induced cytidine deaminase (AID)-deficient mice. AID is responsible both for class-switch recombination (CSR) and somatic hypermutation (SHM) of Ig genes, and thus AID-deficient mice lack the effector function (i.e., CSR) and the antigen-binding specificity (i.e., SHM) of the antibodies (Muramatsu et al. 2000). In the absence of IgA, AID-deficient mice showed marked expansion of anaerobic commensals such as uncultured segmented filamentous bacteria (SFB) (Fagarasan et al. 2002; Suzuki et al. 2004) (Fig. 9.1). AID-deficient mice had hyperplasia of GCs in the whole body including gut and systemic immune system. The hyperplastic GCs disappeared by depleting gut microbiota with the treatment of broad-spectrum antibiotics cocktail. In addition, re-establishment of IgA plasma cells into the gut LP of AID-deficient mice also reduced the hyperplasia of GCs in gut and systemic immune compartments. Thus, gut IgA was shown to have a critical role to suppress over expansion of anaerobic bacteria, thereby regulating activation status both of gut and systemic immune systems (Fagarasan et al. 2002; Suzuki et al. 2004).

The loss of SHM on Ig genes is responsible for the phenotype of AID-deficient mice. The knock-in mice of N-terminal mutant of AID (AID^{G23S}) are unable to sustain efficient SHM, yet keeping CSR activity (Wei et al. 2011). The analysis of AID^{G23S} mice showed that the phenotype of AID-deficient mice was recapitulated in these animals. The phenotype of AID deficiency is likely depending on T cells, because SHM and selection of antigen-specific B cells are mainly a T-cell dependent process. Several key molecules were identified in T cells for the regulation of gut commensals. An inhibitory co-receptor PD-1 is expressed on activated T cells and critical to shut down ineffective immune responses and maintain homeostasis (Okazaki et al. 2013). In the absence of PD-1 expression, the selection of PPs B cells

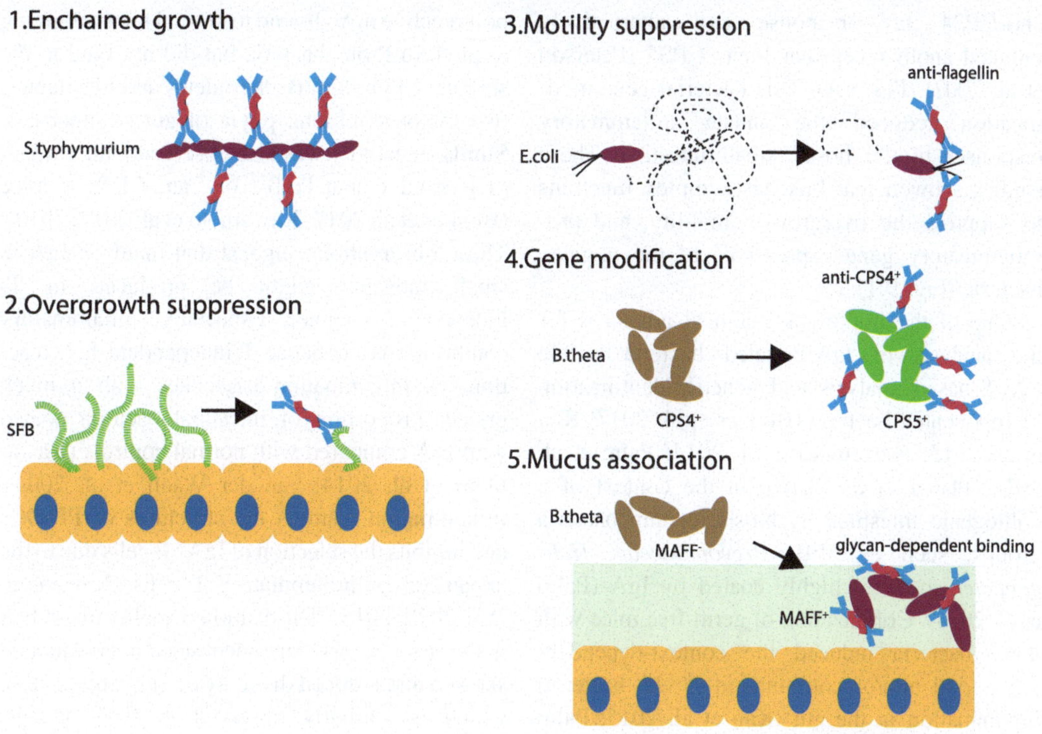

Fig. 9.1 Mechanisms of IgA-mediated regulation of composition and function of gut microbiota. (1) IgA cross-links the dividing cells of *S.typhymurium*, and thus the daughter bacteria cannot separate from the mother bacteria (enchained growth). The bacterial clump is efficiently eliminated from the gut lumen. (2) In the absence of IgA (AID deficiency), SFB undergoes over-expansion in the murine small intestine. (3) Anti-flagellin IgA binds on flagella, thereby suppressing motility of the bacteria. (4) CPS4 and CPS5 are capsular polysaccharide of *B.theta*. *B.theta* evades the molecular targeting of anti-CPS4 IgA, and suppress the gene expression of CPS4 and alternatively induce another CPS5 expression. (5) *B.theta* requires the expression MAFF gene to interact with other bacterial strains belonging to phylum Firmicutes. MAFF gene does not express in the luminal bacteria but induced in the mucus environment. Glycan-dependent IgA binding induces the MAFF gene expression to regulate composition and metabolic function of the total gut microbiome

and the formation of IgA repertoire were disturbed due to the insufficient T-B interactions. As a result, PD-1 deficient mice had dysbiosis with the reduction of "healthy" members of bacteria such as *Bifidobacterium* and the expansion of potentially pathogenic organisms such as *Enterobacteriacheae* in the small intestine (Kawamoto et al. 2012). Similarly, the deletion of innate adaptor MyD88 signaling or ATP-gated ionotropic P2X7 receptor in T cells disturbed the selection of IgA^{+} B cells in PPs and altered the profiles of commensal consortium (Kubinak et al. 2015; Proietti et al. 2014). These observations showed that epitope-specific recognition of bacteria by gut IgA is critical to maintain the diversified community of gut microbiota.

The analysis of TLR5 deficient mice showed that anti-flagellin IgA is required to suppress penetration of potentially pathogenic bacteria by targeting flagella and quench motility of the bacteria (Cullender et al. 2013) (Fig. 9.1). Interestingly, anti-flagellin IgA suppressed the gene-expression level of flagella in *E.Coli* (Cullender et al. 2013). Similar effect of bacterial-gene modification was observed in mono-colonized mice with *Bacteroides thetaiotaomicron* (*B.-theta*). The gene expression of *B.theta* was modified in the presence of a monoclonal IgA that recognizes a capsular polysaccharide CPS4 of the bacteria (Peterson et al. 2007). The *B.theta* specific IgA suppressed the oxidative stress responses of *B.theta*, and the bacteria evaded the anti-CPS4 IgA response and alternatively induced another capsular locus CPS5 (Peterson et al. 2007) (Fig. 9.1). This bacterial gene modification reduced the innate inflammatory responses in the hosts' small intestine. These studies showed that IgA has complex functions to suppress the overgrowth, motility, and pro-inflammatory gene expressions of the targeted bacteria (Fig. 9.1).

One of the important technical advances for the analysis of IgA-targeted bacteria is the FACS-based analysis and genetic identification of IgA-coated bacteria (Bunker et al. 2017; Kau et al. 2015; Kawamoto et al. 2014; Palm et al. 2014; Planer et al. 2016). In the context of a colitogenic intestinal dysbiosis, certain bacteria groups, such as SFB, *Prevotellaceae*, *Helicobacter* sp. were highly coated by IgA (Palm et al. 2014). Colonization of germ-free mice with these bacteria induced the context-dependent (e.g., food and/or combination of the bacteria) inflammation in the gut (Kau et al. 2015; Palm et al. 2014). Some of these bacteria were shown to strongly attach on epithelial cells or invade into inner layer of colonic mucus, which is usually recognized as the bacteria-free region, and strongly stimulate gut immune responses (Ivanov et al. 2009; Lecuyer et al. 2014; Palm et al. 2014; Viladomiu et al. 2017). These studies suggest that the neutralization of bacterial epitopes and suppression of the overgrowth of invasive commensal populations by IgA-coating appears to be important to avoid gut inflammation.

9.3 Polyreactive IgA–Bacteria Bindings

It is generally accepted that antigen-specific and polyreactive IgA are produced in T-dependent and T-independent pathway, respectively. The generation of IgA-derived monoclonal antibodies (mAbs) expressed with human IgG1 constant region showed that more than half of small intestinal IgA bound to multiple bacterial species (Bunker et al. 2017). Interestingly, the polyreactive mAb bound to several taxa belonging to phylum Proteobacteria but did not bind to the surfaces of phylum Bacteroidetes and Firmicutes, two major symbiotic phyla of gut commensals. Similar reactivity was also observed with gut IgA of T-cell deficient $Tcr\beta^{-/-}\delta^{-/-}$ and $CD3\varepsilon^{-/-}$ mice (Bunker et al. 2017; Kawamoto et al. 2012, 2014). These observations suggest that many of IgA in small intestine might be produced in T-independent manner. Especially, inflammatory condition may enhance T-independent IgA reaction, as inflammation associates with a much greater proportion of intestinal bacteria coated with IgA compared with normal controls (Kawamoto et al. 2014; van der Waaij et al. 2004). Inflammation disturbs the structures of PP-GCs and inhibits the selection of IgA^+ B cells due to the expansion of inflammatory T cells (Kawamoto et al. 2012, 2014). The disturbed quality of gut IgA in the absence of T-dependent selection resulted in skewed and reduced diversity of gut commensals, which is similarly observed in IBD patients (Gevers et al. 2014; Kawamoto et al. 2014). These observations suggest that T-independent polyreactive IgA may have a role in inflammatory condition to eliminate the pathogenic bacterial strains, such as Proteobacteria. In agree with this, a monoclonal IgA clone W27 that recognizes multiple bacteria including *E.coli* but not symbiotic strains such as *Lactobacillus casei*, suppressed chemical-induced colitis by removing colitogenic taxa during oral IgA administrations (Okai et al. 2016).

At the steady state, the amount of polyreactive IgA is controlled by the host's genetic factors, and BALB/c mice were shown to have higher abundance of polyreactive IgA than C57BL/6 mice (Fransen et al. 2015). Polyreactive IgA-coating enhanced internalization of the bacteria into PPs, thereby inducing positive-feedback loop of bacteria-specific IgA responses (Fransen et al. 2015). These observations suggest that T-independent and polyreactive IgA have distinct function from T-dependent IgA, and form an evolutionarily primitive system to establish host-bacteria relationship (Macpherson et al. 2000, 2001; Fagarasan et al. 2010; Kawamoto et al. 2014).

9.4 IgA Dependent Mucus Association of Gut Microbiota

The action of gut IgA is not limited to neutralization and elimination of bacterial cells. In the absence of T-dependent IgA, CD3ε$^{-/-}$ mice have significantly reduced diversity of gut microbial communities (Kawamoto et al. 2014). Strikingly, the transfer of CD4^{+}Foxp3^{+} T cells into CD3ε$^{-/-}$ mice rescued PP-GCs and induced well-selected IgA (Kawamoto et al. 2014). Such changes are associated with normalization of diversity and composition of bacterial communities. T-cell dependent and GC-selected IgA efficiently bound on bacteria belonging to phylum Firmicutes and enhanced the diversification of IgA-targeted bacteria. This observation suggests that T-dependent IgA have capacity to support the retention of IgA-coated bacteria, instead of eliminating them from the gut lumen (Kawamoto et al. 2014). Indeed, gut microbiota in luminal contents and those attach on mucus layer showed significantly different consortium, and the composition of IgA-coated bacteria was shown to be similar with that of mucus-attached microbiota (Kubinak et al. 2015). More directly, a study on *Bacteroides fragilis (B.fragilis)* as a model colonic commensal showed that *B. fragilis* could not colonize efficiently in the colon of IgA-deficient mice, indicating that IgA facilitates mucus colonization of certain members of gut bacteria (Donaldson et al. 2018).

IgA may enhance the trapping of bacteria into the mucus layer depending on the glycan moiety. IgA has multiple N- and O-glycosylation sites, which account for up to 25% of the molecular mass of secretory component, and these carbohydrates can mediate epitope-independent bacteria bindings (Mathias and Corthesy 2011; Perrier et al. 2006; Royle et al. 2003). A heavily glycosylated monoclonal anti-ovalbumin IgA (7−6IgA) could bind on various cultured bacterial strains, even after complete block of the antigen recognition site of the antibody (Nakajima et al. 2018). Among many bacterial strains, *B.theta* had a high-binding capacity to 7−6IgA. The RNA-seq analysis of bacteria showed that *B.theta* significantly changed the gene-expression profile under the presence of 7−6IgA in the cecum. Such changes included the induction of functionally unknown genes belonging to starch utilization system (Sus) of *B.theta*, which bind, degrade, and transport glycan into the bacterial cells (Backhed et al. 2005; Koropatkin et al. 2012; Martens et al. 2008). One of the Sus-like genes induced by the 7−6IgA was specifically expressed in the mucus-attached, but not in the luminal *B.theta* (Nakajima et al. 2018) (Fig. 9.1). The orthologs of this gene were widely shared in bacteria belonging to phylum Bacteroidetes. Interestingly, the ortholog genes of *B.fragilis*, *B. vulgatus,* and *Parabacteroides distasonis* were all significantly induced in mucus-attached bacteria, and thus the ortholog genes were provisionally named Mucus-Associated Functional Factor (MAFF) (Nakajima et al. 2018). Deletion of the MAFF gene of *B.theta* resulted in altered morphology (smaller in mutant) in the colon of specific pathogen-free (SPF) mice in the presence of diverse microbiota. Strikingly, the morphology of wild-type *B.theta* in mono-colonized mice was similar with that of MAFF-deletion mutant in SPF mice. In addition, bacterial RNA-seq analysis showed that mono-colonized wild-type *B.theta* and also the MAFF-deletion mutant both in mono-colonized and SPF mice were metabolically insufficient in the cecum. Mono-colonized wild-type *B.theta* expressed very low level of MAFF gene, and the addition of diverse microbiota to the mono-colonized mice significantly increased the gene expression of the MAFF system. Thus, *B.theta* sense other members of bacteria to induce the MAFF gene, and then acquire full metabolic function. In turn, MAFF-dependent function of *B.theta* was required to maintain diversity and numbers of phylum Firmicutes in the colon. In addition, the genes related with metabolic function of Firmicutes, such as the genes related with the production of short-chain fatty acids, were highly increased via the MAFF system. Thus, glycosylated 7−6IgA induced the MAFF system in mucus environment, and regulate the composition and metabolic function of whole gut microbiome (Nakajima et al. 2018) (Fig. 9.1). These observations show that IgA plays an important role to maintain diverse microbiota by inducing bacteria-mucus and bacteria–bacteria interactions within the gut ecosystem.

9.5 Dynamics and Maintenance of Gut IgA

IgA-producing cells are generated upon microbial colonization. SFB provides strong stimuli to the gut immune system (Atarashi et al. 2015; Hirota et al. 2013; Ivanov et al. 2009; Ladinsky et al. 2019), but the secondary colonization of *Morganella morganii* to SFB mono-colonized mice adds *M.morganii*-specific IgA on top of anti-SFB IgA (Talham et al. 1999). This observation suggests that gut immune system responds to newly encountered antigen by adding the novel IgA responses. Strikingly, such additive response of IgA production was also observed with the sequential stimulation of identical bacterial strain (Hapfelmeier et al. 2010). In this study, auxotrophic-deletion mutant of *E.Coli* was mono-colonized into germ-free mice. The mutant *E.Coli* strain could not grow in the gut lumen for more than 48 h and return to germ-free status within 72 h. In this system, repeated colonization of the mutant *E.Coli* added the numbers of IgA plasma cells in a dose-dependent manner (Hapfelmeier et al. 2010). The additive response of gut IgA was clearly different from a rapid and synergistic expansion of memory B cells in systemic immune compartment. Importantly, the number of IgA plasma cells did not decrease for more than 4 months after the disappearance of live bacteria and marked decrease of newly induced GC B cells (Hapfelmeier et al. 2010). Thus, in contrast to short-lived GC B cells, IgA plasma cells are long-lived in gut LP, and the dynamics of IgA response is clearly different from that of systemic IgG responses.

In addition to microbial responses, one of the critical checkpoints for the maintenance of IgA is the antibody-secretion process from the plasma cells. IgA plasma cells release soluble IgA as dimers or larger polymers upon association with the joining chain (J chain). The IgA-J chain complexes are produced in gut LP and then transported to the luminal side via the epithelial cells depend on polymeric Ig receptor (pIgR). pIgR is expressed on the basolateral side of epithelial cells and binds to internalize and transport polymeric IgA to the luminal surface of the epithelium. A part of pIgR molecule is incorporated to IgA after the proteolysis at epithelial surfaces (secretory component). During this process, marginal zone B and B-1 cell-specific protein (MZB1) have been identified in IgA plasma cells as a molecular chaperone that facilitate the formation of polymeric IgA (Xiong et al. 2019) (Fig. 9.2). MZB1 is localized in endoplasmic reticulum (ER) and constitutively expressed in innate-like B cells, such as marginal zone (MZ) B cells and B1 cells, and highly up-regulated during plasma cell differentiation. MZB1 binds to the secretory tailpiece of IgA heavy-chain protein and promotes J-chain incorporation to stabilize heavy-/light-chain complex (Xiong et al. 2019) (Fig. 9.2). Unexpectedly, $Mzb1^{-/-}$ mice had normal levels of fecal IgA at the steady state, but the acute IgA responses upon LPS injection and chemical colitis were disturbed. Also, $Mzb1^{-/-}$ mice had gut dysbiosis and enhanced susceptibility to chemical colitis. The administration of a polyreactive W27IgA in the drinking water ameliorated the colitis induction. Thus, MZB1-dependent IgA secretion is critical to maintain the amount of gut IgA (Xiong et al. 2019).

Another modification of IgA protein occurs after secretion into the gut lumen. The analysis of cage variation in mice colonies for fecal IgA levels revealed that some wild-type mice had very low levels of IgA at the steady state (IgA-low mice) (Moon et al. 2015). The IgA-low phenotype was laterally transferred to IgA-high mice by cohousing. In addition, antibiotics treatment increased the amount of fecal IgA of the IgA-low mice. Thus, IgA-low phenotype was bacteria dependent. In vitro experiments showed that cultured bacteria derived from the gut microbiota of IgA-low mice degraded secretory component and IgA protein itself in a protease-dependent manner (Fig. 9.2). Thus, gut bacteria (*Sutterella* species was specifically identified in IgA-low mice) negatively regulate IgA amount by inducing degradation of the protein (Moon

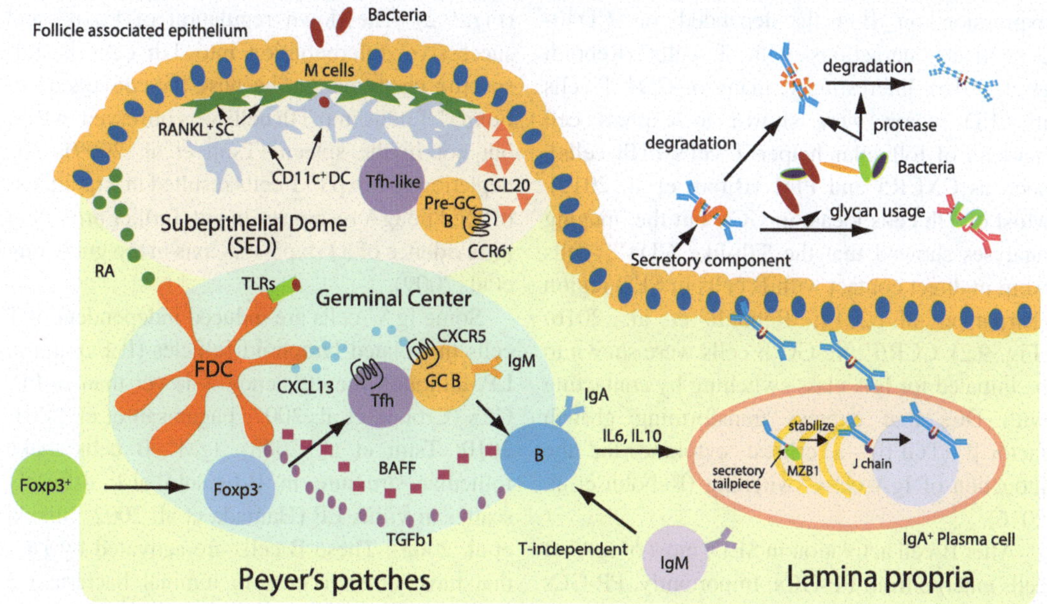

Fig. 9.2 Pathways for induction and maintenance of gut IgA. (left) Cellular responses in PPs: RANKL$^+$ stromal cells (SC) are essential for induction of M cells and CCL20 production from follicle-associated epithelium. CCR6$^+$ pre-germinal center (GC) B cells respond to CCL20, enter into subepithelial dome (SED) and interact with Tfh-like cells within the dense network of CD11c$^+$ dendritic cells (DCs). Tfh cells are derived from Foxp3$^+$CD4$^+$T cells and are essential for GC formation. Both Tfh cells and B cells express CXCR5 and respond to CXCL13 produced by follicular dendritic cells (FDCs). Bacteria and food-derived signals stimulate FDCs via Toll-like receptors (TLRs) and retinoic acid (RA) receptors, respectively, and enhance the production of B-cell activating factor of the tumor-necrosis-factor family (BAFF) and active form of TGFβ. These cytokines induce class switching of B cells from IgM$^+$ to IgA$^+$. (right) In IgA$^+$ plasma cells, MZB1 binds on secretory tailpiece of IgA heavy chain to stabilize IgA heavy-/light-chain complex and enhances the secretion of IgA protein from the plasma cells. Secretory component is added to IgA during the transport via epithelia cells. Some bacteria negatively regulate IgA amount by degrading secretory component and IgA protein itself. Other bacteria have capacity to change glycosylation of IgA protein by using the glycan as bacterial nutrient

et al. 2015). In addition, some bacteria can modify glycosylation pattern of IgA by specifically degrading the peptide of glycosylation site of the antibody, and also by utilizing complex N-glycan on IgA as the bacterial nutrient (Bratanis and Lood 2019; Briliute et al. 2019) (Fig. 9.2). Together, these studies show the unique and complex mechanisms of cellular dynamics and molecular interactions that are required for the maintenance of gut IgA.

9.6 IgA Induction

It is generally accepted that PPs in small intestine are the dominant source of IgA-producing cells (Fig. 9.2). Luminal antigens are internalized into subepithelial dome (SED) of PPs through specialized antigen sampling epithelium called M cells. The analyses of SED B cells showed that B cells enter into SED and communicate with dense CD11c$^+$DCs population depend on a chemokine receptor CCR6 (Reboldi et al. 2016) (Fig. 9.2). CCL20, the ligand of CCR6, was shown to be generated by follicle-associated epithelium under the interaction with mesenchymal cells that express membrane-bound form of receptor activator of nuclear factor-κB ligand (RANKL) (Nagashima et al. 2017) (Fig. 9.2). This study showed that RANKL$^+$ mesenchymal cells also regulate M-cell induction. Thus, mesenchymal-derived RANKL is essential for IgA responses in PPs. In vivo transfer experiments revealed that CCR6 expression on B cells depended on CD40-dependent interactions with T cells (Reboldi et al. 2016). Interestingly, many of CD4$^+$T cells in SED region were shown to express cell markers of follicular helper T cells (Tfh cells), such as CXCR5 and PD1 (Biram et al. 2019). Most of Tfh cells locate in GCs, but the imaging analyses showed that the Tfh-like CD4$^+$T cells were in direct contact with B cells in SED region (Biram et al. 2019; Reboldi et al. 2016) (Fig. 9.2). CCR6$^+$ pre-GC B cells were shown to be initiated for IgA class switching by contacting with DCs that express transforming growth factor-β (TGFβ)—a critical cytokine for the induction of IgA class switching (Reboldi et al. 2016).

After B-cell activation in SED, most of IgA$^+$ B cells emerge from PP-GCs. Importantly, PP-GCs are functionally distinct from systemic GCs present in peripheral lymph nodes or spleen, because PP-GCs generate mainly IgA$^+$ B cells while peripheral GCs mainly induce IgG$^+$ B cells. It has been shown that follicular dendritic cells (FDCs) in PPs support more efficiently the generation of IgA$^+$ B cells than lymph nodes FDCs by producing high amounts of active TGFβ and B-cell activating factor of the tumor-necrosis-factor family (BAFF) (Suzuki et al. 2010) (Fig. 9.2). Interestingly, the purified lymph nodes FDCs produced large amounts of active TGFβ and BAFF when the FDCs were stimulated via Toll-like receptors (TLRs) and retinoic acid receptors (RARs) (Suzuki et al. 2010). Thus, the microenvironment of PP-GCs is induced by sensing the signals both from bacteria-derived (TLR ligands) and food-derived (RA) components (Fig. 9.2). In addition, such FDC activation enhances CXCL13 production to facilitate the encounter of CXCR5$^+$B cells with Tfh cells (Suzuki et al. 2010) (Fig. 9.2). Tfh cells in PPs also acquire the properties to help IgA responses in the context of gut-specific environment. Notably, CD4$^+$Foxp3$^+$ regulatory T cells had capacity to convert into CXCR5$^+$PD1$^+$Tfh cells and supported GC formation and IgA response (Tsuji et al. 2009) (Fig. 9.2). The down regulation of Foxp3 and successive differentiation into Tfh cells is gut-specific phenomenon, because the conversion of Foxp3$^+$ T cells into Tfh cells was observed in PPs, but not in the spleen (Tsuji et al. 2009). The depletion of Foxp3$^+$ T cells resulted in a rapid loss of specific IgA responses in gut, further providing the evidence of a Foxp3-IgA axis in the gut (Cong et al. 2009).

Some IgA$^+$ cells are induced independent of T cells in isolated lymphoid follicles (ILFs) and in LP, although the efficiency is lower than in PP-GCs (Crouch et al. 2007; Fagarasan et al. 2001, 2010; Tsuji et al. 2008). IgM$^+$ B cells make follicular structure in ILFs and also diffusely scatter in villus LP (Hamada et al. 2002; Suzuki et al. 2005). These B cells are activated by DCs that have direct access to luminal bacteria via extended dendrites through the tight junction of the epithelium (Niess et al. 2005; Rescigno et al. 2001). A few distinct subsets of DCs were reported to be involved in this process. CX3CR1$^+$ DCs through BAFF and IL-10, CD103$^+$ DCs through TLR5-dependent production of retinoic acid and a special subset of DCs called Tip-DCs via iNOS and TNFα production (Litinskiy et al. 2002; Murai et al. 2009; Tezuka et al. 2007; Uematsu et al. 2008; Varol et al. 2009). Interestingly, some population of IgA$^+$ plasma cells is also involved in IgA induction by producing iNOS and TNFα (Fritz et al. 2011). After the recognition of gut bacterial antigens, these DCs and IgA$^+$ plasma cells present in ILFs or in LP induce CSR from IgM to IgA even in the absence of T cells. DCs in LP and ILFs were shown to produce large amounts of TNFα and stimulate local stromal cells to release the active form of TGFβ via the function of matrix metalloproteinase 9 (MMP9) and MMP13 (Tsuji et al. 2008). Also, DCs and intestinal epithelial cells produce APRIL to promote T-independent IgA generation in human gut (He et al. 2007; Litinskiy et al. 2002). In addition, eosinophils promote the generation of IgA$^+$ cells by the capacity to release the active form of TGFβ via the function of MMP2 and MMP9, and by the production of APRIL (Chu et al. 2014). Thus, IgA induction requires complex interactions among bacteria, epithelial cells, DCs, eosinophils, stromal cells, and IgA^+ plasma cells both in T-dependent and T-independent mechanisms.

9.7 Conclusion

Recent studies have made significant advances in our understandings of IgA function. Accumulating evidence supports that the function of gut IgA has multidimensional phenomenon such as 1. bacterial clump formation (including enchained growth) 2. overgrowth suppression 3. motility suppression 4. Bacterial-gene modification, and 5. mucus association of the IgA-coated bacteria (Fig. 9.1). Future works need to identify the mechanisms of actions of these IgA functions. For example, it will be important to understand how the T-dependent and GC-selected IgA suppress the overgrowth of certain members of commensals. Does IgA use enchained growth to suppress the overgrowth of commensals? Also, what is the mechanism of IgA to enhance mucus association of symbiotic bacteria? Does IgA-glycan play a major role for this? These are the questions that are required to understand host-bacteria mutualism and may have implications to develop new strategies for mucosal vaccines and also for the therapies of inflammatory bowel diseases.

There are some other important aspects of gut IgA biology. For example, how maternal IgA influences the microbiota development in neonates and immune system maturation is an important issue to establish a better intervention for newborn health (Sutherland et al. 2016). In addition, detailed evaluation of the gut-derived IgA^+ cells will be another interesting field for future studies. For example, a fraction of B-lineage cells, such as LPS-stimulated B cells and IgA^+ plasma cells, elicit suppressive function by expressing IL10 and PD-L1 (Rojas et al. 2019; Shalapour et al. 2015; Shen et al. 2014). These B cells and IgA^+ plasma cells inhibit autoimmunity such as experimental autoimmune encephalomyelitis (EAE) and also modulate the efficacy of cancer therapies (Rojas et al. 2019; Shalapour et al. 2015; Shen et al. 2014). Also, metabolic changes induced by gut immune system need to be studied more in detail. B-cells-deficient mice were reported to have less fat due to the reduced lipid absorption by gut epithelial cells (Shulzhenko et al. 2011). Furthermore, secretory antibodies were shown to regulate host responses by limiting the penetration of microbial metabolites to systemic tissues (Uchimura et al. 2018). Future studies related with the impact of gut-derived immune cells and secretory IgA within and beyond the gut tissues will provide important implications to minimize the risk of diseases related with microbial dysregulation and immune deficiencies.

References

Atarashi K, Tanoue T, Ando M, Kamada N, Nagano Y, Narushima S et al (2015) Th17 cell induction by adhesion of microbes to intestinal epithelial cells. Cell 163:367–380

Backhed F, Ley RE, Sonnenburg JL, Peterson DA, Gordon JI (2005) Host-bacterial mutualism in the human intestine. Science 307:1915–1920

Biram A, Stromberg A, Winter E, Stoler-Barak L, Salomon R, Addadi Y et al (2019) BCR affinity differentially regulates colonization of the subepithelial dome and infiltration into germinal centers within Peyer's patches. Nat Immunol 20:482–492

Brandtzaeg P, Baekkevold ES, Farstad IN, Jahnsen FL, Johansen FE, Nilsen EM et al (1999) Regional specialization in the mucosal immune system: what happens in the microcompartments? Immunol Today 20:141–151

Bratanis E, Lood R (2019) A novel broad-spectrum elastase-like serine protease from the predatory bacterium bdellovibrio bacteriovorus facilitates elucidation of site-specific IgA glycosylation pattern. Front Microbiol 10:971

Briliute J, Urbanowicz PA, Luis AS, Basle A, Paterson N, Rebello O et al (2019) Complex N-glycan breakdown by gut Bacteroides involves an extensive enzymatic apparatus encoded by multiple co-regulated genetic loci. Nat Microbiol 4:1571–1581

Bunker JJ, Erickson SA, Flynn TM, Henry C, Koval JC, Meisel M et al (2017) Natural polyreactive IgA antibodies coat the intestinal microbiota. Science 358

Chu VT, Beller A, Rausch S, Strandmark J, Zanker M, Arbach O et al (2014) Eosinophils promote generation and maintenance of immunoglobulin-A-expressing plasma cells and contribute to gut immune homeostasis. Immunity 40:582–593

Cong Y, Feng T, Fujihashi K, Schoeb TR, Elson CO (2009) A dominant, coordinated T regulatory cell-IgA response to the intestinal microbiota. Proc Natl Acad Sci USA 106:19256–19261

Crouch EE, Li Z, Takizawa M, Fichtner-Feigl S, Gourzi P, Montano C et al (2007) Regulation of AID expression in the immune response. J Exp Med 204:1145–1156

Cullender TC, Chassaing B, Janzon A, Kumar K, Muller CE, Werner JJ et al (2013) Innate and adaptive immunity interact to quench microbiome flagellar motility in the gut. Cell Host Microbe 14:571–581

Donaldson GP, Ladinsky MS, Yu KB, Sanders JG, Yoo BB, Chou WC et al (2018) Gut microbiota utilize immunoglobulin A for mucosal colonization. Science 360:795–800

Fadlallah J, El Kafsi H, Sterlin D, Juste C, Parizot C, Dorgham K et al (2018) Microbial ecology perturbation in human IgA deficiency. Sci Transl Med 10

Fagarasan S, Honjo T (2003) Intestinal IgA synthesis: regulation of front-line body defences. Nat Rev Immunol 3:63–72

Fagarasan S, Kawamoto S, Kanagawa O, Suzuki K (2010) Adaptive immune regulation in the gut: T cell-dependent and T cell-independent IgA synthesis. Annu Rev Immunol 28:243–273

Fagarasan S, Kinoshita K, Muramatsu M, Ikuta K, Honjo T (2001) In situ class switching and differentiation to IgA-producing cells in the gut lamina propria. Nature 413:639–643

Fagarasan S, Muramatsu M, Suzuki K, Nagaoka H, Hiai H, Honjo T (2002) Critical roles of activation-induced cytidine deaminase in the homeostasis of gut flora. Science 298:1424–1427

Fransen F, Zagato E, Mazzini E, Fosso B, Manzari C, El Aidy S et al (2015) BALB/c and C57BL/6 mice differ in polyreactive IgA abundance, which impacts the generation of antigen-specific IgA and microbiota diversity. Immunity 43:527–540

Fritz JH, Rojas OL, Simard N, McCarthy DD, Hapfelmeier S, Rubino S et al (2011) Acquisition of a multifunctional IgA+ plasma cell phenotype in the gut. Nature 481:199–203

Gevers D, Kugathasan S, Denson LA, Vazquez-Baeza Y, Van Treuren W, Ren B et al (2014) The treatment-naive microbiome in new-onset Crohn's disease. Cell Host Microbe 15:382–392

Hamada H, Hiroi T, Nishiyama Y, Takahashi H, Masunaga Y, Hachimura S et al (2002) Identification of multiple isolated lymphoid follicles on the antimesenteric wall of the mouse small intestine. J Immunol 168:57–64

Hapfelmeier S, Lawson MA, Slack E, Kirundi JK, Stoel M, Heikenwalder M et al (2010) Reversible microbial colonization of germ-free mice reveals the dynamics of IgA immune responses. Science 328:1705–1709

He B, Xu W, Santini PA, Polydorides AD, Chiu A, Estrella J et al (2007) Intestinal bacteria trigger T cell-independent immunoglobulin A(2) class switching by inducing epithelial-cell secretion of the cytokine APRIL. Immunity 26:812–826

Hirota K, Turner JE, Villa M, Duarte JH, Demengeot J, Steinmetz OM et al (2013) Plasticity of Th17 cells in Peyer's patches is responsible for the induction of T cell-dependent IgA responses. Nat Immunol 14: 372–379

Ivanov II, Atarashi K, Manel N, Brodie EL, Shima T, Karaoz U et al (2009) Induction of intestinal Th17 cells by segmented filamentous bacteria. Cell 139:485–498

Kau AL, Planer JD, Liu J, Rao S, Yatsunenko T, Trehan I et al (2015) Functional characterization of IgA-targeted bacterial taxa from undernourished Malawian children that produce diet-dependent enteropathy. Sci Transl Med 7:276ra224

Kawamoto S, Maruya M, Kato LM, Suda W, Atarashi K, Doi Y et al (2014) Foxp3(+) T cells regulate immunoglobulin a selection and facilitate diversification of bacterial species responsible for immune homeostasis. Immunity 41:152–165

Kawamoto S, Tran TH, Maruya M, Suzuki K, Doi Y, Tsutsui Y et al (2012) The inhibitory receptor PD-1 regulates IgA selection and bacterial composition in the gut. Science 336:485–489

Koropatkin NM, Cameron EA, Martens EC (2012) How glycan metabolism shapes the human gut microbiota. Nat Rev Microbiol 10:323–335

Kubinak JL, Petersen C, Stephens WZ, Soto R, Bake E, O'Connell RM et al (2015) MyD88 signaling in T cells directs IgA-mediated control of the microbiota to promote health. Cell Host Microbe 17:153–163

Ladinsky MS, Araujo LP, Zhang X, Veltri J, Galan-Diez M, Soualhi S et al (2019) Endocytosis of commensal antigens by intestinal epithelial cells regulates mucosal T cell homeostasis. Science 363

Lecuyer E, Rakotobe S, Lengline-Garnier H, Lebreton C, Picard M, Juste C et al (2014) Segmented filamentous bacterium uses secondary and tertiary lymphoid tissues to induce gut IgA and specific T helper 17 cell responses. Immunity 40:608–620

Litinskiy MB, Nardelli B, Hilbert DM, He B, Schaffer A, Casali P et al (2002) DCs induce CD40-independent immunoglobulin class switching through BLyS and APRIL. Nat Immunol 3:822–829

Macpherson AJ, Gatto D, Sainsbury E, Harriman GR, Hengartner H, Zinkernagel RM (2000) A primitive T cell-independent mechanism of intestinal mucosal IgA responses to commensal bacteria. Science 288:2222–2226

Macpherson AJ, Lamarre A, McCoy K, Harriman GR, Odermatt B, Dougan G et al (2001) IgA production without mu or delta chain expression in developing B cells. Nat Immunol 2:625–631

Martens EC, Chiang HC, Gordon JI (2008) Mucosal glycan foraging enhances fitness and transmission of a saccharolytic human gut bacterial symbiont. Cell Host Microbe 4:447–457

Mathias A, Corthesy B (2011) Recognition of gram-positive intestinal bacteria by hybridoma- and colostrum-derived secretory immunoglobulin A is mediated by carbohydrates. J Biol Chem 286:17239–17247

Moon C, Baldridge MT, Wallace MA, Burnham DCA, Virgin HW et al (2015) Vertically transmitted faecal IgA levels determine extra-chromosomal phenotypic variation. Nature 521:90–93

Moor K, Diard M, Sellin ME, Felmy B, Wotzka SY, Toska A et al (2017) High-avidity IgA protects the intestine by enchaining growing bacteria. Nature 544:498–502

Murai M, Turovskaya O, Kim G, Madan R, Karp CL, Cheroutre H et al (2009) Interleukin 10 acts on regulatory T cells to maintain expression of the transcription factor Foxp3 and suppressive function in mice with colitis. Nat Immunol 10:1178–1184

Muramatsu M, Kinoshita K, Fagarasan S, Yamada S, Shinkai Y, Honjo T (2000) Class switch recombination and hypermutation require activation-induced cytidine deaminase (AID), a potential RNA editing enzyme. Cell 102:553–563

Nagashima K, Sawa S, Nitta T, Tsutsumi M, Okamura T, Penninger JM et al (2017) Identification of subepithelial mesenchymal cells that induce IgA and diversify gut microbiota. Nat Immunol 18:675–682

Nakajima A, Vogelzang A, Maruya M, Miyajima M, Murata M, Son A et al (2018) IgA regulates the composition and metabolic function of gut microbiota by promoting symbiosis between bacteria. J Exp Med 215:2019–2034

Niess JH, Brand S, Gu X, Landsman L, Jung S, McCormick BA et al (2005) CX3CR1-mediated dendritic cell access to the intestinal lumen and bacterial clearance. Science 307:254–258

Okai S, Usui F, Yokota S, Hori IY, Hasegawa M, Nakamura T et al (2016) High-affinity monoclonal IgA regulates gut microbiota and prevents colitis in mice. Nat Microbiol 1:16103

Okazaki T, Chikuma S, Iwai Y, Fagarasan S, Honjo T (2013) A rheostat for immune responses: the unique properties of PD-1 and their advantages for clinical application. Nat Immunol 14:1212–1218

Palm NW, de Zoete MR, Cullen TW, Barry NA, Stefanowski J, Hao L et al (2014) Immunoglobulin A coating identifies colitogenic bacteria in inflammatory bowel disease. Cell 158:1000–1010

Perrier C, Sprenger N, Corthesy B (2006) Glycans on secretory component participate in innate protection against mucosal pathogens. J Biol Chem 281:14280–14287

Peterson DA, McNulty NP, Guruge JL, Gordon JI (2007) IgA response to symbiotic bacteria as a mediator of gut homeostasis. Cell Host Microbe 2:328–339

Planer JD, Peng Y, Kau AL, Blanton LV, Ndao IM, Tarr PI et al (2016) Development of the gut microbiota and mucosal IgA responses in twins and gnotobiotic mice. Nature 534:263–266

Proietti M, Cornacchione V, Rezzonico Jost T, Romagnani A, Faliti CE, Perruzza L et al (2014) ATP-gated ionotropic P2X7 receptor controls follicular T helper cell numbers in Peyer's patches to promote host-microbiota mutualism. Immunity 41:789–801

Reboldi A, Arnon TI, Rodda LB, Atakilit A, Sheppard D, Cyster JG (2016) IgA production requires B cell interaction with subepithelial dendritic cells in Peyer's patches. Science 352:aaf4822

Rescigno M, Urbano M, Valzasina B, Francolini M, Rotta G, Bonasio R et al (2001) Dendritic cells express tight junction proteins and penetrate gut epithelial monolayers to sample bacteria. Nat Immunol 2:361–367

Rojas OL, Probstel AK, Porfilio EA, Wang AA, Charabati M, Sun T et al (2019) Recirculating intestinal IgA-producing cells regulate neuroinflammation via IL-10. Cell 177:492–493

Royle L, Roos A, Harvey DJ, Wormald MR, van Gijlswijk-Janssen D, el Redwan RM et al (2003) Secretory IgA N- and O-glycans provide a link between the innate and adaptive immune systems. J Biol Chem 278:20140–20153

Shalapour S, Font-Burgada J, Di Caro G, Zhong Z, Sanchez-Lopez E, Dhar D et al (2015) Immunosuppressive plasma cells impede T-cell-dependent immunogenic chemotherapy. Nature 521:94–98

Shen P, Roch T, Lampropoulou V, O'Connor RA, Stervbo U, Hilgenberg E et al (2014) IL-35-producing B cells are critical regulators of immunity during autoimmune and infectious diseases. Nature 507:366–370

Shulzhenko N, Morgun A, Hsiao W, Battle M, Yao M, Gavrilova O et al (2011) Crosstalk between B lymphocytes, microbiota and the intestinal epithelium governs immunity versus metabolism in the gut. Nat Med 17:1585–1593

Singh K, Chang C, Gershwin ME (2014) IgA deficiency and autoimmunity. Autoimmun Rev 13:163–177

Stokes CR, Soothill JF, Turner MW (1975) Immune exclusion is a function of IgA. Nature 255:745–746

Sutherland DB, Suzuki K, Fagarasan S (2016) Fostering of advanced mutualism with gut microbiota by Immunoglobulin A. Immunol Rev 270:20–31

Suzuki K, Maruya M, Kawamoto S, Sitnik K, Kitamura H, Agace WW et al (2010) The sensing of environmental stimuli by follicular dendritic cells promotes immunoglobulin a generation in the gut. Immunity 33:71–83

Suzuki K, Meek B, Doi Y, Honjo T, Fagarasan S (2005) Two distinctive pathways for recruitment of naive and primed IgM^+ B cells to the gut lamina propria. Proc Natl Acad Sci USA 102:2482–2486

Suzuki K, Meek B, Doi Y, Muramatsu M, Chiba T, Honjo T et al (2004) Aberrant expansion of segmented filamentous bacteria in IgA-deficient gut. Proc Natl Acad Sci USA 101:1981–1986

Talham GL, Jiang HQ, Bos NA, Cebra JJ (1999) Segmented filamentous bacteria are potent stimuli of a physiologically normal state of the murine gut mucosal immune system. Infect Immun 67:1992–2000

Tezuka H, Abe Y, Iwata M, Takeuchi H, Ishikawa H, Matsushita M et al (2007) Regulation of IgA production by naturally occurring TNF/iNOS-producing dendritic cells. Nature 448:929–933

Tsuji M, Komatsu N, Kawamoto S, Suzuki K, Kanagawa O, Honjo T et al (2009) Preferential generation of follicular B helper T cells from Foxp3+ T cells in gut Peyer's patches. Science 323:1488–1492

Tsuji M, Suzuki K, Kitamura H, Maruya M, Kinoshita K, Ivanov II et al (2008) Requirement for lymphoid tissue inducer cells in isolated follicle formation and T cell-independent immunoglobulin a generation in the gut. Immunity 29:261–271

Uchimura Y, Fuhrer T, Li H, Lawson MA, Zimmermann M, Yilmaz B et al (2018) Antibodies set boundaries limiting microbial metabolite penetration and the resultant mammalian host response. Immunity 49:545–559 e545

Uematsu S, Fujimoto K, Jang MH, Yang BG, Jung YJ, Nishiyama M et al (2008) Regulation of humoral and cellular gut immunity by lamina propria dendritic cells expressing Toll-like receptor 5. Nat Immunol 9:769–776

van der Waaij LA, Kroese FG, Visser A, Nelis GF, Westerveld BD, Jansen PL et al (2004) Immunoglobulin coating of faecal bacteria in inflammatory bowel disease. Eur J Gastroenterol Hepatol 16:669–674

Varol C, Vallon-Eberhard A, Elinav E, Aychek T, Shapira Y, Luche H et al (2009) Intestinal lamina propria dendritic cell subsets have different origin and functions. Immunity 31:502–512

Viladomiu M, Kivolowitz C, Abdulhamid A, Dogan B, Victorio D, Castellanos JG et al (2017) IgA-coated E. coli enriched in Crohn's disease spondyloarthritis promote TH17-dependent inflammation. Sci Transl Med 9

Wei M, Shinkura R, Doi Y, Maruya M, Fagarasan S, Honjo T (2011) Mice carrying a knock-in mutation of Aicda resulting in a defect in somatic hypermutation have impaired gut homeostasis and compromised mucosal defense. Nat Immunol 12:264–270

Williams RC, Gibbons RJ (1972) Inhibition of bacterial adherence by secretory immunoglobulin A: a mechanism of antigen disposal. Science 177:697–699

Wu HJ, Ivanov II, Darce J, Hattori K, Shima T, Umesaki Y et al (2010) Gut-residing segmented filamentous bacteria drive autoimmune arthritis via T helper 17 cells. Immunity 32:815–827

Xiong E, Li Y, Min Q, Cui C, Liu J, Hong R et al (2019) MZB1 promotes the secretion of J-chain-containing dimeric IgA and is critical for the suppression of gut inflammation. Proc Natl Acad Sci USA 116:13480–13489

Yel L (2010) Selective IgA deficiency. J Clin Immunol 30:10–16

Primary Antibody Deficiencies

10

Qing Min, Xin Meng, and Ji-Yang Wang

Abstract

Primary antibody deficiencies (PADs) are the most common types of inherited primary immunodeficiency diseases (PIDs) presenting at any age, with a broad spectrum of clinical manifestations including susceptibility to infections, autoimmunity and cancer. Antibodies are produced by B cells, and consequently, genetic defects affecting B cell development, activation, differentiation or antibody secretion can all lead to PADs. Whole exome and whole genome sequencing approaches have helped identify genetic defects that are involved in the pathogenesis of PADs. Here, we summarize the clinical manifestations, causal genes, disease mechanisms and clinical treatments of different types of PADs.

Keywords

Primary antibody deficiencies · B cell development · B cell activation and differentiation · Class-switch recombination · T-B interaction

10.1 Introduction

Antibodies (Abs) are circulating proteins that are produced in vertebrates spontaneously (natural Abs) or in response to foreign antigens (specific Abs) and protect bodies from an almost unlimited variety of pathogens. B lymphocytes are the only cells that secrete Abs. Intrinsic defects in B cell development, activation, differentiation or Ab secretion can all lead to primary antibody deficiencies (PADs). PADs can also result from functional impairments in T lymphocytes or other cells that cooperate with or provide "help" to B cells for Ab production. Studying the etiology of PADs provides us with unique opportunities to reveal new important molecular pathways involved in B cell development and function (Durandy et al. 2013; Pieper et al. 2013; Conley et al. 2009).

PADs are the most common types of primary immunodeficiency diseases (PIDs), accounting for approximately half of the diseases (Pieper et al. 2013). PADs consist of a heterogeneous group of disorders, ranging from patients with a severe reduction of all serum immunoglobulin (Ig) classes and absence of B cells to patients who have a selective deficiency in a particular Ab isotype with relatively normal levels of other Abs. Genetic analysis of PADs revealed complicated genotype-phenotype correlation. Different mutations in the same gene may present striking variability in clinical and laboratory findings and can even have different patterns of

Q. Min · X. Meng · J.-Y. Wang (✉)
Department of Immunology, School of Basic Medical Sciences, Fudan University, Shanghai, China
e-mail: wang@fudan.edu.cn

J.-Y. Wang (ed.), *B Cells in Immunity and Tolerance*, Advances in Experimental Medicine and Biology 1254, https://doi.org/10.1007/978-981-15-3532-1_10

inheritance (Bogaert et al. 2016). In addition to genetic defects, environmental factors also affect the pathogenesis of PADs. Genetic and immunological features of monogenic forms of PADs are summarized in Table 10.1.

10.2 Defects in Early B Cell Development

B lymphocytes develop in the bone marrow (BM) from hematopoietic precursor cells. Developing B lymphocytes acquire functional antigen receptor through DNA rearrangement events that bring randomly chosen V, (D) and J gene segments into contiguity. Based on the status of heavy chain (HC) and light chain (LC) gene rearrangements, three early B cell developmental stages are defined. The first is pro-B stage, where Ig gene HC undergoes D to J and then V to DJ rearrangements. If successful, the HC together with the surrogate light chains (VpreB and Lambda 5) and the signal-transducing components Igα and Igβ form a pre-BCR and pro-B cells become pre-B cells. Pre-BCR transmits an autologous signal to shut down further rearrangement of the HC locus and initiates V to J rearrangement of LC. If the LC rearrangement is successful, the expressed LC associates with HC to form an IgM molecule on the cell surface, and cells thus become immature B cells (Pieper et al. 2013). Genetic defects affecting V(D)J gene rearrangements or the expression of the pre-BCR components or downstream signaling molecules can all cause severe defects in B cell development, resulting in agammaglobulinemia due to the absence of circulating B cells and recurrent bacterial infections in the first 5 years of life. However, clinical course may vary dependent on different genetic defects (Conley et al. 2009).

10.2.1 Defects in Pre-BCR Component

Pre-BCR consists of two μ heavy chains, two λ5, two VpreB and one co-receptor complex, Igα and Igβ. To date, genetic defects in μ heavy chains (*IGHM*), λ5 (*IGLL1*), Igα (*CD79A*) and Igβ (*CD79B*) have been described to be associated with autosomal recessive agammaglobulinemia (AR-agammaglobulinemia) (Yel et al. 1996; Minegishi et al. 1998; 1999; Ferrari et al. 2007), a rare form of PAD characterized by severe reduction of all Ig isotypes and absence of peripheral B cells. Defects in *IGHM* account for approximately half of the AR-agammaglobulinemia. Most IGHM-deficient patients resulted from gross deletions ranging in size from 40 to 732 kb, which encompassed the *IGHM* gene, or a single base pair substitution at the splice site, which would inhibit production of the membrane form of the μ chain (Yel et al. 1996; Silva et al. 2017). All the reported patients showed less than 0.01% of $CD19^+$ B cells in the peripheral circulation and had a high incidence of enteroviral infection and *Pseudomonas* sepsis with neutropenia (Conley et al. 2009). Similar to patients with defects in *IGHM*, patients with defects in *IGLL1*, *CD79A* and *CD79B* also suffered from early-onset severe infections, but less severe than those with IGHM deficiency.

10.2.2 Defects in Pre-BCR Signaling

Pre-BCR initiates downstream signaling by triggering tyrosine phosphorylation of ITAMs by LYN and the activation of the spleen tyrosine kinase SYK. LYN and SYK then together phosphorylate the adaptor protein B cell linker (BLNK) and Bruton's tyrosine kinase (BTK), leading to the activation of phospholipase Cγ2 (PLCγ2) and the phosphoinositide 3-kinase (PI3K) pathway (Durandy et al. 2013).

The most common PAD is X-linked agammaglobulinemia (XLA), which is caused by mutations in the *BTK* gene and accounts for 85% of the patients with agammaglobulinemia (Vetrie et al. 1993). BTK deficiency is the first identified immunological disorder for which the genetic cause was discovered (Tsukada et al. 1993; Vetrie et al. 1993). BTK consists of five domains: PH, TH, SH3, SH2 and TK. In addition to mutations that cause frameshift or premature stop codon, missense mutations in PH, TH, SH2 and

Table 10.1 Genes associated with monogenic forms of PADs: summary of genetic and immunological features

Causal gene	Effect on protein	Inheritance	Onset	Affected cells	Ig level	Other manifestations
Defects in early B cell development						
Defects in pre-BCR component						
IGHM (μ heavy chain)	LOF	AR	Within the first year of life	Absent peripheral B cells, normal numbers of pro-B cells	All isotypes decreased	
IGLL1 (λ5)	LOF	AR	Early childhood to adulthood	Absent or less than 0.1% of peripheral B cells; normal numbers of pro-B cells	All isotypes decreased	
CD79A (Igα)	LOF	AR	Within the first year of life	Absent or less than 0.3% of peripheral B cells; normal numbers of pro-B cells	All isotypes decreased	
CD79B (Igβ)	LOF	AR	Within the first year of life	Absent or less than 1% of peripheral B cells; normal numbers of pro-B cells	All isotypes decreased	
Defects in pre-BCR signaling						
BTK	LOF	X-linked	Early childhood to adulthood	Absent peripheral B cells in majority of patients; some patients present with slightly low or even normal numbers of B lymphocytes; normal numbers of pro-B cells	All isotypes decreased in majority of patients; some patients have detectable immunoglobulins	
BLNK	LOF	AR	Early childhood to adulthood	Absent peripheral B cells; normal numbers of pro-B cells	All isotypes decreased	
Other forms of early B cell development deficiency						
PIK3R1 (p85α)	LOF	AR	Within the first year of life	Absence of peripheral B cells and bone marrow pro-B cells	All isotypes decreased	
TCF3 (E47 transcription factor)	LOF/GOF (dominant negative)	AD/AR	Early childhood	Reduced peripheral B cells and bone marrow pro-B cells; residual peripheral B cells had increased CD19 but no BCR expression	All isotypes decreased	Some patients accompanied with B-ALL

(continued)

Table 10.1 (continued)

Causal gene	Effect on protein	Inheritance	Onset	Affected cells	Ig level	Other manifestations
AK2	LOF	AR	Within the first month of life	Severe neutropenia; T and NK cell lymphopenia; variable peripheral B cells	All isotypes decreased	Bilateral sensorineural deafness
ADA	LOF	AR	Within the first year of life in majority of patients	Absent T, B, NK cells in majority of patients	All isotypes decreased	Neurologic abnormalities
Defects in B cell survival, activation and differentiation						
Defects in B cell survival						
TNFRSF13B (TACI)	LOF	AD/AR	Early childhood to adulthood	Variable in total B cells and memory B cells	Low IgG and IgA and/or IgM	
TNFRSF13C (BAFFR)	LOF/GOF	AD/AR	Within the first year of life to late adulthood	Variable in total B, transitional B and memory B cells	Low IgG and low to normal IgA and IgM	
TNFSF12 (TWEAK)	LOF	AD	Early childhood	Variable in total B, transitional B and memory B cells	Low IgG and undetectable to normal IgA and IgM	
Defects in B cell activation						
CD19	LOF	AR	Within the first year of life to early childhood	Normal $CD20^{+}$ B cells; reduced memory B cells	Low IgG and undetectable to normal IgA and IgM	
CD21	LOF	AR	Early childhood to childhood	Normal total B cells; reduced memory B cells	Low IgG and IgA; low to normal IgM	
CD81	LOF	AR	Within the first year of life	Normal $CD20^{+}$ B cells; reduced memory B cells; absent CD19 expression	Low IgG; normal IgM and low to normal IgA	
CD20	LOF	AR	Within the first year of life	Normal total B cells; reduced memory B cells	Low IgG; normal IgM and IgA	
TNFRSF7 (CD27)	LOF	AR	Within the first year of life to childhood	Decreased to normal total B cells; absent memory B cells; variable in T cells and NK cells	Low to normal IgG, IgM and IgA	EBV-induced lymphoproliferation
TNFSF7 (CD70)	LOF	AR	Within the first year of life to early childhood	Reduced switched memory B cells; variable in T cells and NK cells	Reduced IgG, IgM and IgA in majority of patients	EBV-induced lymphoproliferation

(continued)

Table 10.1 (continued)

Causal gene	Effect on protein	Inheritance	Onset	Affected cells	Ig level	Other manifestations
LRBA	LOF	AR	Within the first year of life to childhood	Decreased or normal total B cells; decreased or normal $CD4^+$ T cells	Reduced IgG and IgA in majority of patients	
CTLA4	LOF	AD	Within the first year of life to adulthood	Decreased or normal total B and T cells; impaired function of Tregs	Low to normal IgG, IgM and IgA	
IL21	LOF	AR	Within the first year of life	Decreased total and switched memory B cells; increased transitional B cells	Low IgG; high IgE	Inflammatory bowel disease
IL21R	LOF	AR	Within the first year of life to early childhood	Normal numbers of total B and T cells; abnormal T cell proliferation	High IgE	
PLCG2 (PLCγ2)	GOF	AD	Within the first year of life to childhood	Normal numbers of total B cells; reduced to normal memory B cells; reduced or normal NK cells	Low to normal IgG, IgM and IgA	Cold urticarial; granulomatous rash
PRKCD (PKCδ)	LOF	AR	Within the first year of life to early childhood	Variable in total B, T and NK cells; reduced memory B cells	Variable in IgG, IgM and IgA	
PIK3CD	GOF	AD	Within the first year of life to early childhood	Decreased total B cells while increased transitional B cells in majority of patients; variable in T cells	Low IgG while increased IgM in majority of patients	
PIK3R1	LOF	AD	Within the first year of life to childhood	Decreased total B cells while increased transitional B cells in majority of patients; variable in T cells	Low IgG while increased IgM in majority of patients	
PTEN	LOF	AD	Early childhood to childhood	Reduced memory B cells	Low IgG, IgM and IgA	Autoimmunity; peripheral lymphoid hyperplasia
NFKB1	LOF	AD	Early childhood to adulthood	Decreased to normal numbers of total B cells; impaired early and late B cell development in several patients	Low to normal IgG, IgM and IgA	EBV-driven lymphoproliferation; autoimmunity; autoinflammatory disease

(continued)

Table 10.1 (continued)

Causal gene	Effect on protein	Inheritance	Onset	Affected cells	Ig level	Other manifestations
CARD11	LOF	AR/AD	Within the first year	Increased transitional B cells	Low IgG; low to normal IgA, IgM	Opportunistic infections; severe atopic disease
BCL10	LOF	AR	Within the first year	Reduced memory B and T cells; fibroblast deficiency	Low IgG	
MALT1	LOF	AR	Within the first year	Reduced memory B cells	High IgE in some patients	Autoimmunity; autoinflammation
NFKB2	LOF/GOF	AD	Within the first year of life to childhood	Absent to normal total B cells; decreased or normal memory B cells; variable in T cells	Low to normal IgG, IgM and IgA	Adrenal insufficiency
IKZF1 (IKAROS)	LOF	AD	Early childhood to late adulthood	Progressive loss of peripheral B cells; variable in T cells and NK cells	Low IgG; low to normal IgM and IgA	SLE; APLS
RAC2	LOF/GOF	AR/AD	Within the first year of life to childhood	Decreased or normal B cells	Low IgG; low to normal IgM and IgA	
BLK	LOF	AR	Within the first year of life	Decreased or normal total B and memory B cells; normal or increased T cells	Low IgG; low to normal IgM and IgA	SLE; rheumatoid arthritis
Defects in B cell differentiation						
IRF2BP2	GOF	AD	Early childhood to childhood	Decreased switched memory B cells	Low IgG and IgM; absent IgA	
SEC61A1	GOF	AD	Within the first year of life to adulthood	Reduced plasma cells	Low IgG, IgA and IgM in majority of patients	
MOGS	LOF	AR	Childhood	Normal or increased numbers of B cells	Low IgG, IgM and IgA	Multiple neurologic complications
Defects in antibody secreting						
ATP6AP1	LOF	XL	Childhood to adulthood	Increased naïve B and reduced memory B cells	Low IgG; low to normal IgM and IgA	Hepatopathy; neurocognitive abnormalities
Other genetic defects involved in CVID						
TRNT1	LOF	AR	Within the first year of life	Absent or low total B cells	Low IgG, IgM and IgA	Sideroblastic anemia; developmental delay

(continued)

Table 10.1 (continued)

Causal gene	Effect on protein	Inheritance	Onset	Affected cells	Ig level	Other manifestations
TTC37	LOF	AR	Within the first year of life	Reduced memory B cells in majority of patients	Low IgG, IgM and IgA in majority of patients	Life-threatening diarrhea; liver disease; trichorrhexis nodosa; facial dysmorphism; hypopigmentation; cardiac defects
Defects in class-switch recombination						
Defects in T cells						
CD40LG (*CD154*, *TNFSF5*)	LOF	XL	Within the first year of life to adulthood	Absent $sIgG^+$, $sIgA^+$, $sIgE^+$ B cells; reduced to normal T cells	Low or absent IgG, IgA and IgE; normal or high IgM	Opportunistic infections; neutropenia; neuroendocrine tumors
Defects in B cells						
CD40 (*TNFRSF5*)	LOF	AR	Within the first year of life	Absent $sIgG^+$, $sIgA^+$, $sIgE^+$ B cells	Low or absent IgG, IgA and IgE; normal or high IgM	Opportunistic infections; neutropenia
AICDA (*AID*)	LOF	AR/AD	Within the first year of life to adulthood	Absent $sIgG^+$, $sIgA^+$, $sIgE^+$ B cells	Low or absent IgG, IgA and IgE; high IgM	Lymphoid hyperplasia; lymphadenopathy; autoimmune cytopenias
UNG	LOF	AR	Childhood to adulthood	Absent $sIgG^+$, $sIgA^+$, $sIgE^+$ B cells	Low or absent IgG, IgA and IgE; high IgM	Lymphoid hyperplasia
ION80	LOF	AR	Childhood to adulthood	Absent $sIgG^+$, $sIgA^+$, $sIgE^+$ B cells	Low IgG, IgA and IgE; high IgM	
MSH6	LOF	AR	Childhood to adulthood	Reduced switched memory B cells	High IgM in majority of patients; low to normal IgG and IgA	Cancer
PMS2	LOF	AR	Early childhood	Reduced switched memory B cells	High IgM; low IgG and IgA	Cancer; hereditary non-polyposis
Hyper-IgE syndrome						
STAT3 associated HIES						
STAT3	LOF	AD	Within the first year of life to adulthood	Reduced memory B cells	High IgE	Eczema; connective tissue; skeletal; dental abnormalities
IL6ST (*GP130*)	LOF	AR	Within the first year of life	Progressive decline total B cells	High IgE; low or normal IgG	Atopic dermatitis; eczema; skeletal abnormalities
IL6R	LOF	AR	Within the first year of life	Normal total B and T cells	High IgE; low IgM, IgG and IgA	Atopic dermatitis

(continued)

Table 10.1 (continued)

Causal gene	Effect on protein	Inheritance	Onset	Affected cells	Ig level	Other manifestations
ZNF431	LOF	AR	Within the first year of life	Reduced Th17 $CD4^+$ T cells	High IgE and IgG	Atopic dermatitis; connective tissue abnormalities
Autosomal recessive HIES						
DOCK8	LOF	AR	Childhood to adulthood	Low total and memory B cells; low T cells; low NK cells	Low IgM; normal to high IgG and IgA; high IgE	Atopic dermatitis; allergy
PGM3	LOF	AR	Within the first year of life to childhood	Low total and memory B cells; low T cells	Normal to high IgG and IgA; high IgE	Glomerulonephritis; allergies; eczema; severe congenital glycosylation disorders; neurologic manifestations
SPINK5 (*LEKTI*)	LOF	AR	Within the first year of life	Low memory B cells	High IgE and IgG_4	Skin barrier defect; dermatitis; Neurologic abnormalities

TK domains can also lead to XLA. XLA is a leaky defect in B cell development. Unlike the complete absence of peripheral B cells caused by *IGHM* mutations, mutations in *BTK* usually result in a developmental arrest at the pro-B to pre-B stage, with less than 1% of mature B cells detectable in the periphery of the patients and very low levels of all Ig isotypes. Patients with "atypical" XLA were also reported (Saffran et al. 1994). Some of these patients had reduced or abnormal BTK expression and presented with slightly low or even normal numbers of B lymphocytes and not very low levels of Ig (Saffran et al. 1994; Mitsuiki et al. 2015).

Defects in *BLNK* also have been reported to be associated with AR-agammaglobulinemia. Immunological analysis of BLNK-deficient patients revealed that B cell development was blocked at the pro-B to pre-B stage, and the phenotype was similar to that seen in patients with mutations in *BTK*, with only a small number of circulating B cells (Conley et al. 2009). Moreover, additional experiments suggest that BLNK is essential for further B cell development after the pre-BCR is expressed (Rezaei et al. 2017).

10.2.3 Other Forms of Early B Cell Development Deficiency

More recently, two independent patients with null mutations in *PIK3R1*, which encodes the p85α regulatory subunit of class I PI3K, have been described as AR-agammaglobulinemia (Conley et al. 2012; Tang et al. 2018). They presented with recurrent pneumonia and colitis associated with decreased Ig levels of all isotypes (Conley et al. 2012). B cell development in patients with PIK3R1 deficiency was blocked at the earliest stage of B-lineage commitment, much earlier than the genetic defects described above.

Five patients with transcription factor 3 gene (*TCF3*) mutations have been reported to show decreased peripheral B cell numbers and agammaglobulinemia (Ben-Ali et al. 2017; Boisson et al. 2013). TCF3 (E47) is a broadly expressed transcription factor and is required for B cell development in mice (Bain et al. 1994). Boisson and colleagues found four unrelated patients who had the same de novo missense heterozygous mutation in *TCF3*, which led to markedly decreased numbers of peripheral B cells and agammaglobulinemia (Boisson et al. 2013). Residual B cells that could be detected had an increased expression of CD19 but absence of B cell receptor (Boisson et al. 2013). Recently, Meriem Ben-Ali found a patient who had a novel homozygous nonsense mutation in the *TCF3* gene, resulting in the expression of a truncated protein. This patient presented with severe hypogammaglobulinemia and had B cell acute lymphoblastic leukemia (B-ALL), but his younger sister who had the same mutation exhibited slightly lower peripheral B cell numbers, borderline low IgG and significantly decreased IgA and IgM levels (Ben-Ali et al. 2017). Therefore, the phenotypes of *TCF3* mutations seem to be variable, and more patients need to be analyzed to determine TCF3 function in humans.

In addition to PADs caused by genetic defects mainly affecting B cells, several combined immunodeficiency (CID) syndromes are also associated with defects in early B cell development. The proteins encoded by recombination-activating gene *RAG1* and *RAG2* initiate the V(D)J recombination process by introducing DNA double-strand breaks (DSBs) adjacent to the V, D or J gene segment, resulting in the formation of sealed hairpin coding ends and blunt signal ends, which are eventually processed and joined by the non-homologous end-joining pathway (NHEJ pathway). Successful V(D)J recombination is essential for normal B and T cell development. Genetic defects affecting the expression or function of RAG1 or RAG2 lead to a broad spectrum of clinical phenotypes, including severe combined immunodeficiency (SCID) with lack of T and B cells as well as all classes of Abs, Omenn syndrome with oligoclonal, activated and anergic autologous T cells that infiltrate target tissues, leaky SCID, and combined immunodeficiency with granulomas or autoimmunity (CID-G/AI). Several missense mutations in *RAG1* gene have been reported to cause marked decrease of B cells and agammaglobulinemia (Hedayat et al. 2014; Cifaldi et al. 2016). Genetic defects in the components of NHEJ pathway, such as Artemis (*DCLRE1C*), DNA-PKcs (*PRKDC*), *LIG4* and XLF (*NHEJ1*), can also lead to absence of B and T lymphocytes and all Ig isotypes (Moshous et al. 2001; van der Burg et al. 2009; O'Driscoll et al. 2001; Buck et al. 2006).

Adenylate kinase 2 (*AK2*) deficiency (also known as reticular dysgenesis) is an autosomal recessive form of human SCID characterized by an early differentiation arrest in the myeloid lineage and impaired lymphocyte maturation, leading to early-onset, recurrent and overwhelming infections (Lagresle-Peyrou et al. 2009; Rissone et al. 2015). It is the most severe form of SCID with severe neutropenia and T and NK cell lymphopenia, while the B cell lineage could variably be affected.

Biallelic mutations in adenosine deaminase (*ADA*) result in accumulation of toxic metabolites which disturb cellular functions in numerous tissues and particularly impair lymphocyte development, viability and function (Cagdas et al. 2018; Giblett et al. 1972). ADA deficiency not only partially blocks B cell development at later developmental stages, but also affects V(D)J recombination, resulting in peripheral lymphopenia and reduced B cell proliferation (Cagdas et al. 2018).

Among PADs, some genetic defects specifically affect early B cell development, in particular pro-B to pre-B transition, whereas other defects not only affect the development of B cells but also other haematopoietic cell lineages, leading to multiple cell defects. Among patients with agammaglobulinemia and absent B cells, the vast majority ($\sim$85%) are caused by mutations in *BTK* but the genetic defects for the remaining cases are still unknown.

10.3 Defects in B Cell Survival, Activation and Differentiation

Common variable immunodeficiency (CVID) is a heterogeneous group of disorders characterized by hypogammaglobulinemia, defective specific Ab production and increased susceptibility to recurrent and chronic infections. Patients with CVID also have increased incidence of autoimmune disorders and cancers (Rezaei et al. 2017). CVID is the most common PAD with an estimated prevalence ranging from 1/10,000 to 1/50,000 in Caucasians and affects males and females equally. The clinical spectrum of CVID is broad, and it may present at any age but with a peak incidence in childhood and early adult life (Bogaert et al. 2016). CVID has a complex genetic basis. To date, a monogenic cause has been identified only in 2-10% of patients, and most cases are likely in polygenic inheritance (Bonilla et al. 2016). All CVIDs are associated with B cell intrinsic defects in survival, activation, differentiation or Ab production.

10.3.1 Defects in B Cell Survival

Immature B cells leave the BM and migrate to the spleen, where they mature into naïve B cells. During these processes, BAFF (B cell activating factor) and APRIL (a proliferation-inducing ligand) are required for B cells to maintain their viability and homeostasis. BAFF could bind to three types of receptors expressed by B cells, namely B cell activating factor belonging to the TNF family receptor (BAFFR, encoded by *TNFRSF13C*), transmembrane activator and calcium modulator and cyclophilin ligand interactor (TACI, encoded by *TNFRSF13B*) and B cell maturation antigen (BCMA, encoded by *TNFRSF17*), whereas APRIL only binds to TACI and BCMA (Rickert et al. 2011).

Biallelic and monoallelic loss-of-function mutations in *TNFRSF13B* (*TACI*) have been described to be associated with CVID, which lead to various degrees of Ab deficiency. Nearly all patients with biallelic mutations presented with hypogammaglobulinemia, variable levels of IgM and IgA and impaired Ab responses to vaccination (Salzer et al. 2009; Bogaert et al. 2016). The monoallelic C104R and A181E variants account for 80% of all *TNFRSF13B* mutations in patients with CVID (Bogaert et al. 2016). C104R mutation dominantly interferes with ligand binding, and A181E affects receptor oligomerization. Moreover, CVID patients with monoallelic C104R mutations had a higher risk of developing benign lymphoproliferation and autoantibody-mediated autoimmunity, but the mechanism remains unclear (Salzer et al. 2009). However, monoallelic *TNFRSF13B* mutations have also been detected in asymptomatic relatives and in 1-2% of the general population, which suggests that these variants alone cannot explain the clinical phenotype in patients with CVID (Bogaert et al. 2016).

Biallelic and monoallelic mutations in *TNFRSF13C* (*BAFFR*) have also been identified in more than 80 patients with CVID (Bogaert et al. 2016). Complete BAFFR deficiency is rare, as only two adult-onset patients have been reported so far, who showed impaired B cell development, severely decreased circulating B cells and low IgG and IgM but normal IgA concentrations (Warnatz et al. 2009). Interestingly, only one of them presented with recurrent infections (Warnatz et al. 2009). The majority of patients carried heterozygous or compound heterozygous mutations in *TNFRSF13C* and displayed variable immunological abnormalities (Lougaris et al. 2016). Most variants do not affect or only reduce the BAFFR expression (Lougaris et al. 2016; Bogaert et al. 2016). P21R mutation is the most common variant in reported cases, which reduces BAFF ligand binding (Pieper et al. 2013). Similar to *TNFRSF13B* variants, an abnormal BAFFR function predisposes to but does not suffice for CVID development (Pieper et al. 2013).

Heterozygous missense mutation in *TNFSF12*, the gene encoding TNF-like weak inducer of apoptosis (TWEAK), is associated with an autosomal dominant hypogammaglobulinemia (Wang et al. 2013). The R145C TWEAK mutant described in the patients formed both intramolecular complexes of TWEAK and TWEAK/BAFF protein complexes via intermolecular disulfide bridges. The TWEAK/BAFF protein complexes showed slightly enhanced binding to BAFFR, but the signaling was impaired (Wang et al. 2013). Consequently, BAFF-dependent B cell survival and proliferation were impaired in the patients.

10.3.2 Defects in B Cell Activation

B cell activation is initiated by specific recognition of antigens by the surface BCR, along with other stimuli, including complement, pathogen-associated molecular patterns (PAMPs) and signals from helper T cells, leading to their proliferation and differentiation into memory B cells or Ab-secreting plasma cells.

BCR co-receptor (consisting of CD19, CD21, CD81 and CD225) initiates Ca^{2+} signaling following BCR stimulation and lowers the threshold for B cell activation upon antigen binding to the BCR (van Zelm et al. 2006). To date, defects in *CD19*, *CD81* and *CD21* (*CR2*) have been identified in patients with early childhood-onset, autosomal recessive form of CVID (van Zelm et al. 2006; van Zelm et al. 2010; Thiel et al. 2012). Patients with defects in *CD19* and *CD81* had normal $CD20^+$ B cell numbers, but reduced $CD27^+$ B cells, and defective somatic hypermutation (SHM) and class-switch recombination (CSR) (which indicates impaired germinal center reaction) (van Zelm et al. 2014). Compared with patients with defects in *CD19* and *CD81*, four patients from three unrelated families with homozygous mutations in *CD21* had a later onset age, milder infections and less pronounced humoral immune defects. This might suggest that CD21 may be more redundant than CD19 and CD81 in regulating B cell activation (Thiel et al. 2012; Wentink et al. 2015; Rosain et al. 2017).

CD20 is a component of B cell surface complex and is involved in a signal transduction cascade that regulates B cell activation, adhesion and proliferation (Kuijpers et al. 2010). Biallelic mutations in *CD20* have been reported in a patient with complete loss of CD20 surface expression. This patient presented with early-onset recurrent pulmonary infections and impaired T-cell independent Ab responses to polysaccharides. Immunological analysis revealed decreased serum IgG but normal IgM and IgA levels and markedly reduced numbers of class-switched memory B cells (Kuijpers et al. 2010).

CD27 is a transmembrane receptor encoded by *TNFRSF7*. Through interaction with its ligand CD70 (encoded by *TNFSF7*), CD27 provides costimulatory signals for T, B and NK cell activation and regulates their survival, function and differentiation (van Montfrans et al. 2012). Biallelic *TNFRSF7* mutations have been reported in patients with various phenotypes. Most of them had persistent hypogammaglobulinemia, low levels of IgA and IgM and recurrent pneumonia, and thus diagnosed as CVID (Alkhairy et al. 2015a). Furthermore, almost all CD27-deficient patients suffered from severe and/or atypical EBV-associated lymphoproliferative disease/hemophagocytic lymphohistiocytosis (van Montfrans et al. 2012; Alkhairy et al. 2015a). However, given that CD27 deficiency is associated with T cell dysfunction and impaired T-cell dependent B cell responses, it is currently considered as a lymphoproliferative syndrome. Similarly, CD70 deficiency due to homozygous mutations in *TNFSF7* gene has been reported in five patients, and the majority of them presented with reduced memory B cells, decreased serum IgG, IgM and IgA levels and chronic EBV infection and lymphoma (Izawa et al. 2017; Abolhassani et al. 2017). At present, CD27 deficiency and CD70 deficiency are considered as immune dysregulation syndrome (Picard et al. 2018).

Biallelic loss-of-function mutations in the gene encoding lipopolysaccharide-responsive beige-like anchor protein (LRBA) have been identified in several patients affected by CVID-like disease, some accompanied with autoimmune lymphoproliferative syndrome or immune dysregulation, polyendocrinopathy and enteropathy (Bogaert et al. 2016). B cell survival, plasmablast generation and Ig secretion are all impaired under in vitro conditions. The phenotype of LRBA deficiency is very similar to that of cytotoxic T lymphocyte antigen 4 (CTLA-4) insufficiency, which is caused by heterozygous mutations in *CTLA4* (D'Elios and Rizzi 2019). Recent study has shown that LRBA is required for the post-translational expression and trafficking of CTLA-4 (Lo et al. 2015). Many LRBA and CTLA-4-deficient patients were clinically diagnosed with CVID. However, CTLA-4 and LRBA are crucial for quantitative regulation of immune homeostasis and tolerance, and their defects are currently considered as immune dysregulation syndrome (Picard et al. 2018).

Defects in cytokines and cytokine receptors affecting the cytokine signaling can also result in CVID-like disease. Homozygous mutations in *IL21* and *IL21R* were correlated with both Ab deficiency and autoimmune manifestations (Rezaei et al. 2017). IL21-IL21R signaling is involved in germinal center (GC) formation, which is critical for the generation of high-affinity Ab, and in the survival of memory B cells and plasma cells (Avery et al. 2010). The typical phenotypes of IL21 and IL21R deficiency were respiratory tract infections, inflammatory complications and/or opportunistic infections, such as *Cryptosporidiosis* and *Pneumocystis jirovecii* pneumonia (Salzer et al. 2014). IL21 deficiency led to decreased numbers of B cells and switched memory B cells while increased transitional B cells. Ig test revealed reduced IgG but elevated IgE levels (Salzer et al. 2014). IL21R deficiency, however, showed normal T and B cell counts, but abnormal T cell proliferation to specific stimuli. The serum Ig levels were normal except for high total IgE, and the patients had impaired specific Ab responses (Kotlarz et al. 2013, 2014). In addition, some patients demonstrated functional defects in T and NK cells (Bogaert et al. 2016).

Following antigen binding to BCR, B cells collect bound antigen in a central aggregate and form the immunological synapse. BCR aggregation rapidly activates the Src family kinases LYN, BTK, PLCγ2 and FYN as well as the SYK and B-lymphoid tyrosine kinases (BLK). After several minutes, microsignalosomes (probably including CD19, SYK, PLCγ2, PI3K and VAV) dissociate from the BCR clusters, and activate IκB kinase (IKK) and extracellular signal-related kinase (ERK) (Kurosaki et al. 2010). Among them, PLCγ2 promotes the generation of diacylglycerol (DAG) and the influx of Ca^{2+}, which in turn activates protein kinase Cβ (PKCβ) and the CARMA1-, BCL10- and MALT1-containing (CBM) complex. IKK activation leads to the activation of the canonical nuclear factor of kappa light chain enhancer of activated B cell (NF-κB) pathway and regulates downstream gene expression (Rickert 2013).

Monoallelic gain-of-function mutations in *PLCG2*, which encodes PLCγ2, result in autosomal dominant Ab deficiency and immune dysregulation (PLAID) (Ombrello et al. 2012; Zhou et al. 2012). All reported PLAID patients carried deletion or missense mutations within the autoinhibitory domain, which resulted in constitutive activation of the mutant PLCγ2 (Ombrello et al. 2012). PLAID is characterized by CVID-like phenotype (low levels of serum IgM and IgA and reduced memory B cells), cold urticarial, granulomatous rash, autoimmune thyroiditis, ocular inflammation, sinopulmonary infections and enterocolitis. Given that the main clinical presentation was autoinflammation, PLCG2 deficiency is currently considered as an autoinflammatory disorder (Picard et al. 2018).

Recently, eight patients from five unrelated families with autosomal recessive mutations in *PRKCD*, which encodes protein kinase c delta (PKCδ), have been identified (Salzer et al. 2013; Kuehn et al. 2013; Belot et al. 2013; Kiykim et al. 2015; Nanthapisal et al. 2017). In B cells, PKCδ is involved in BCR-mediated signaling downstream of BTK and PLCγ2 (Salzer et al. 2013). PKCδ has several tyrosine residues that can be phosphorylated by different tyrosine kinases in response to specific stimuli (Salzer et al. 2016). PKCδ deficiency causes variable phenotypes, only the first reported patient presented with a CVID-like phenotype with decreased peripheral B cells, low numbers of memory B cells, increased $CD21^{low}$ B cells and hypogammaglobulinemia (Salzer et al. 2013). Among the remaining patients, one patient was diagnosed as autoimmune lymphoproliferative syndrome (ALPS)-like disease (Kuehn et al. 2013), and the other six patients were initially diagnosed as early-onset systemic lupus erythematosus (SLE). All eight described patients showed symptoms before the age of 10 and presented with hepatosplenomegaly, lymphoproliferation, autoreactive Abs, and SLE or SLE-like autoimmunity.

Heterozygous mutations in the gene encoding the PI3K catalytic subunit p110δ (*PIK3CD*) have been demonstrated to cause activated PI3Kδ syndrome (APDS) (Lucas et al. 2016). These mutations result in the overactivation of PI3K pathway leading to increased downstream AKT/mTOR signaling activation, which results in immune dysregulation and immunodeficiency, characterized by respiratory infections, bronchiectasis and autoimmune cytopenias (Elgizouli et al. 2016). Immunological analysis showed hypogammaglobulinemia but increased IgM levels in most patients, and reduced peripheral B cell counts with relatively increased transitional B cells. Overall, approximately 80% of the patients identified carried the E1021K variant, which affected the highly conserved residue in the C-terminus of p110δ (Tangye et al. 2019). Importantly, these mutations increased the risk of lymphoma (Bogaert et al. 2016).

Loss-of-function monoallelic mutations in *PIK3R1* encoding the p85α regulatory subunit of PI3K also result in overactivation of PI3K pathway with the same phenotype caused by *PIK3CD* gain-of-function mutations. To our knowledge, all reported mutations in *PIK3R1* were splice site mutations resulting in the skipping of exon 11 encoding for the domain that inhibits p110δ catalytic activity (Bogaert et al. 2016; Bravo Garcia-Morato et al. 2017). Homozygous PIK3R1 deficiency resulting in agammaglobulinemia was mentioned above.

Phosphoinositide 3-kinase and phosphatase and tensin homolog (encoded by *PTEN*) is a phosphatase antagonising the signaling cascades downstream of receptor tyrosine kinases and PI3K (Browning et al. 2015). Heterozygous loss-of-function mutations in *PTEN* are associated with PTEN hamartoma tumor syndromes (PHTS) (Marsh et al. 1998). Recently, several PHTS patients have been identified as CVID and presented with hypogammaglobulinemia, recurrent pulmonary infections, impaired memory B response and impaired CSR and SHM, which are similar to patients with activation mutations in *PIK3CD* (Driessen et al. 2016; Browning et al. 2015). Moreover, autoimmunity and peripheral lymphoid hyperplasia have been found in approximately half of the PHTS patients (Chen et al. 2017).

Impairment of the canonical NF-κB pathway also leads to abnormal B cell activation. Heterozygous loss-of-function mutations affecting the *NFKB1* (encoding NF-κB1) gene have been identified in a part of CVID patients (Fliegauf et al. 2015; Boztug et al. 2016; Schipp et al. 2016; Maffucci et al. 2016; Lougaris et al. 2017; Kaustio et al. 2017; B. Keller et al. 2017; Tuijnenburg et al. 2018). Initially, haploinsufficiency of NF-κB1 was demonstrated as a causative gene for CVID and hypogammaglobulinemia characterized by recurrent infections, decreased serum Ig levels and reduced numbers of memory B cells. Recent evidence indicates that NF-κB1 haploinsufficiency underlies a variable type of combined immunodeficiency (CID) affecting both B and T lymphocyte compartments, with a broadened spectrum of disease manifestations, including EBV-induced lymphoproliferative disease, autoimmune and autoinflammatory disease (Kaustio et al. 2017). Furthermore, an impairment of early (bone marrow) and late (periphery) B cell development upon monoallelic loss of *NFKB1* was identified, with partial arrest at the pre-BI stage during B cell development and decreased peripheral B cells (Kaustio et al. 2017).

CARD11/BCL10/MALT1 complex plays a crucial role in the activation of NF-κB pathway in adaptive immunity (Ruland and Hartjes 2019). Homozygous or heterozygous mutations in *CARD11* (caspase recruitment domain family, member 11), a scaffold for NF-κB activity, lead to CID (Dadi et al. 2018; Ma et al. 2017; Stepensky et al. 2013; Greil et al. 2013). Immunological analysis revealed hypogammaglo bulinemia with normal numbers of peripheral B and T cells while impaired T cell proliferation after in vitro stimulation and partial developmental blockage of B cell at transitional B stage. Apart from recurrent bacterial infections, some CARD11-deficient patients also presented with opportunistic infections and severe atopic disease. Patients deficient in BCL10 or MALT1 had similar impairments in adaptive immunity. The loss of BCL10 expression resulted in hypogammaglobulinemia and a profound defects in memory T and B cells, which led to uncontrolled gastrointestinal, central nervous system and respiratory tract infections with various bacteria and viruses (Torres et al. 2014). Patients with homozygous deficiency of MALT1 suffered from gastrointestinal, respiratory tract and systemic infections with multiple bacterial, viral and fungal species (Jabara et al. 2013; McKinnon et al. 2014; Ruland and Hartjes 2019). Serum Ig levels were normal in all MALT1-deficient patients, except elevated serum IgE found in some of them (Charbit-Henrion et al. 2017; Jabara et al. 2013; McKinnon et al. 2014).

Heterozygous *NFKB2* mutations have been identified in an autosomal dominant type of CVID, complicated with autoimmunity and endocrine deficiency. The patients were characterized by early-onset recurrent infections, hypogammaglobulinemia, variable B cell lymphopenia and impaired terminal B cell development (Chen et al. 2013; Lee et al. 2014). Alopecia areata, autoimmune features and adrenal insufficiency as well as impaired TCR-mediated T cell proliferation were also found in some patients (Chen et al. 2013; Lindsley et al. 2014). Most of the NFKB2-deficient patients have loss-of-function *NFKB2* mutations. In contrast, three patients from two families have been detected with novel heterozygous nonsense gain-of-function mutations in *NFKB2,* which are associated with a CID phenotype (Kuehn et al. 2017). However, two related individuals who carried the same nonsense mutations were asymptomatic, suggesting that these mutations alone are not sufficient to cause diseases or the asymptomatic individuals might develop phenotype in later lives.

Ikaros family zinc finger 1 (IKAROS, encoded by *IKZF1*) is a haematopoietic transcription factor required for mammalian B cell development. Recently, loss-of-function mutations in *IKZF1* have been reported to be associated with CVID, and with autoimmunity in the forms of SLE, immune thrombocytopenic purpura and antiphospholipid syndrome (APLS) (Kuehn et al. 2016; Hoshino et al. 2017; Van Nieuwenhove et al. 2018). Most of the patients showed a progressive loss of peripheral B cells and serum Ig, and some of them had markedly decreased early B cell precursors and normal development of pro-B to pre-B cells (Kuehn et al. 2016; Hoshino et al. 2017). Furthermore, seven unrelated patients with an early-onset CID phenotype were discovered to have unique heterozygous mutations in single amino acid site N159 of *IKZF1* gene, which resulted in a dominant-negative effect (Boutboul et al. 2018).

Ras related C3 botulinum toxin substrate 2 (RAC2, encoded by *RAC2*), a hematopoietic-specific member of the Rho family of guanosine triphosphatases (Rho GTPase), is a crucial regulator of cell signaling. A homozygous null mutation in *RAC2* has been identified in two siblings born from consanguineous parents. Both of them were diagnosed as CVID with decreased serum Ig levels, recurrent infections, reduced memory B cells and gradually reduced B cell numbers (Alkhairy et al. 2015b). Interestingly, heterozygous dominant-negative mutations affecting *RAC2* was associated with neutrophil dysfunction (Ambruso et al. 2000) or with $CD4^+$ T cell lymphopenia, and reduced serum IgA and IgM (Accetta et al. 2011). More recently, a dominant gain-of-function mutation in *RAC2* has been identified in three patients presented with severe T and B cell lymphopenia, myeloid dysfunction and recurrent respiratory infections (Hsu et al. 2019). With the discovery of new cases, the phenotype of RAC2 deficiency has been broadened. Thus, RAC2 deficiency should be considered as CID, not phagocyte dysregulation or CVID.

A heterozygous loss-of-function mutation in *BLK* gene variant L3P was identified in two CVID patients from a single family, which caused suppressed B cell proliferation and reduced ability of B cells to present antigen and elicit T cell responses (Compeer et al. 2015). However, some evidence indicated that variants of *BLK* were associated with autoimmune diseases, including SLE, rheumatoid arthritis (RA) and several other B cell associated autoimmune disorders (Jiang et al. 2019; Simpfendorfer et al. 2015). More patients will need to be identified to determine whether BLK deficiency should be considered as CVID or immune dysregulation disease.

10.3.3 Defects in B Cell Differentiation

B cell activation induces the expression of specific transcription factors, leading to B cell proliferation and differentiation into memory B cells or Ab-secreting plasma cells. Some genetic defects affecting this differentiation process also result in PAD, and most of them presented as CVID.

Three patients from a single family with an autosomal dominant CVID were identified. These patients had a heterozygous missense *IRF2BP2* (IFN regulatory factor 2 binding protein 2) mutation (M. D. Keller et al. 2016). All affected patients presented with hypogammaglobulinemia with low IgM and absent IgA, poor specific Ab production after vaccination and remarkably reduced switched memory B cells. The expression of IRF2BP2 was increased in these patients, which suggested a gain-of-function effect of the mutant *IRF2BP2*. The adverse effect of the mutant *IRF2BP2* on differentiation of plasmablasts was demonstrated by in vitro transfection of mutant *IRF2BP2* to healthy B cells (M. D. Keller et al. 2016).

Most recently, heterozygous mutations in *SEC61A1* (Sec61 translocon alpha 1 subunit) have been described to be associated with reduced plasma cells in two unrelated families. Patients presented with early-onset hypogammaglobulinemia and severe recurrent respiratory tract infections. *SEC61A1* is a target gene of XBP1 during plasma cell differentiation. In vivo and in vitro analysis revealed that heterozygous *SEC61A1* mutation specifically impaired plasma cell homeostasis in a dominant-negative mode without interfering with B cell and T cell development, activation and memory formation (Schubert et al. 2018).

Two siblings with severe hypogammaglobulinemia and type II congenital disorders of glycosylation (CDG-IIb) were identified with genetic deficiency in the gene encoding mannosyl-oligosaccharide glucosidase (MOGS) (Sadat et al. 2014). Immunological analysis revealed normal B and T cells but impaired plasma cell differentiation. However, they do not have recurrent infections. Further studies revealed that a shortened Ig half-life due to altered processing of N-linked glycans attached to Ig was the mechanism underlying the hypogammaglobulinemia. The impaired N-linked glycan processing cannot support cellular entry, and efficient replication of viruses is one of the explanations of decreased susceptibility to infections (Sadat et al. 2014).

10.3.4 Defects in Ab Secretion

ATP6AP1, encoding the accessory protein Ac45 of the V-ATPase, is located on the X chromosome. Hemizygous missense mutations in *ATP6AP1* were identified in 11 male patients displaying an immunodeficiency phenotype associated with hypogammaglobulinemia, increased naïve B and reduced memory B cells as well as hepatopathy (as Ac45 is mainly expressed in liver, brain and B cells) (Jansen et al. 2016). Some of them had poor response to vaccinations. *ATP6AP1* mutations result in abnormal protein glycosylation. In vitro analysis suggested that the phenotypes of the patients could be related to aberrant acidification caused by dysfunction of the V-ATPase, which led to impaired membrane trafficking and fusion and thus affected B cell differentiation, antigen processing and Ab production. However, the deeper relationship between Ac45 deficiency and CVID remains to be investigated (Jansen et al. 2016).

10.3.5 Other Genetic Defects Involved in CVID

CAA-adding enzyme (encoded by *TRNT1*) is a template-independent RNA polymerase required for the maturation of cytosolic and mitochondrial transfer RNAs (tRNAs) (Shi et al. 1998). Biallelic loss-of-function mutations in *TRNT1* are associated with sideroblastic anemia with immunodeficiency, periodic fevers and developmental delay (SIFD) in childhood (Chakraborty et al. 2014; Wedatilake et al. 2016). The presentation of patients varies depending on the degrees of CCA-adding enzyme activity (Chakraborty et al. 2014). Some mutations which retained certain CCA-adding enzyme activity or which occurred in less conserved domain resulted in less severe phenotype and longer survival compared with mutations that severely impaired the enzyme activity (Chakraborty et al. 2014; Frans et al. 2017). All of the reported patients displayed early-onset hypogammaglobulinemia with low levels of serum IgM and IgA, and some of them developed diarrhea and inflammatory bowel disease (IBD).

Biallelic loss-of-function mutations in the gene encoding the tetratricopeptide repeat domain-containing protein 37 (TTC37) have been demonstrated in patients with tricho-hepato-enteric syndrome (THES) characterized by life-threatening diarrhea in infancy, immunodeficiency, liver disease, trichorrhexis nodosa, facial dysmorphism, hypopigmentation and cardiac defects (Hartley et al. 2010). Immunological characteristics were described in about half of the clinically explored patients. Most of them presented with low concentrations of Ig of all isotypes, reduced number of memory B cells and an impaired response to vaccination (Hartley et al. 2010; Vely et al. 2018; Bourgeois et al. 2018). Some THES patients were diagnosed as CID (Vely et al. 2018). However, the pathogenesis of TTC37 deficiency still remains largely unclear.

10.4 Defects in Class-Switch Recombination

Antigen-induced T-cell dependent B cell activation takes place in GCs in the spleen and lymph nodes. Two key molecular events occur in GCs, namely class-switch recombination (CSR) and somatic hypermutation (SHM), which change the Ab isotypes and specificity, respectively. B cells that have acquired high affinity for the antigen are selected to differentiate into Ab-secreting plasma cells or switched memory B cells. GC reaction requires the cognate interaction between follicular helper T cells (TFH) and follicular B cells (FOB) and CD40L expressed by activated TFH and CD40 constitutively expressed by B cells are essential for T-B interaction (Dominique Gatto, JACI, 2010). B cells in GCs are induced to express the activation-induced cytidine deaminase (AID), which creates DNA lesions by catalyzing the deamination of cytosine and generating a uracil in the switch (S) region and the variable (V) region. The resulting U:G lesions in the S region are further processed by the uracil DNA glycosylase (UNG), which removes the uracil residues and produces an abasic site, and AP endonucleases, which creates DSBs. The repair of the DSBs by NHEJ pathway eventually results in CSR (Pieper et al. 2013).

Defects in this process can lead to very low levels of switched Ig, including IgG, IgA and IgE, but with normal and frequently increased levels of serum IgM. Given that both T and B cells are required for GC reaction, the defects in CSR can be divided into two groups, namely B cell intrinsic and T cell intrinsic defects.

10.4.1 Defects in T Cells

The most common and well-recognized form of deficiency in CSR is the mutations in the CD40 ligand gene (*CD40LG*), which is located on the X chromosome. Defects in this gene account for about half of the CSR deficiencies (de la Morena 2016; Korthauer et al. 1993). CD40 ligand deficiency disturbs T-B cooperation and GC formation and thus affects both CSR and SHM. Absence of CD40L-CD40 interaction also impairs antigen priming of T cells and causes defective T cell responses. Therefore, CD40 ligand deficiency leads to CID. Patients with CD40 ligand deficiency usually had early-onset recurrent bacterial infections and opportunistic infections, such as *Pjirovecii*, *Cryptosporidium* and *Sclerosing cholangitis*, and clinical phenotypes also include chronic diarrhea and neuroendocrine tumors (de la Morena 2016).

10.4.2 Defects in B Cells

CD40 (TNFRSF5) is a member of the tumor necrosis factor receptor superfamily. Mutations in *CD40* lead to a very rare autosomal recessive deficiency that is characterized by defects in both CSR and SHM (Ferrari et al. 2001; Lougaris et al. 2005; de la Morena 2016). Immunological studies of these patients revealed low levels of serum IgG and IgA, normal to high levels of IgM, absent or impaired vaccine responses, absent switched memory B cells with a low or normal IgM memory B cells carrying a mutated Ig receptor (Lougaris et al. 2005). The phenotypes are quite similar to CD40 ligand deficiency (de la Morena 2016).

Intriguingly, while absence of AID results in complete lack of both CSR and SHM, mutations located in the carboxyl terminus of AID abolish CSR but do not affect SHM (Durandy et al. 2013). Patients with complete AID deficiency have two different $CD27^+$ B cell subsets in the peripheral blood, IgM^+IgD^+ and IgM^+IgD^-, both of which carried remarkably fewer mutations in Ig receptors (Lougaris et al. 2005). In addition to recurrent infection, lymphadenopathy and autoimmune cytopenias can occur in AID-deficient patients (de la Morena 2016). In contrast to CD40-deficient patients, opportunistic infections are not commonly observed in AID-deficient patients. Notably, several mutations located in the C-terminus lead to an autosomal dominant CSR deficiency (Rezaei et al. 2017).

Biallelic mutations in the gene encoding UNG also resulted in profound impairment in CSR but retained an abnormal pattern of SHM (Imai et al. 2003; de la Morena 2016). The clinical characteristics of UNG-deficient patients are similar to AID defects. Autosomal recessive mutations in *INO80*, which encodes a catalytic ATPase subunit of the chromatin remodeling complex (INO80 chromatin remodeling complex), led to impaired CSR but did not affect SHM (Kracker et al. 2015). However, the reported patients who carried *INO80* mutations were diagnosed as CVID based on the clinical phenotypes. Defects in mismatch repair complex have been shown to be associated with CSR deficiency that mainly affects IgG and IgA subclass. A partial defect in CSR and an abnormal SHM were found in patients with mutations in Mutator S homolog 6 (*MSH6*) and *PMS2* (Gardes et al. 2012; Peron et al. 2008). Moreover, dominant mutations in *PI3KCD* could also lead to defective CSR but normal SHM (Angulo et al. 2013).

In addition, some syndromic PIDs are also associated with defects in CSR. A variable CSR deficiency can develop in patients with ataxia telangiectasia caused by recessive mutations in *ATM*, Nijmegen breakage syndrome resulted from recessive mutations in *NBS1* and Cernunnos/XRCC4-like factor deficiency due to mutations in the non-homologous end-joining 1 gene (*NHEJ1*), as well as in patients with mutations in nuclear factor kappa B essential modulator (*NEMO*) (de la Morena 2016). However, approximately 60% of the patients with CSR deficiency are caused by intrinsic B cell defects, but the causal genes remain to be identified (Rezaei et al. 2017).

10.5 IgA Deficiency

IgA deficiency (IgAD) consists of selective IgA deficiency (SIgAD) and partial IgA deficiency. SIgAD is the most common PAD in humans (Yazdani et al. 2017) and is defined by very low levels of serum IgA (<0.07 g/L) but normal levels of serum IgG and IgM and normal IgG Ab response to all vaccinations in a patient older than 4 years (exclusion of other causes of hypogammaglobulinemia and T cell defect). Partial IgA deficiency is defined as decreased IgA levels that are more than two standard deviations below the normal age-adjusted means (Rezaei et al. 2017). The worldwide incidence of SIgAD varies, ranging from 1:142 to 1:18,000, depending on ethnic background, which suggests a genetic basis for the disorder. An impaired terminal differentiation of B cells and defect in switching to IgA-producing plasma cells are presumed to be the cause of SIgAD. Nevertheless, the genetic defects and exact pathogenesis of SIgAD are still not well understood. Some family members of CVID patients were diagnosed as SIgAD, which suggested a genetic association between IgAD and CVID (Hammarstrom et al. 2000). Furthermore, CVID may develop from IgAD. Defects in TACI have been identified in a few patients with IgAD and CVID. Studies based on a large number of multiple-case families suggested that MHC class II or class III region may be a predisposing locus (Vorechovsky et al. 1999). Many SIgAD patients show simultaneous change in the IgG subclass pattern, mainly with reduced IgG_2 and IgG_4, indicating that SIgAD is partly associated with impaired CSR downstream of the $\gamma 1$ (Hammarstrom et al. 2000).

In symptomatic IgA-deficient patients, recurrent sinopulmonary infections are the most frequent symptoms. SIgAD with an associated IgG subclass deficiency and/or defects in specific Ab production against polysaccharide antigens is more prone to develop recurrent otitis media and sinopulmonary infections. Gastrointestinal diseases also occurred frequently in SIgAD patients, including giardiasis, nodular lymphoid hyperplasia, celiac disease and IBD. Moreover, SIgAD patients were at high risk for autoimmune disorders, allergy and malignancies (Valizadeh et al. 2017). Remarkably, approximately two-thirds of the SIgAD remain asymptomatic. One possibility is that the function of IgA in the gut may be compensated for by IgM.

Recently, we have found that the marginal zone B and B-1 cell-specific protein (MZB1) promotes J-chain binding to IgA and dimeric IgA secretion. MZB1-deficient mice are impaired in secreting IgA and IgM into the gut under inflammatory conditions and are highly susceptible to DSS-induced colitis (Xiong et al. 2019). It remains to be determined whether mutations in *MZB1* can result in IgAD and cause IBD in humans.

10.6 Hyper-IgE Syndrome

Hyper-IgE syndrome (HIES) is a rare PID, classically presenting with high serum IgE levels, elevated eosinophilia, recurrent bacterial and fungal infections, and various non-hematopoietic developmental manifestations, such as retained primary dentition and bone abnormalities (Holland et al. 2007; Heimall et al. 2010; Zhang et al. 2018). To date, several genetic defects have been identified as the underlying causes of HIES and can be divided into STAT3-associated HIES and autosomal recessive HIES (AR-HIES)

10.6.1 STAT3-Associated HIES

Autosomal dominant hyper-IgE syndrome (AD-HIES) or Job's syndrome is the first described HIES (Davis et al. 1966). In 2007, heterozygous dominant-negative mutations in signal transducer and activator of transcription 3 (*STAT3*) were identified in patients with AD-HIES (Holland et al. 2007). Mutations in *STAT3* account for the vast majority of autosomal dominant and sporadic HIES cases (Heimall et al. 2010). AD-HIES has been recognized as multiorgan dysfunction characterized by both immunological and non-immunological manifestations. Immunological studies revealed reduced circulating memory B cells, elevated IgE levels and poor specific Ab response. Patients presented with eczematoid rashes, skin abscesses, recurrent sinopulmonary infections and increased incidence of lymphoma. Non-immunological presentations include connective tissue, skeletal and dental abnormalities (Freeman and Holland 2010). STAT3 is a transcription factor that transmits signals to the nucleus after activation by a number of cytokines and growth factors. As a consequence, cells that require a stronger STAT3 signal for their normal function are affected by STAT3 deficiency, which explains the multisystem involvement in these patients.

Several patients with clinical manifestations similar to AD-HIES but with autosomal recessive inheritance were described, and several causal genes have been identified, including interleukin 6 signal transducer (*IL6ST*, also called *GP130*) (Schwerd et al. 2017), interleukin-6 receptor (*IL6R*) (Spencer et al. 2019) and transcription factor ZNF431 (*ZNF431*) (Beziat et al. 2018; Frey-Jakobs et al. 2018). GP130 and IL6R are central elements in IL-6 signaling. IL-6/IL-6R complex ligates GP130, leading to JAK activation and STAT (predominantly STAT3) phosphorylation. Loss-of-function in GP130 or IL6R resulted in remarkably reduced or absence of pSTAT3, which led to the AD-HIES phenotype. ZNF431 is a nuclear transcription factor, which binds to a specific DNA motif found in various genes, including the STAT3 promoter (Beziat et al. 2018; Frey-Jakobs et al. 2018). ZNF431-deficient patients presented with reduced STAT3 mRNA expression without *STAT3* mutations. Slightly different from AD-HIES, patients with null *ZNF431* mutations showed stronger inflammatory responses and fewer extra-hematopoietic manifestations (Frey-Jakobs et al. 2018).

10.6.2 Autosomal Recessive HIES

Biallelic loss-of-function mutations in dedicator of cytokinesis 8 (*DOCK8*) are associated with AR-HIES and CID (Zhang et al. 2009). *DOCK8* deficiency shares some similarities with AD-HIES, including eczema, sinopulmonary infections, elevated serum IgE and eosinophilia. Since DOCK8 deficiency affects B cells, NK cells and various T cell subsets, some other clinical features are different from AD-HIES. Patients harboring *DOCK8* mutations usually presented with severe cutaneous viral infections, pulmonary infections and predisposition to malignancies at a young age. However, the connective tissue, skeletal and dental abnormalities were rarely observed in DOCK8-deficient patients (Freeman and Holland 2010; Aydin et al. 2015).

Recently, autosomal recessive defects in phosphoglucomutase 3 (*PGM3*) have been reported in AR-HIES patients. PGM3 is an enzyme required for the synthesis of UDP-GlcNAc in the hexosamine biosynthesis pathway, which is essential for the assembly of N-glycans, O-glycans, proteoglycans and glycolipids (Yang et al. 2014). As a consequence, in addition to recurrent respiratory infections, glomerulonephritis, allergies and eczema, PGM3-deficient patients showed multiple severe congenital glycosylation disorders and neurologic manifestations (Yang et al. 2014; Sassi et al. 2014; Zhang et al. 2018). Reduced number of circulating B cells and memory B cells were found in PGM3-deficient patients. However, the mechanism by which this glycosylation defect results in HIES remains to be elucidated.

Deficiency in serine protease inhibitor LEKTI (lymphoepithelial Kazal-type-related inhibitor), encoded by *SPINK5*, underlies a rare life-threatening syndrome, called Netherton syndrome (NS) (Chavanas et al. 2000). NS patients presented with skin barrier defect and elevated serum IgE with atopic manifestations. Immunologically, in addition to high serum IgE levels, NS patients showed reduced memory B cells and elevated serum IgG_4, and impaired development and function of NK cells (Hannula-Jouppi et al. 2016). The precise mechanism of the immunological dysfunction in NS has not been fully elucidated.

Many other genetic defects leading to high serum IgE levels and severe infections are not categorized as HIES, including Wiskott-Aldrich syndrome (*WAS* or *WIPF1* mutations), DiGeorge syndrome (22q11.2DS), Omenn syndrome (hypomorphic mutations in genes for which null alleles underlie SCID), and immune dysregulation, polyendocrinopathy, enteropathy, X-linked syndrome (*IPEX*, *FOXP3* mutations) (Zhang et al. 2018).

10.7 Other Ab Deficiencies

10.7.1 Isolated IgG Subclass Deficiency

IgG subclass deficiency is defined as a deficiency of one or more IgG subclasses (less than 2SD below the mean normal level for their age), in the presence of a normal level of total IgG (Rezaei et al. 2017). In some patients, IgG subclass deficiency was associated with low serum IgA levels and may be also observed in conjunction with other PIDs including ataxia telangiectasia and Wiskott-Aldrich syndrome (Kutukculer et al. 2007). Deficiencies in IgG_4 are most common, followed by IgG_2, IgG_3 and IgG_1. Most patients with IgG subclass deficiency were asymptomatic but some suffered from recurrent respiratory tract infections. A few patients have been reported with homozygous deletions of the constant region genes of specific IgG subclasses. The pathogenesis of IgG subclass deficiencies is not fully understood.

10.7.2 κ Light Chain Deficiency

Biallelic mutations in the Ig kappa constant region gene are associated with κ light chain deficiency. All Ig of these patients have λ light chain. κ light chain deficiency may be associated with some conditions, including recurrent infections (Bernier et al. 1972), cystic fibrosis, diabetes mellitus and IgA deficiency (Zegers et al. 1976), but can also be asymptomatic.

10.7.3 Specific Ab Deficiency with Normal Ig Concentrations

Specific Ab deficiency (SAD) is characterized by abnormal IgG Ab responses to a majority of polysaccharide antigens and increased susceptibility to recurrent bacterial infections in subjects over the age of 2 years. Most of these patients were between 3 and 6 years of age (Ballow et al. 2012), and mainly presented with recurrent bacterial respiratory infections, such as sinusitis, otitis media and bronchitis. Moreover, SAD is associated with allergic diseases, particularly allergic rhinitis (Boyle et al. 2006). Patients with SAD were heterogeneous in the integrity of their B cell activation pathways (McGeady et al. 2019), and also defective in B cell repertoire and marginal zone of the spleen (Rezaei et al. 2017), but the basic origin of SAD remains unclear.

10.8 Clinical Features Associated with PADs

10.8.1 Infections

Chronic and recurrent infections are the predominant symptoms of PADs. *Streptococcus pneumoniae*, *Haemophilus influenza* and Gram-negative bacteria are the most commonly isolated pathogens, while fungal or viral infections are rare. The infections mainly occur in the respiratory and gastrointestinal tracts, although skin is also vulnerable. Patients with PADs predominantly present with otitis media, sinusitis and pneumonia, and chronic or recurrent diarrhea is also a common feature. Some patients with agammaglobulinemia also suffer from severe, chronic enteroviral infections and show a critical role of Abs in preventing enteroviruses. A small part of CVID, XLA and CSR defective patients (caused by CD40, CD40L or NEMO deficiency) may also suffer from opportunistic infections. The pathogens include *Pneumocystis jirovecii* and *Cryptosporidium* (Fried and Bonilla 2009; de la Morena 2016).

10.8.2 Autoimmunity

Several studies revealed that PAD patients are vulnerable to autoimmune disorders (Sarmiento et al. 2005; Azizi et al. 2016). Immunodeficiency and autoimmune manifestations may occur concomitantly in the same individual, which seems paradoxical, but may not be implausible considering the complex nature of immune cells, signaling pathways and their interactions. Immune thrombocytopenic purpura (ITP) and autoimmune hemolytic anemia (AIHA) are the most common autoimmune disorders found in PADs. In addition, type 1 diabetes (T1D), RA, SLE, dermatomyositis and IBD are also frequently observed. Moreover, autoinflammation and granulomas also occur frequently in PADs, especially in CVID and CSR deficiencies.

The mechanisms are not yet well elucidated. Some suggest that impaired Treg development and function are the main factors leading to autoimmune complications in PADs (Arandi et al. 2013). Defective checkpoints in the control of self-reactive B cells can also cause Ab-mediated autoimmune disorders (Meffre 2011). Furthermore, insufficient elimination of self-reactive T cells, expansion of $CD21^{low}$ B cells and impaired activation-induced cell death are also considered to be the cause of autoimmunity.

10.8.3 Malignancy

The risk of malignancy in PAD patients increases by 1.8- to 13-folds, which seems more specifically related to Ab deficiencies rather than to genetic background (Wood 2010). Lymphomas are the most common malignancies found in PAD patients and are particularly frequent in CVID. The incidence of epithelial malignancies is also increased in PADs. The development of cancer is a significant cause of premature death. Defective DNA damage response (DDR) and a dysregulated immune response may be responsible for the development of tumors.

10.9 Treatment

Treatments of patients with PADs include Ig replacement therapy, administration of antibiotics, hematopoietic stem cell transplantation (HSCT) and more recently gene therapy. Almost all PAD patients require Ig replacement therapy, with either intravenous or subcutaneous delivery (IVIg and SCIg, respectively). The use of Ig replacement therapy significantly reduced the rate of bacterial infections and chronic lung lesions (Wood 2010). Prophylactic antibiotics and good pulmonary hygiene measures as important supportive care are also required in the treatment of PADs. Infections are usually well controlled with IVIg/SCIg and prophylactic antibiotics. In a small portion of patients with life-threatening complications and resistance to treatment, HSCT should be considered as the only curative therapy. Most importantly, some CID and CVID patients with severe complications, such as LRBA deficiency, might benefit more from early HSCT (D'Elios and Rizzi 2019). More recently, gene therapy has been shown to be effective in murine models (Kerns et al. 2010; Hubbard et al. 2016), but clinical applications have yet to be developed and need to be strictly assessed for safety issues. In addition, immunosuppressive, anti-inflammatory, cytotoxic and antineoplastic therapies are also used for the treatment of autoimmune or malignant complications of PADs.

10.10 Conclusion

There has been tremendous progress in our understanding of the clinical manifestations and the genetic defects of PADs. Investigation of consanguineous family with multiple affected individuals has greatly helped the identification of the causal genes. However, the genetic defects of many PADs still remain unknown, and it is conceivable that some PADs may be caused by the dysfunction of more than one genes. It is thus challenging to uncover the genetic defects responsible for PADs in sporadic cases. It may be necessary to develop new bioinformatic tools to more efficiently narrow down the mutated genes that are more likely to be involved in the diseases. In addition, it will also be important to establish new in vitro and in vivo analytical methods to pinpoint the biological basis of abnormalities in B cells of the patients. With the development of new technologies, more casual genes for PADs will be identified, which should greatly facilitate the diagnosis and treatment of PADs.

Acknowledgements We thank Luming Zhang for secretarial assistance, Fudan University Animal Facility for maintaining the mice and the members in Wang Lab for helpful suggestions. This work was supported by the Major Research Plan of the National Natural Science Foundation of China (91942302 to J.Y.W.), the National Key R & D Plan of the Ministry of Science and Technology (SQ2019YFE0100600 to J.Y.W.), the National

Natural Science Foundation of China (81571529 and 31870898 to J.Y.W), Projects of International Cooperation and Exchanges NSFC (to J.Y.W.) and a grant-in-aid for scientific research (C) from Japan Society for the Promotion of Science (17K08878 to J.Y.W).

References

Abolhassani H, Edwards ES, Ikinciogullari A, Jing H, Borte S, Buggert M et al (2017) Combined immunodeficiency and Epstein-Barr virus-induced B cell malignancy in humans with inherited CD70 deficiency. J Exp Med 214(1):91–106. https://doi.org/10.1084/jem.20160849

Accetta D, Syverson G, Bonacci B, Reddy S, Bengtson C, Surfus J et al (2011) Human phagocyte defect caused by a Rac2 mutation detected by means of neonatal screening for T-cell lymphopenia. J Allergy Clin Immunol 127(2), 535–538.e1–2. https://doi.org/10.1016/j.jaci.2010.10.013

Alkhairy OK, Perez-Becker R, Driessen GJ, Abolhassani H, van Montfrans J, Borte S et al (2015a) Novel mutations in TNFRSF7/CD27: clinical, immunologic, and genetic characterization of human CD27 deficiency. J Allergy Clin Immunol 136(3):703–712 e10. https://doi.org/10.1016/j.jaci.2015.02.022

Alkhairy OK, Rezaei N, Graham RR, Abolhassani H, Borte S, Hultenby K et al (2015b) RAC2 loss-of-function mutation in 2 siblings with characteristics of common variable immunodeficiency. J Allergy Clin Immunol 135(5):1380–134 e1-5. https://doi.org/10.1016/j.jaci.2014.10.039

Ambruso DR, Knall C, Abell AN, Panepinto J, Kurkchubasche A, Thurman G et al (2000) Human neutrophil immunodeficiency syndrome is associated with an inhibitory Rac2 mutation. Proc Natl Acad Sci U S A 97(9):4654–4659. https://doi.org/10.1073/pnas.080074897

Angulo I, Vadas O, Garcon F, Banham-Hall E, Plagnol V, Leahy TR et al (2013) Phosphoinositide 3-kinase delta gene mutation predisposes to respiratory infection and airway damage. Science 342(6160):866–871. https://doi.org/10.1126/science.1243292

Arandi N, Mirshafiey A, Jeddi-Tehrani M, Abolhassani H, Sadeghi B, Mirminachi B et al (2013) Evaluation of CD4+ CD25+ FOXP3+ regulatory T cells function in patients with common variable immunodeficiency. Cell Immunol 281(2):129–133. https://doi.org/10.1016/j.cellimm.2013.03.003

Avery DT, Deenick EK, Ma CS, Suryani S, Simpson N, Chew GY et al (2010) B cell-intrinsic signaling through IL-21 receptor and STAT3 is required for establishing long-lived antibody responses in humans. J Exp Med 207(1):155–171. https://doi.org/10.1084/jem.20091706

Aydin SE, Kilic SS, Aytekin C, Kumar A, Porras O, Kainulainen L et al (2015) DOCK8 deficiency: clinical and immunological phenotype and treatment options—a review of 136 patients. J Clin Immunol 35 (2):189–198. https://doi.org/10.1007/s10875-014-0126-0

Azizi G, Ahmadi M, Abolhassani H, Yazdani R, Mohammadi H, Mirshafiey A et al (2016) Autoimmunity in primary antibody deficiencies. Int Arch Allergy Immunol 171(3–4):180–193. https://doi.org/10.1159/000453263

Bain G, Maandag EC, Izon DJ, Amsen D, Kruisbeek AM, Weintraub BC et al (1994) E2A proteins are required for proper B cell development and initiation of immunoglobulin gene rearrangements. Cell 79 (5):885–892. https://doi.org/10.1016/0092-8674(94)90077-9

Ballow M, Akdis CA, Casale TB, Wardlaw AJ, Wenzel SE, Ballas Z et al (2012) Immune response modifiers in the treatment of asthma: a PRACTALL document of the American Academy of Allergy, Asthma & Immunology and the European Academy of Allergy and Clinical Immunology. J Allergy Clin Immunol 130(2):311–324. https://doi.org/10.1016/j.jaci.2012.04.046

Belot A, Kasher PR, Trotter EW, Foray AP, Debaud AL, Rice GI et al (2013) Protein kinase cdelta deficiency causes mendelian systemic lupus erythematosus with B cell-defective apoptosis and hyperproliferation. Arthritis Rheum 65(8):2161–2171. https://doi.org/10.1002/art.38008

Ben-Ali M, Yang J, Chan KW, Ben-Mustapha I, Mekki N, Benabdesselem C et al (2017) Homozygous transcription factor 3 gene (TCF3) mutation is associated with severe hypogammaglobulinemia and B-cell acute lymphoblastic leukemia. J Allergy Clin Immunol 140(4):1191–1194.e4. https://doi.org/10.1016/j.jaci.2017.04.037

Bernier GM, Gunderman JR, Ruymann FB (1972) Kappa-chain deficiency. Blood 40(6):795–805

Beziat V, Li J, Lin JX, Ma CS, Li P, Bousfiha A et al (2018) A recessive form of hyper-IgE syndrome by disruption of ZNF341-dependent STAT3 transcription and activity. Sci Immunol 3(24). https://doi.org/10.1126/sciimmunol.aat4956

Bogaert DJ, Dullaers M, Lambrecht BN, Vermaelen KY, De Baere E, Haerynck F (2016) Genes associated with common variable immunodeficiency: one diagnosis to rule them all? J Med Genet 53(9):575–590. https://doi.org/10.1136/jmedgenet-2015-103690

Boisson B, Wang YD, Bosompem A, Ma CS, Lim A, Kochetkov T et al (2013) A recurrent dominant negative E47 mutation causes agammaglobulinemia and BCR(-) B cells. J Clin Invest 123(11):4781–4785. https://doi.org/10.1172/jci71927

Bonilla FA, Barlan I, Chapel H, Costa-Carvalho BT, Cunningham-Rundles C, de la Morena MT et al (2016) International Consensus Document (ICON): common variable immunodeficiency disorders. J Allergy Clin Immunol Pract 4(1):38–59. https://doi.org/10.1016/j.jaip.2015.07.025

Bourgeois P, Esteve C, Chaix C, Beroud C, Levy N, consortium Tc et al (2018) Tricho-Hepato-Enteric Syndrome mutation update: mutations spectrum of TTC37 and SKIV2L, clinical analysis and future prospects. Hum Mutat 39(6):774–789. https://doi.org/10.1002/humu.23418

Boutboul D, Kuehn HS, Van de Wyngaert Z, Niemela JE, Callebaut I, Stoddard J et al (2018) Dominant-negative IKZF1 mutations cause a T, B, and myeloid cell combined immunodeficiency. J Clin Invest 128 (7):3071–3087. https://doi.org/10.1172/jci98164

Boyle RJ, Le C, Balloch A, Tang ML (2006) The clinical syndrome of specific antibody deficiency in children. Clin Exp Immunol 146(3):486–492. https://doi.org/10.1111/j.1365-2249.2006.03242.x

Boztug H, Hirschmugl T, Holter W, Lakatos K, Kager L, Trapin D et al (2016) NF-kappaB1 haploinsufficiency causing immunodeficiency and EBV-driven lymphoproliferation. J Clin Immunol 36(6):533–540. https://doi.org/10.1007/s10875-016-0306-1

Bravo Garcia-Morato M, Garcia-Minaur S, Molina Garicano J, Santos Simarro F, Del Pino Molina L, Lopez-Granados E et al (2017) Mutations in PIK3R1 can lead to APDS2, SHORT syndrome or a combination of the two. Clin Immunol 179:77–80. https://doi.org/10.1016/j.clim.2017.03.004

Browning MJ, Chandra A, Carbonaro V, Okkenhaug K, Barwell J (2015) Cowden's syndrome with immunodeficiency. J Med Genet 52(12):856–859. https://doi.org/10.1136/jmedgenet-2015-103266

Buck D, Malivert L, de Chasseval R, Barraud A, Fondaneche MC, Sanal O et al (2006) Cernunnos, a novel nonhomologous end-joining factor, is mutated in human immunodeficiency with microcephaly. Cell 124(2):287–299. https://doi.org/10.1016/j.cell.2005.12.030

Cagdas D, Gur Cetinkaya P, Karaatmaca B, Esenboga S, Tan C, Yilmaz T et al (2018) ADA deficiency: evaluation of the clinical and laboratory features and the outcome. J Clin Immunol 38(4):484–493. https://doi.org/10.1007/s10875-018-0496-9

Chakraborty PK, Schmitz-Abe K, Kennedy EK, Mamady H, Naas T, Durie D et al (2014) Mutations in TRNT1 cause congenital sideroblastic anemia with immunodeficiency, fevers, and developmental delay (SIFD). Blood 124(18):2867–2871. https://doi.org/10.1182/blood-2014-08-591370

Charbit-Henrion F, Jeverica AK, Begue B, Markelj G, Parlato M, Avcin SL et al (2017) Deficiency in mucosa-associated lymphoid tissue lymphoma translocation 1: a novel cause of IPEX-like syndrome. J Pediatr Gastroenterol Nutr 64(3):378–384. https://doi.org/10.1097/mpg.0000000000001262

Chavanas S, Bodemer C, Rochat A, Hamel-Teillac D, Ali M, Irvine AD et al (2000) Mutations in SPINK5, encoding a serine protease inhibitor, cause Netherton syndrome. Nat Genet 25(2):141–142. https://doi.org/10.1038/75977

Chen HH, Handel N, Ngeow J, Muller J, Huhn M, Yang HT et al (2017) Immune dysregulation in patients with PTEN hamartoma tumor syndrome: analysis of FOXP3 regulatory T cells. J Allergy Clin Immunol 139(2):607–620.e15. https://doi.org/10.1016/j.jaci.2016.03.059

Chen K, Coonrod EM, Kumanovics A, Franks ZF, Durtschi JD, Margraf RL et al (2013) Germline mutations in NFKB2 implicate the noncanonical NF-kappaB pathway in the pathogenesis of common variable immunodeficiency. Am J Hum Genet 93 (5):812–824. https://doi.org/10.1016/j.ajhg.2013.09.009

Cifaldi C, Scarselli A, Petricone D, Di Cesare S, Chiriaco M, Claps A et al (2016) Agammaglobulinemia associated to nasal polyposis due to a hypomorphic RAG1 mutation in a 12 years old boy. Clin Immunol 173:121–123. https://doi.org/10.1016/j.clim.2016.09.013

Compeer EB, Janssen W, van Royen-Kerkhof A, van Gijn M, van Montfrans JM, Boes M (2015) Dysfunctional BLK in common variable immunodeficiency perturbs B-cell proliferation and ability to elicit antigen-specific CD4+ T-cell help. Oncotarget 6 (13):10759–10771. https://doi.org/10.18632/oncotarget.3577

Conley ME, Dobbs AK, Farmer DM, Kilic S, Paris K, Grigoriadou S et al (2009) Primary B cell immunodeficiencies: comparisons and contrasts. Annu Rev Immunol 27:199–227. https://doi.org/10.1146/annurev.immunol.021908.132649

Conley ME, Dobbs AK, Quintana AM, Bosompem A, Wang YD, Coustan-Smith E et al (2012) Agammaglobulinemia and absent B lineage cells in a patient lacking the p85alpha subunit of PI3K. J Exp Med 209 (3):463–470. https://doi.org/10.1084/jem.20112533

D'Elios MM, Rizzi M (2019) Humoral primary immunodeficiencies. Springer. https://doi.org/10.1007/978-3-319-91785-6

Dadi H, Jones TA, Merico D, Sharfe N, Ovadia A, Schejter Y et al (2018) Combined immunodeficiency and atopy caused by a dominant negative mutation in caspase activation and recruitment domain family member 11 (CARD11). J Allergy Clin Immunol 141 (5):1818–1830.e2. https://doi.org/10.1016/j.jaci.2017.06.047

Davis SD, Schaller J, Wedgwood RJ (1966) Job's syndrome. recurrent, "cold", staphylococcal abscesses. Lancet 1(7445):1013–1015. https://doi.org/10.1016/s0140-6736(66)90119-x

de la Morena MT (2016) Clinical phenotypes of hyper-IgM syndromes. J Allergy Clin Immunol Pract 4(6):1023–1036. https://doi.org/10.1016/j.jaip.2016.09.013

Driessen GJ, IJspeert H, Wentink M, Yntema HG, van Hagen PM, van Strien A et al (2016) Increased PI3K/Akt activity and deregulated humoral immune response in human PTEN deficiency. J Allergy Clin Immunol 138(6):1744–1747.e5. https://www.doi.org/10.1016/j.jaci.2016.07.010

Durandy A, Kracker S, Fischer A (2013) Primary antibody deficiencies. Nat Rev Immunol 13(7):519–533. https://doi.org/10.1038/nri3466

Elgizouli M, Lowe DM, Speckmann C, Schubert D, Hulsdunker J, Eskandarian Z et al (2016) Activating PI3Kdelta mutations in a cohort of 669 patients with primary immunodeficiency. Clin Exp Immunol 183 (2):221–229. https://doi.org/10.1111/cei.12706

Ferrari S, Giliani S, Insalaco A, Al-Ghonaium A, Soresina AR, Loubser M et al (2001) Mutations of CD40 gene cause an autosomal recessive form of immunodeficiency with hyper IgM. Proc Natl Acad Sci U S A 98(22):12614–12619. https://doi.org/10.1073/pnas.221456898

Ferrari S, Lougaris V, Caraffi S, Zuntini R, Yang J, Soresina A et al (2007) Mutations of the Igbeta gene cause agammaglobulinemia in man. J Exp Med 204 (9):2047–2051. https://doi.org/10.1084/jem.20070264

Fliegauf M, Bryant VL, Frede N, Slade C, Woon ST, Lehnert K et al (2015) Haploinsufficiency of the NF-kappaB1 subunit p50 in common variable immunodeficiency. Am J Hum Genet 97(3):389–403. https://doi.org/10.1016/j.ajhg.2015.07.008

Frans G, Moens L, Schaballie H, Wuyts G, Liston A, Poesen K et al (2017) Homozygous N-terminal missense mutation in TRNT1 leads to progressive B-cell immunodeficiency in adulthood. J Allergy Clin Immunol 139(1):360–363 e6. https://doi.org/10.1016/j.jaci.2016.06.050

Freeman AF, Holland SM (2010) Clinical manifestations of hyper IgE syndromes. Dis Markers 29(3–4):123–30. https://doi.org/10.3233/DMA-2010-0734

Frey-Jakobs S, Hartberger JM, Fliegauf M, Bossen C, Wehmeyer ML, Neubauer JC et al (2018) ZNF341 controls STAT3 expression and thereby immunocompetence. Sci Immunol 3(24). https://doi.org/10.1126/sciimmunol.aat4941

Fried AJ, Bonilla FA (2009) Pathogenesis, diagnosis, and management of primary antibody deficiencies and infections. Clin Microbiol Rev 22(3):396–414. https://doi.org/10.1128/CMR.00001-09

Gardes P, Forveille M, Alyanakian MA, Aucouturier P, Ilencikova D, Leroux D et al (2012) Human MSH6 deficiency is associated with impaired antibody maturation. J Immunol 188(4):2023–2029. https://doi.org/10.4049/jimmunol.1102984

Giblett ER, Anderson JE, Cohen F, Pollara B, Meuwissen HJ (1972) Adenosine-deaminase deficiency in two patients with severely impaired cellular immunity. Lancet 2(7786):1067–1069. https://doi.org/10.1016/s0140-6736(72)92345-8

Greil J, Rausch T, Giese T, Bandapalli OR, Daniel V, Bekeredjian-Ding I et al (2013) Whole-exome sequencing links caspase recruitment domain 11 (CARD11) inactivation to severe combined immunodeficiency. J Allergy Clin Immunol 131(5):1376–83.e3. https://doi.org/10.1016/j.jaci.2013.02.012

Hammarstrom L, Vorechovsky I, Webster D (2000) Selective IgA deficiency (SIgAD) and common variable immunodeficiency (CVID). Clin Exp Immunol 120(2):225–231. https://doi.org/10.1046/j.1365-2249.2000.01131.x

Hannula-Jouppi K, Laasanen SL, Ilander M, Furio L, Tuomiranta M, Marttila R et al (2016) Intrafamily and interfamilial phenotype variation and immature immunity in patients with Netherton syndrome and Finnish SPINK5 founder mutation. JAMA Dermatol 152 (4):435–442. https://doi.org/10.1001/jamadermatol.2015.5827

Hartley JL, Zachos NC, Dawood B, Donowitz M, Forman J, Pollitt RJ et al (2010) Mutations in TTC37 cause trichohepatoenteric syndrome (phenotypic diarrhea of infancy). Gastroenterology 138 (7):2388–2398, 2398.e1–2. https://doi.org/10.1053/j.gastro.2010.02.010

Hedayat M, Massaad MJ, Lee YN, Conley ME, Orange JS, Ohsumi TK et al (2014) Lessons in gene hunting: a RAG1 mutation presenting with agammaglobulinemia and absence of B cells. J Allergy Clin Immunol 134(4):983–985.e1. https://doi.org/10.1016/j.jaci.2014.04.037

Heimall J, Freeman A, Holland SM (2010) Pathogenesis of hyper IgE syndrome. Clin Rev Allergy Immunol 38 (1):32–38. https://doi.org/10.1007/s12016-009-8134-1

Holland SM, DeLeo FR, Elloumi HZ, Hsu AP, Uzel G, Brodsky N et al (2007) STAT3 mutations in the hyper-IgE syndrome. N Engl J Med 357(16):1608–1619. https://doi.org/10.1056/NEJMoa073687

Hoshino A, Okada S, Yoshida K, Nishida N, Okuno Y, Ueno H et al (2017) Abnormal hematopoiesis and autoimmunity in human subjects with germline IKZF1 mutations. J Allergy Clin Immunol 140(1):223–231. https://doi.org/10.1016/j.jaci.2016.09.029

Hsu AP, Donko A, Arrington ME, Swamydas M, Fink D, Das A et al (2019) Dominant activating RAC2 mutation with lymphopenia, immunodeficiency, and cytoskeletal defects. Blood 133(18):1977–1988. https://doi.org/10.1182/blood-2018-11-886028

Hubbard N, Hagin D, Sommer K, Song Y, Khan I, Clough C et al (2016) Targeted gene editing restores regulated CD40L function in X-linked hyper-IgM syndrome. Blood 127(21):2513–2522. https://doi.org/10.1182/blood-2015-11-683235

Imai K, Slupphaug G, Lee WI, Revy P, Nonoyama S, Catalan N et al (2003) Human uracil-DNA glycosylase deficiency associated with profoundly impaired immunoglobulin class-switch recombination. Nat Immunol 4(10):1023–1028. https://doi.org/10.1038/ni974

Izawa K, Martin E, Soudais C, Bruneau J, Boutboul D, Rodriguez R et al (2017) Inherited CD70 deficiency in humans reveals a critical role for the CD70-CD27 pathway in immunity to Epstein-Barr virus infection. J Exp Med 214(1):73–89. https://doi.org/10.1084/jem.20160784

Jabara HH, Ohsumi T, Chou J, Massaad MJ, Benson H, Megarbane A et al (2013) A homozygous mucosa-associated lymphoid tissue 1 (MALT1) mutation in a family with combined immunodeficiency. J Allergy Clin Immunol 132(1):151–158. https://doi.org/10.1016/j.jaci.2013.04.047

Jansen EJ, Timal S, Ryan M, Ashikov A, van Scherpenzeel M, Graham LA et al (2016) ATP6AP1 deficiency causes an immunodeficiency with hepatopathy, cognitive impairment and abnormal protein glycosylation. Nat Commun 7:11600. https://doi.org/10.1038/ncomms11600

Jiang SH, Athanasopoulos V, Ellyard JI, Chuah A, Cappello J, Cook A et al (2019) Functional rare and low frequency variants in BLK and BANK1 contribute to human lupus. Nat Commun 10(1):2201. https://doi.org/10.1038/s41467-019-10242-9

Kaustio M, Haapaniemi E, Goos H, Hautala T, Park G, Syrjanen J et al (2017) Damaging heterozygous mutations in NFKB1 lead to diverse immunologic phenotypes. J Allergy Clin Immunol 140(3):782–796. https://doi.org/10.1016/j.jaci.2016.10.054

Keller B, Cseresnyes Z, Stumpf I, Wehr C, Fliegauf M, Bulashevska A et al (2017) Disturbed canonical nuclear factor of kappa light chain signaling in B cells of patients with common variable immunodeficiency. J Allergy Clin Immunol 139(1):220–231.e8. https://doi.org/10.1016/j.jaci.2016.04.043

Keller MD, Pandey R, Li D, Glessner J, Tian L, Henrickson SE et al (2016) Mutation in IRF2BP2 is responsible for a familial form of common variable immunodeficiency disorder. J Allergy Clin Immunol 138(2):544–550 e4. https://doi.org/10.1016/j.jaci.2016.01.018

Kerns HM, Ryu BY, Stirling BV, Sather BD, Astrakhan A, Humblet-Baron S et al (2010) B cell-specific lentiviral gene therapy leads to sustained B-cell functional recovery in a murine model of X-linked agammaglobulinemia. Blood 115(11):2146–2155. https://doi.org/10.1182/blood-2009-09-241869

Kiykim A, Ogulur I, Baris S, Salzer E, Karakoc-Aydiner E, Ozen AO et al (2015) Potentially beneficial effect of hydroxychloroquine in a patient with a novel mutation in protein kinase cdelta deficiency. J Clin Immunol 35(6):523–526. https://doi.org/10.1007/s10875-015-0178-9

Korthauer U, Graf D, Mages HW, Briere F, Padayachee M, Malcolm S et al (1993) Defective expression of T-cell CD40 ligand causes X-linked immunodeficiency with hyper-IgM. Nature 361(6412):539–541. https://doi.org/10.1038/361539a0

Kotlarz D, Zietara N, Milner JD, Klein C (2014) Human IL-21 and IL-21R deficiencies: two novel entities of primary immunodeficiency. Curr Opin Pediatr 26(6):704–712. https://doi.org/10.1097/mop.0000000000000160

Kotlarz D, Zietara N, Uzel G, Weidemann T, Braun CJ, Diestelhorst J et al (2013) Loss-of-function mutations in the IL-21 receptor gene cause a primary immunodeficiency syndrome. J Exp Med 210(3):433–443. https://doi.org/10.1084/jem.20111229

Kracker S, Di Virgilio M, Schwartzentruber J, Cuenin C, Forveille M, Deau MC et al (2015) An inherited immunoglobulin class-switch recombination deficiency associated with a defect in the INO80 chromatin remodeling complex. J Allergy Clin Immunol 135(4):998–1007 e6. https://doi.org/10.1016/j.jaci.2014.08.030

Kuehn HS, Boisson B, Cunningham-Rundles C, Reichenbach J, Stray-Pedersen A, Gelfand EW et al (2016) Loss of B cells in patients with heterozygous mutations in IKAROS. N Engl J Med 374(11):1032–1043. https://doi.org/10.1056/NEJMoa1512234

Kuehn HS, Niemela JE, Rangel-Santos A, Zhang M, Pittaluga S, Stoddard JL et al (2013) Loss-of-function of the protein kinase C delta (PKCdelta) causes a B-cell lymphoproliferative syndrome in humans. Blood 121(16):3117–3125. https://doi.org/10.1182/blood-2012-12-469544

Kuehn HS, Niemela JE, Sreedhara K, Stoddard JL, Grossman J, Wysocki CA et al (2017) Novel nonsense gain-of-function NFKB2 mutations associated with a combined immunodeficiency phenotype. Blood 130(13):1553–1564. https://doi.org/10.1182/blood-2017-05-782177

Kuijpers TW, Bende RJ, Baars PA, Grummels A, Derks IA, Dolman KM et al (2010) CD20 deficiency in humans results in impaired T cell-independent antibody responses. J Clin Invest 120(1):214–222. https://doi.org/10.1172/JCI40231

Kurosaki T, Shinohara H, Baba Y (2010) B cell signaling and fate decision. Annu Rev Immunol 28:21–55. https://doi.org/10.1146/annurev.immunol.021908.132541

Kutukculer N, Karaca NE, Demircioglu O, Aksu G (2007) Increases in serum immunoglobulins to age-related normal levels in children with IgA and/or IgG subclass deficiency. Pediatr Allergy Immunol 18(2):167–173. https://doi.org/10.1111/j.1399-3038.2006.00491.x

Lagresle-Peyrou C, Six EM, Picard C, Rieux-Laucat F, Michel V, Ditadi A et al (2009) Human adenylate kinase 2 deficiency causes a profound hematopoietic defect associated with sensorineural deafness. Nat Genet 41(1):106–111. https://doi.org/10.1038/ng.278

Lee CE, Fulcher DA, Whittle B, Chand R, Fewings N, Field M et al (2014) Autosomal-dominant B-cell deficiency with alopecia due to a mutation in NFKB2 that results in nonprocessable p100. Blood 124(19):2964–2972. https://doi.org/10.1182/blood-2014-06-578542

Lindsley AW, Qian Y, Valencia CA, Shah K, Zhang K, Assa'ad A (2014) Combined immune deficiency in a patient with a novel NFKB2 mutation. J Clin Immunol 34(8):910–915. https://doi.org/10.1007/s10875-014-0095-3

Lo B, Zhang K, Lu W, Zheng L, Zhang Q, Kanellopoulou C et al (2015) Patients with LRBA deficiency show CTLA4 loss and immune dysregulation responsive to abatacept therapy. Science 349(6246):436–440. https://doi.org/10.1126/science.aaa1663

Lougaris V, Badolato R, Ferrari S, Plebani A (2005) Hyper immunoglobulin M syndrome due to CD40 deficiency: clinical, molecular, and immunological features. Immunol Rev 203:48–66. https://doi.org/10.1111/j.0105-2896.2005.00229.x

Lougaris V, Baronio M, Moratto D, Cardinale F, Plebani A (2016) Monoallelic BAFFR P21R/H159Y mutations and familiar primary antibody deficiencies. J Clin Immunol 36(1):1–3. https://doi.org/10.1007/s10875-015-0217-6

Lougaris V, Moratto D, Baronio M, Tampella G, van der Meer JWM, Badolato R et al (2017) Early and late B-cell developmental impairment in nuclear factor kappa B, subunit 1-mutated common variable immunodeficiency disease. J Allergy Clin Immunol 139(1):349–352.e1. https://doi.org/10.1016/j.jaci.2016.05.045

Lucas CL, Chandra A, Nejentsev S, Condliffe AM, Okkenhaug K (2016) PI3Kdelta and primary immunodeficiencies. Nat Rev Immunol 16(11):702–714. https://doi.org/10.1038/nri.2016.93

Ma CA, Stinson JR, Zhang Y, Abbott JK, Weinreich MA, Hauk PJ et al (2017) Corrigendum: germline hypomorphic CARD11 mutations in severe atopic disease. Nat Genet 49(11):1661. https://doi.org/10.1038/ng1117-1661b

Maffucci P, Filion CA, Boisson B, Itan Y, Shang L, Casanova JL et al (2016) Genetic diagnosis using whole exome sequencing in common variable immunodeficiency. Front Immunol 7:220. https://doi.org/10.3389/fimmu.2016.00220

Marsh DJ, Coulon V, Lunetta KL, Rocca-Serra P, Dahia PL, Zheng Z et al (1998) Mutation spectrum and genotype-phenotype analyses in Cowden disease and Bannayan-Zonana syndrome, two hamartoma syndromes with germline PTEN mutation. Hum Mol Genet 7(3):507–515. https://doi.org/10.1093/hmg/7.3.507

McGeady SJ (2019) B cell activation in specific polysaccharide antibody deficiency. J Allergy Clin Immunol 143(2):AB78. https://doi.org/10.1016/j.jaci.2018.12.244

McKinnon ML, Rozmus J, Fung SY, Hirschfeld AF, Del Bel KL, Thomas L et al (2014) Combined immunodeficiency associated with homozygous MALT1 mutations. J Allergy Clin Immunol 133(5):1458–1462, 1462.e1–7. https://doi.org/10.1016/j.jaci.2013.10.045

Meffre E (2011) The establishment of early B cell tolerance in humans: lessons from primary immunodeficiency diseases. Ann N Y Acad Sci 1246:1–10. https://doi.org/10.1111/j.1749-6632.2011.06347.x

Minegishi Y, Coustan-Smith E, Rapalus L, Ersoy F, Campana D, Conley ME (1999) Mutations in Igalpha (CD79a) result in a complete block in B-cell development. J Clin Invest 104(8):1115–1121. https://doi.org/10.1172/jci7696

Minegishi Y, Coustan-Smith E, Wang YH, Cooper MD, Campana D, Conley ME (1998) Mutations in the human lambda5/14.1 gene result in B cell deficiency and agammaglobulinemia. J Exp Med 187(1):71–77. https://doi.org/10.1084/jem.187.1.71

Mitsuiki N, Yang X, Bartol SJ, Grosserichter-Wagener C, Kosaka Y, Takada H et al (2015) Mutations in Bruton's tyrosine kinase impair IgA responses. Int J Hematol 101(3):305–313. https://doi.org/10.1007/s12185-015-1732-1

Moshous D, Callebaut I, de Chasseval R, Corneo B, Cavazzana-Calvo M, Le Deist F et al (2001) Artemis, a novel DNA double-strand break repair/V(D)J recombination protein, is mutated in human severe combined immune deficiency. Cell 105(2):177–186. https://doi.org/10.1016/s0092-8674(01)00309-9

Nanthapisal S, Omoyinmi E, Murphy C, Standing A, Eisenhut M, Eleftheriou D et al (2017) Early-onset juvenile SLE associated with a novel mutation in protein kinase C delta. Pediatrics 139(1). https://doi.org/10.1542/peds.2016-0781

O'Driscoll M, Cerosaletti KM, Girard PM, Dai Y, Stumm M, Kysela B et al (2001) DNA ligase IV mutations identified in patients exhibiting developmental delay and immunodeficiency. Mol Cell 8(6):1175–85. https://doi.org/10.1016/s1097-2765(01)00408-7

Ombrello MJ, Remmers EF, Sun G, Freeman AF, Datta S, Torabi-Parizi P et al (2012) Cold urticaria, immunodeficiency, and autoimmunity related to PLCG2 deletions. N Engl J Med 366(4):330–8. https://doi.org/10.1056/NEJMoa1102140

Peron S, Metin A, Gardes P, Alyanakian MA, Sheridan E, Kratz CP et al (2008) Human PMS2 deficiency is associated with impaired immunoglobulin class switch recombination. J Exp Med 205(11):2465–72. https://doi.org/10.1084/jem.20080789

Picard C, Bobby Gaspar H, Al-Herz W, Bousfiha A, Casanova JL, Chatila T et al (2018) International union of immunological societies: 2017 primary immunodeficiency diseases committee report on inborn errors of immunity. J Clin Immunol 38(1):96–128. https://doi.org/10.1007/s10875-017-0464-9

Pieper K, Grimbacher B, Eibel H (2013) B-cell biology and development. J Allergy Clin Immunol 131(4):959–71. https://doi.org/10.1016/j.jaci.2013.01.046

Rezaei N et al (2017) Primary immunodeficiency diseases. https://doi.org/10.1007/978-3-662-52909-6

Rickert RC (2013) New insights into pre-BCR and BCR signalling with relevance to B cell malignancies. Nat Rev Immunol 13(8):578–91. https://doi.org/10.1038/nri3487

Rickert RC, Jellusova J, Miletic AV (2011) Signaling by the tumor necrosis factor receptor superfamily in B-cell biology and disease. Immunol Rev 244(1):115–33. https://doi.org/10.1111/j.1600-065X.2011.01067.x

Rissone A, Weinacht KG, la Marca G, Bishop K, Giocaliere E, Jagadeesh J et al (2015) Reticular dysgenesis-associated AK2 protects hematopoietic stem and progenitor cell development from oxidative stress. J Exp Med 212(8):1185–202. https://doi.org/10.1084/jem.20141286

Rosain J, Miot C, Lambert N, Rousselet MC, Pellier I, Picard C (2017) CD21 deficiency in 2 siblings with recurrent respiratory infections and hypogammaglobulinemia. J Allergy Clin Immunol Pract 5(6):1765–1767 e3. https://doi.org/10.1016/j.jaip.2017.04.011

Ruland J, Hartjes L (2019) CARD-BCL-10-MALT1 signalling in protective and pathological immunity.

Nat Rev Immunol 19(2):118–134. https://doi.org/10.1038/s41577-018-0087-2

Sadat MA, Moir S, Chun TW, Lusso P, Kaplan G, Wolfe L et al (2014) Glycosylation, hypogammaglobulinemia, and resistance to viral infections. N Engl J Med 370(17):1615–1625. https://doi.org/10.1056/NEJMoa1302846

Saffran DC, Parolini O, Fitch-Hilgenberg ME, Rawlings DJ, Afar DE, Witte ON et al (1994) Brief report: a point mutation in the SH2 domain of Bruton's tyrosine kinase in atypical X-linked agammaglobulinemia. N Engl J Med 330(21):1488–91. https://doi.org/10.1056/nejm199405263302104

Salzer E, Kansu A, Sic H, Majek P, Ikinciogullari A, Dogu FE et al (2014) Early-onset inflammatory bowel disease and common variable immunodeficiency-like disease caused by IL-21 deficiency. J Allergy Clin Immunol 133(6):1651–1659.e12. https://doi.org/10.1016/j.jaci.2014.02.034

Salzer E, Santos-Valente E, Keller B, Warnatz K, Boztug K (2016) Protein kinase C delta: a gatekeeper of immune homeostasis. J Clin Immunol 36(7):631–40. https://doi.org/10.1007/s10875-016-0323-0

Salzer E, Santos-Valente E, Klaver S, Ban SA, Emminger W, Prengemann NK et al (2013) B-cell deficiency and severe autoimmunity caused by deficiency of protein kinase C delta. Blood 121(16):3112–6. https://doi.org/10.1182/blood-2012-10-460741

Salzer U, Bacchelli C, Buckridge S, Pan-Hammarstrom Q, Jennings S, Lougaris V et al (2009) Relevance of biallelic versus monoallelic TNFRSF13B mutations in distinguishing disease-causing from risk-increasing TNFRSF13B variants in antibody deficiency syndromes. Blood 113(9):1967–76. https://doi.org/10.1182/blood-2008-02-141937

Sarmiento E, Mora R, Rodriguez-Mahou M, Rodriguez-Molina J, Fernandez-Cruz E, Carbone J (2005) Autoimmune disease in primary antibody deficiencies. Allergol Immunopathol (Madr) 33(2):69–73. https://doi.org/10.1157/13072916

Sassi A, Lazaroski S, Wu G, Haslam SM, Fliegauf M, Mellouli F et al (2014) Hypomorphic homozygous mutations in phosphoglucomutase 3 (PGM3) impair immunity and increase serum IgE levels. J Allergy Clin Immunol 133(5):1410–1419, 1419.e1–13. https://doi.org/10.1016/j.jaci.2014.02.025

Schipp C, Nabhani S, Bienemann K, Simanovsky N, Kfir-Erenfeld S, Assayag-Asherie N et al (2016) Specific antibody deficiency and autoinflammatory disease extend the clinical and immunological spectrum of heterozygous NFKB1 loss-of-function mutations in humans. Haematologica 101(10):e392–e396. https://doi.org/10.3324/haematol.2016.145136

Schubert D, Klein MC, Hassdenteufel S, Caballero-Oteyza A, Yang L, Proietti M et al (2018) Plasma cell deficiency in human subjects with heterozygous mutations in Sec61 translocon alpha 1 subunit (SEC61A1). J Allergy Clin Immunol 141 (4):1427–1438. https://doi.org/10.1016/j.jaci.2017.06.042

Schwerd T, Twigg SRF, Aschenbrenner D, Manrique S, Miller KA, Taylor IB et al (2017) A biallelic mutation in IL6ST encoding the GP130 co-receptor causes immunodeficiency and craniosynostosis. J Exp Med 214 (9):2547–2562. https://doi.org/10.1084/jem.20161810

Shi PY, Maizels N, Weiner AM (1998) CCA addition by tRNA nucleotidyltransferase: polymerization without translocation? EMBO J 17(11):3197–206. https://doi.org/10.1093/emboj/17.11.3197

Silva P, Justicia A, Regueiro A, Farina S, Couselo JM, Loidi L (2017) Autosomal recessive agammaglobulinemia due to defect in mu heavy chain caused by a novel mutation in the IGHM gene. Genes Immun 18 (3):197–199. https://doi.org/10.1038/gene.2017.14

Simpfendorfer KR, Armstead BE, Shih A, Li W, Curran M, Manjarrez-Orduno N et al (2015) Autoimmune disease-associated haplotypes of BLK exhibit lowered thresholds for B cell activation and expansion of Ig class-switched B cells. Arthritis Rheumatol 67 (11):2866–76. https://doi.org/10.1002/art.39301

Spencer S, Kostel Bal S, Egner W, Lango Allen H, Raza SI, Ma CA et al (2019) Loss of the interleukin-6 receptor causes immunodeficiency, atopy, and abnormal inflammatory responses. J Exp Med 216(9):1986–1998. https://doi.org/10.1084/jem.20190344

Stepensky P, Keller B, Buchta M, Kienzler AK, Elpeleg O, Somech R et al (2013) Deficiency of caspase recruitment domain family, member 11 (CARD11), causes profound combined immunodeficiency in human subjects. J Allergy Clin Immunol 131(2):477–85.e1. https://doi.org/10.1016/j.jaci.2012.11.050

Tang P, Upton JEM, Barton-Forbes MA, Salvadori MI, Clynick MP, Price AK et al (2018) Autosomal recessive agammaglobulinemia due to a homozygous mutation in PIK3R1. J Clin Immunol 38(1):88–95. https://doi.org/10.1007/s10875-017-0462-y

Tangye SG, Bier J, Lau A, Nguyen T, Uzel G, Deenick EK (2019) Immune dysregulation and disease pathogenesis due to activating mutations in PIK3CD-the Goldilocks' effect. J Clin Immunol 39(2):148–158. https://doi.org/10.1007/s10875-019-00612-9

Thiel J, Kimmig L, Salzer U, Grudzien M, Lebrecht D, Hagena T, et al (2012) Genetic CD21 deficiency is associated with hypogammaglobulinemia. J Allergy Clin Immunol 129(3):801–810 e6. https://doi.org/10.1016/j.jaci.2011.09.027

Torres JM, Martinez-Barricarte R, Garcia-Gomez S, Mazariegos MS, Itan Y, Boisson B et al (2014) Inherited BCL10 deficiency impairs hematopoietic and nonhematopoietic immunity. J Clin Invest 124 (12):5239–48. https://doi.org/10.1172/jci77493

Tsukada S, Saffran DC, Rawlings DJ, Parolini O, Allen RC, Klisak I et al (1993) Deficient expression of a B cell cytoplasmic tyrosine kinase in human X-linked agammaglobulinemia. Cell 72(2):279–90. https://doi.org/10.1016/0092-8674(93)90667-f

Tuijnenburg P, Lango Allen H, Burns SO, Greene D, Jansen MH, Staples E et al (2018) Loss-of-function nuclear factor kappaB subunit 1 (NFKB1) variants are the most common monogenic cause of common variable immunodeficiency in Europeans. J Allergy Clin Immunol 142(4):1285–1296. https://doi.org/10.1016/j.jaci.2018.01.039

Valizadeh A, Yazdani R, Azizi G, Abolhassani H, Aghamohammadi A (2017) A comparison of clinical and immunologic phenotypes in familial and sporadic forms of common variable immunodeficiency. Scand J Immunol 86(4):239–247. https://doi.org/10.1111/sji.12593

van der Burg M, Ijspeert H, Verkaik NS, Turul T, Wiegant WW, Morotomi-Yano K et al (2009) A DNA-PKcs mutation in a radiosensitive T-B- SCID patient inhibits Artemis activation and nonhomologous end-joining. J Clin Invest 119(1):91–8. https://doi.org/10.1172/jci37141

van Montfrans JM, Hoepelman AI, Otto S, van Gijn M, van de Corput L, de Weger RA, et al (2012) CD27 deficiency is associated with combined immunodeficiency and persistent symptomatic EBV viremia. J Allergy Clin Immunol 129(3):787–793 e6. https://doi.org/10.1016/j.jaci.2011.11.013

Van Nieuwenhove E, Garcia-Perez JE, Helsen C, Rodriguez PD, van Schouwenburg PA, Dooley J et al (2018) A kindred with mutant IKAROS and autoimmunity. J Allergy Clin Immunol 142(2):699–702.e12. https://doi.org/10.1016/j.jaci.2018.04.008

van Zelm MC, Bartol SJ, Driessen GJ, Mascart F, Reisli I, Franco JL et al (2014) Human CD19 and CD40L deficiencies impair antibody selection and differentially affect somatic hypermutation. J Allergy Clin Immunol 134(1):135–44. https://doi.org/10.1016/j.jaci.2013.11.015

van Zelm MC, Reisli I, van der Burg M, Castano D, van Noesel CJ, van Tol MJ et al (2006) An antibody-deficiency syndrome due to mutations in the CD19 gene. N Engl J Med 354(18):1901–12. https://doi.org/10.1056/NEJMoa051568

van Zelm MC, Smet J, Adams B, Mascart F, Schandene L, Janssen F et al (2010) CD81 gene defect in humans disrupts CD19 complex formation and leads to antibody deficiency. J Clin Invest 120(4):1265–74. https://doi.org/10.1172/JCI39748

Vely F, Barlogis V, Marinier E, Coste ME, Dubern B, Dugelay E et al (2018) Combined immunodeficiency in patients with trichohepatoenteric syndrome. Front Immunol 9:1036. https://doi.org/10.3389/fimmu.2018.01036

Vetrie D, Vorechovsky I, Sideras P, Holland J, Davies A, Flinter F et al (1993) The gene involved in X-linked agammaglobulinaemia is a member of the src family of protein-tyrosine kinases. Nature 361(6409):226–33. https://doi.org/10.1038/361226a0

Vorechovsky I, Webster AD, Plebani A, Hammarstrom L (1999) Genetic linkage of IgA deficiency to the major histocompatibility complex: evidence for allele segregation distortion, parent-of-origin penetrance differences, and the role of anti-IgA antibodies in disease predisposition. Am J Hum Genet 64(4):1096–109. https://doi.org/10.1086/302326

Wang HY, Ma CA, Zhao Y, Fan X, Zhou Q, Edmonds P et al (2013) Antibody deficiency associated with an inherited autosomal dominant mutation in TWEAK. Proc Natl Acad Sci U S A 110(13):5127–32. https://doi.org/10.1073/pnas.1221211110

Warnatz K, Salzer U, Rizzi M, Fischer B, Gutenberger S, Bohm J et al (2009) B-cell activating factor receptor deficiency is associated with an adult-onset antibody deficiency syndrome in humans. Proc Natl Acad Sci U S A 106(33):13945–50. https://doi.org/10.1073/pnas.0903543106

Wedatilake Y, Niazi R, Fassone E, Powell CA, Pearce S, Plagnol V et al (2016) TRNT1 deficiency: clinical, biochemical and molecular genetic features. Orphanet J Rare Dis 11(1):90. https://doi.org/10.1186/s13023-016-0477-0

Wentink MW, Lambeck AJ, van Zelm MC, Simons E, van Dongen JJ, IJspeert H, et al. (2015). CD21 and CD19 deficiency: Two defects in the same complex leading to different disease modalities. Clin Immunol 161(2):120–127. https://doi.org/10.1016/j.clim.2015.08.010

Wood PM (2010) Primary antibody deficiency syndromes. Curr Opin Hematol 17(4):356–61. https://doi.org/10.1097/MOH.0b013e328338f69e

Xiong E, Li Y, Min Q, Cui C, Liu J, Hong R et al (2019) MZB1 promotes the secretion of J-chain-containing dimeric IgA and is critical for the suppression of gut inflammation. Proc Natl Acad Sci U S A 116(27):13480–13489. https://doi.org/10.1073/pnas.1904204116

Yang L, Fliegauf M, Grimbacher B (2014) Hyper-IgE syndromes: reviewing PGM3 deficiency. Curr Opin Pediatr 26(6):697–703. https://doi.org/10.1097/MOP.0000000000000158

Yazdani R, Azizi G, Abolhassani H, Aghamohammadi A (2017) Selective IgA deficiency: Epidemiology, pathogenesis, clinical phenotype, diagnosis, prognosis and management. Scand J Immunol 85(1):3–12. https://doi.org/10.1111/sji.12499

Yel L, Minegishi Y, Coustan-Smith E, Buckley RH, Trubel H, Pachman LM et al (1996) Mutations in the mu heavy-chain gene in patients with agammaglobulinemia. N Engl J Med 335(20):1486–93. https://doi.org/10.1056/nejm199611143352003

Zegers BJ, Maertzdorf WJ, Van Loghem E, Mul NA, Stoop JW, Van Der Laag J, et al (1976) Kappa-chain deficiency: an immunoglobulin disorder. N Engl J Med 294(19):1026–1030. https://doi.org/10.1056/nejm197605062941902

Zhang Q, Boisson B, Beziat V, Puel A, Casanova JL (2018) Human hyper-IgE syndrome: singular or plural? Mamm Genome 29(7–8):603–617. https://doi.org/10.1007/s00335-018-9767-2

Zhang Q, Davis JC, Lamborn IT, Freeman AF, Jing H, Favreau AJ et al (2009) Combined immunodeficiency associated with DOCK8 mutations. N Engl J Med 361(21):2046–55. https://doi.org/10.1056/NEJMoa0905506

Zhou Q, Lee GS, Brady J, Datta S, Katan M, Sheikh A et al (2012) A hypermorphic missense mutation in PLCG2, encoding phospholipase Cgamma2, causes a dominantly inherited autoinflammatory disease with immunodeficiency. Am J Hum Genet 91(4):713–20. https://doi.org/10.1016/j.ajhg.2012.08.006

11 B Cell-Mediated Autoimmune Diseases

Xiang Lin and Liwei Lu

Abstract

Extensive studies have suggested a central role of B cells in the autoimmune pathogenesis, as loss of B cell tolerance results in increased serum levels of autoantibodies, enhanced effector T cell response and tissue damages. Here, we provide an overview of dysregulated B cell responses in the development of autoimmunity. In addition to their presence in the target organs, autoreactive B cells can promote the formation of ectopic lymphoid structures and differentiate into plasma cells that produce large amounts of autoantibodies and cytokines. In animal models that recapitulate the key features of human autoimmune disease, mechanistic studies have indicated two categories of autoantibodies: (1) serological markers for disease diagnosis and prognosis; (2) effector molecules that induce organ hypofunction or damage directly in an epitope-specific manner, or indirectly by activating other immune cell subsets. Moreover, B cell-derived cytokines usually promote the autoreactive T cell response during autoimmune development, but there is compelling evidence that a subpopulation of B cells negatively regulates immune responses, also known as regulatory B cells via secreting anti-inflammatory cytokines (IL-10, IL-35, etc.) or a contact-dependent fashion. Although B cell depletion could eliminate most circulating B cells in the periphery, the clinical outcomes of B cell depletion therapy for autoimmune diseases vary among individuals due to differential activation or survival signals for B cells provided by tissue microenvironment. Thus, therapeutic combinations that target immune checkpoints and B cell activation may represent a promising strategy for the effective treatment of human autoimmune diseases.

Keywords

Autoimmune diseases · B cell tolerance · Autoantibodies · Inflammatory cytokines

X. Lin
Department of Pathology and Shenzhen Institute of Research and Innovation, The University of Hong Kong, Hong Kong, China

L. Lu (✉)
Department of Pathology, The University of Hong Kong, Pokfulam, Hong Kong, China
e-mail: liweilu@hku.hk

11.1 Introduction

B cell tolerance is established throughout B cell developmental stages both in the bone marrow and peripheral lymphoid organs. Emerging evidence has suggested that B cells play a central

J.-Y. Wang (ed.), *B Cells in Immunity and Tolerance*, Advances in Experimental Medicine and Biology 1254, https://doi.org/10.1007/978-981-15-3532-1_11

role in the autoimmune pathogenesis and inflammatory response. Although approximately 55–75% early immature B cells exhibit self-reactivity, most autoreactive B cells are eliminated by multiple checkpoints accordingly (Wardemann et al. 2003). The defects in immune tolerance have been observed in patients with autoimmune diseases, including rheumatoid arthritis (RA), systemic lupus erythematosus (SLE), Sjogren's syndrome (SS) and type 1 diabetes (T1D) (Rubin et al. 2019). Histopathologically, massive B cells are detected in the aggregates of lymphocytic infiltrations and may even form ectopic germinal centers in the inflamed tissues upon the disease progression, which is strongly associated with the disease activities and severity. Currently, the detailed nature of defects in immune checkpoints during B cell development in autoimmune disorders remains largely unclear. However, B cell depletion therapy in both humans and mouse models with autoimmune diseases results in attenuated clinical manifestations and ameliorated disease progression, suggesting a critical role of B cells in the autoimmune pathogenesis.

11.2 B Cell Tolerance Checkpoints in Autoimmune Disease

B cell activation and effector functions are important for both innate and adaptive immune responses. However, dysregulations at various immune checkpoints may lead to B cell hyperactivation and autoimmunity.

BAFF. B cell stimulatory checkpoints are closely associated with B cell tolerance. Upon the elimination of immature B cells bearing an autoreactive B cell receptor in the bone marrow, newly generated B cells migrate into the spleen via the terminal branches of the central arteriole that drains into sinusoids of the marginal zone (MZ) (Cyster 1999), while the non-self-reactive IgM^+/IgD^- immature B cells penetrate the MZ sinus to migrate through the interface between the periarteriolar lymphoid sheaths and B cell follicles, and eventually become naive mature B cells. Notably, this process is highly dependent on B cell activating factor (BAFF; also known as *TNFSF13B*), a cytokine discovered by Tschopp and colleagues, that belongs to the TNF family and promotes B cell survival, activation and maturation (Ng et al. 2004). BAFF is produced by various types of immune cells including follicular dendritic cells and monocytes, which can regulate B cell functions through interactions with three different receptors: transmembrane activator and calcium modulator (TACI; also known as *TNFRSF13B*), the predominant BAFF receptor on splenic transitional type 2 and MZ B cells; B cell maturation antigen (BCMA; also known as *TNFRSF17*), the predominant BAFF receptor on germinal center B cells; and BAFF receptor (BAFFR), the predominant BAFF receptor on peripheral B cells. BAFF concentrations are often increased in the serum of patients with SLE, SS and other autoimmune conditions (Vincent et al. 2014), which are also positively correlated with serum levels of autoantibodies, including anti-dsDNA and anti-SSA IgG. Moreover, a variant of *TNFSF13B* is strongly associated with multiple sclerosis (MS), SS and SLE. This variant encodes a truncated mRNA, which escapes microRNA-mediated inhibition, resulting in enhanced BAFF production (Steri et al. 2017). Interestingly, BAFF-transgenic mice spontaneously develop features of SLE and SS, among which skewed development of MZ B cells is observed in the spleen and found predominantly in the lymphocytic infiltrates of the target organs (Groom et al. 2002). In addition, compared with their wild-type littermates, BAFF-transgenic mice possess an increased risk of lymphoma as they age, which is further boosted in the absence of TNF expression (Batten et al. 2004). Thus, the above evidence suggests that BAFF serves as a critical immune checkpoint in B cell survival and maturation in autoimmune pathogenesis.

CD40. CD40 also belongs to the TNF superfamily and serves as a co-stimulatory molecule found on numerous cell types, including B cells, monocytes and dendritic cells via CD40 ligand (CD40L, also known as CD154). The CD40/CD40L axis is strongly involved in T cell-mediated cognate B cell help, which significantly promotes plasma cell differentiation. In contrast, in the absence of CD40 signaling, B cell receptor (BCR)-mediated activation can lead to B cell apoptosis, instead of activation (Hokazono et al. 2003). T–B interactions are involved in the loss of tolerance to self-antigens, as increased CD40L-expressing T cells and soluble CD40L have been frequently observed in patients with autoimmune disorders, including Graves' disease (GD), RA, MS, SLE and Crohn's disease, which usually positively correlated with disease activities. These observations are further exemplified by the findings from CD40-transgenic mice with spontaneous production of antinuclear, antiDNA and antihistone autoantibodies (Higuchi et al. 2002). In addition, it is reported that tissue-specific CD40 also serves as an immune checkpoint, as thyroidal CD40 deficiency leads to autoimmune GD development in mice.

Toll-like receptors. Apart from T cell-dependent activation, B cells can also recognize antigens independently of T cells via dual stimulations of BCR and Toll-like receptors (TLRs). It has been well demonstrated that TLRs can recognize pathogen-associated molecular patterns (PAMPs) and damage-associated molecular patterns (DAMPs) in both host defense and wound healing. However, upon the exposure of intracellular components after cell death, TLRs are also capable of binding self-ligands or DAMPs, which promotes pathogenic autoimmune responses under inflammatory conditions. In 2002, Marshak-Rothstein and colleagues have reported that dual stimulation of BCR and TLR9 by self-DNA-containing immune complexes promotes autoreactive B cell response in patients with SLE (Leadbetter et al. 2002). Moreover, together with BCR engagement, other TLR members such as TLR7 and TLR8 that bind single-strand DNA, RNA or immune complexes containing small nuclear ribonucleoproteins are also closely involved in the autoreactive B cell activation and autoantibodies productions, which is important in the pathogenesis of autoimmune hepatitis, SS, RA and autoimmune myositis (Moritoki et al. 2006; Pelka et al. 2016).

CD19. In addition to the co-stimulatory signals of TLRs and CD40, CD19 also serves as a co-receptor that mediates B cell activation. CD19 is an immunoglobulin superfamily glycoprotein expressed from pre-B cell stage to mature B cell stage during differentiation. B cells are largely eliminated in the absence of CD19 in mice, suggesting an essential role of CD19 in B cell development and activation, while stimulation of CD19 or BCR alone leads to apoptosis. Indeed, mice deficient for CD19 exhibit diminished MZ B cells and are resistant to autoimmune induction, while mice with slight overexpression of CD19 develop spontaneous autoimmunity (Hasegawa et al. 2001; Sato et al. 2000). Similarly, a subpopulation of $CD19^{hi}$ B cells has been found increased in patients with pemphigus and SLE. Thus, CD19 is considered as a crucial checkpoint and potential target for the treatment of autoimmune diseases.

Thymic B cells. In addition to the importance of self-tolerance in B cells, recent studies also implicate a non-redundant role of B cells in the central tolerance of T cells. In 1987, Addis and colleagues first identified thymic B cells in humans (Isaacson et al. 1987), which is subsequently found in mice. Thymic B cells represent approximately 0.3% of the thymic population. Similar to those mice lack dendritic cells, mice with B cell deficiency exhibited increased frequencies of the CD4 single-positive population in the thymus. In addition, accumulated thymic B cells are observed in BAFF-transgenic mice, resulting in increased thymic regulatory T (Treg) cells. Unlike resting B cells in spleen and lymph nodes, thymic B cells express high levels of MHC class II, co-stimulatory molecules CD80 and CD86, which may facilitate the deletion of autoreactive T cells (Kleindienst et al. 2000). Further studies have shown that B cells with engineered BCR against autoantigen also contribute to cognate T cell licensing in the thymus (Perera et al. 2013). Although thymic B cells express an unusual autoimmune regulator (Aire) gene, little is known whether their function of an immune checkpoint is Aire-dependent. Interestingly, an age-associated decline has been observed in both cell count and Aire expression of thymic B cells (Cepeda et al. 2018), which may be considered as a risk factor of autoimmunity within the elderly.

11.3 B Cells in the Target Tissues During Autoimmune Development

Histological assessment of biopsies from patients with autoimmune disorders has revealed the presence of massive B cells in the targeted organs, including renal biopsies of SLE patients, synovial biopsies from RA patients and labial biopsies from SS patients, etc., which is correlated with disease activities. A key feature of local inflammation in the target organ is the interaction between tissue stromal cells and immune cells. Moreover, focal T and B cell aggregates can be segregated to form ectopic lymphoid structure (ELS) in the presence of follicular dendritic cells (FDCs) upon disease progression (Pitzalis et al. 2014). It has been reported that activated T and B cells at the site of infiltrates express membrane-bound lymphotoxin $\alpha 1\beta 2$ ($LT\alpha 1\beta 2$), while persistent exposure to $LT\alpha 1\beta 2$ leads to differentiation of resident stromal cells into FDCs (Ware 2005), which secrete CXCL13 to recruit $CXCR5^{+}$ B cells and promote pathogenic B cell differentiation. Infiltrating B cells also reciprocally interact with tissue cells such as BAFF-producing epithelial and stromal cells to maintain their homeostasis in situ. In addition to $CD23^{+}$ follicular-like B cells are found in the ELS, many studies also report the presence of $CD21^{+}$ marginal zone-like B cells within the lymphocytic foci at chronic stages of both humans and mouse models with autoimmune disorders. Furthermore, FDCs secrete other chemokines including CCL19/CCL21 to promote T cell chemotaxis and CXCL12 to promote plasma cell retention. The residing plasma cells subsequently produce large amounts of autoantibodies and participate in tissue damages. In patients with RA, in addition to chemokine productions, synovial fibroblasts also secret IL-7 that contributes to ectopic lymphoid neogenesis. Moreover, infiltrating T cells in the ELS can produce key cytokines including IL-21, IL-4 and BAFF to synergize the development of effector B cells within the inflamed tissues. ELS formed during autoimmune progression is not only structurally reminiscent of secondary lymphoid organs, but also functionally active with germinal centers (GCs). Indeed, B cells isolated from ELS in autoimmune conditions display somatically hypermutated Ig VH and VL regions in line with a local antigen-driven process. Consistently, focal B cells in the ELS exhibit clonal diversification and express activation-induced cytidine deaminase, an enzyme regulating both somatic hypermutation and isotype class-switch of the Ig genes (Humby et al. 2009). Thus, antigens from local tissues can drive autoreactive B cell selection and differentiation in a disease-specific manner. Formation of ELS is widely observed in patients with autoimmune disorders, which allows the generation of high-affinity plasma cells that produce autoantibodies including anti-citrullinated proteins in RA; anti-SSA and anti-SSB in SS; anti-thyroglobulin in autoimmune thyroiditis and anti-insulin in T1D (Corsiero et al. 2016). Notably, accompanied by chronic inflammation, patients with ELS are more likely to develop B cell lymphoma (Theander et al. 2011).

11.4 Antibody-Dependent B Cell Functions in Autoimmune Diseases

Autoantibodies are produced by B cells and serve historically as the *sine qua non* of disease diagnostic and prognostic criteria. Apart from being the biomarkers, some identified autoantibodies are pathogenic and closely involved in the disease pathology (Fig. 11.1).

Autoantibodies are highly prevalent in the peripheral circulation and detectable during various disease stages, rendering them favorable markers in diagnosis. Given the diversification of autoreactive BCR, autoantibodies can provide relatively high sensitivity and specificity for the presence of clinical syndromes. It has been well recognized that seropositivity of antinuclear antibodies (ANA) is most prevalent in patients

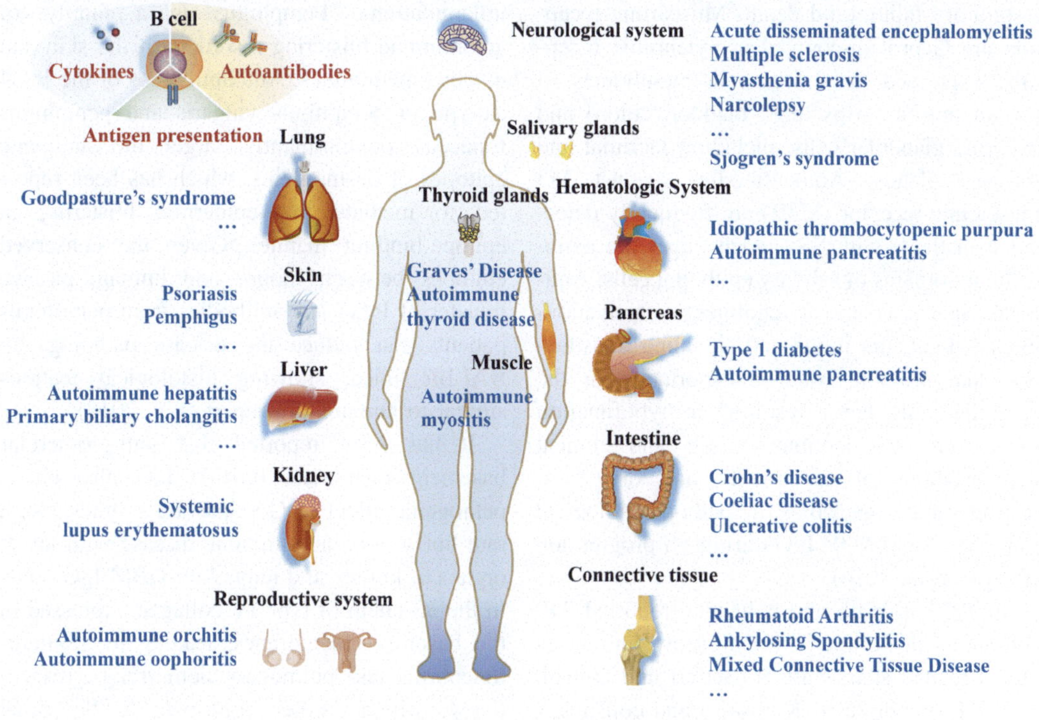

Fig. 11.1 Diagram of B cell-mediated organ-specific autoimmune diseases

with SLE, which leads to immune complex (IC) formation in various organs including skin, kidney, lung and even nervous system. However, clinical observations suggest that serum titers of ANA do not correlate with the disease activities or severity. By contrast, relapse SLE patients do not exhibit significant changes of ANA levels during flares. Some other autoantibodies including anti-Sm, anti-RNP and anti-phospholipid antibodies, on the contrary, are more specific and indicative for both disease diagnosis and prognosis of SLE. In particular, seropositivity of anti-RNP IgG identifies a subpopulation of cohort with clinical complications of mixed connective tissue diseases, while anti-phospholipid IgG is more associated with thrombotic development. In addition, anti-SSA autoantibodies can be detected in a large population of patients with SLE and SS, but have been reported to be associated with the increased risk of congenital heart block in the newborns of patients (Buyon and Clancy 2003). Notably, emerging evidence suggests that in patients with SS, anti-SSA autoantibodies are detectable years before the onset of clinical symptoms (Jonsson et al. 2013), indicating the importance of early humoral autoimmunity in disease development. Indeed, seropositivity of anti-SSA has gained increased attention in the consensus classification criteria of SS approved by the American College of Rheumatology (ACR) and the European League Against Rheumatism (EULAR) in 2016. Moreover, autoantibodies against the adrenal cortex serve as serological markers in the diagnosis of autoimmune Addison's disease and autoimmune oophoritis, which are correlated with the degree of adrenal dysfunction. However, these autoantibodies target 21-hydroxylase do not seem to inhibit the activity of 21-hydroxylase in vivo.

Apart from being serological markers, autoantibodies are found to possess pathogenic functions in the target organs during autoimmune inflammation. For example, anti-acetylcholine receptor (AChR) IgG can bind to the cell surface and block acetylcholine neurotransmission by altering the signaling within the postsynaptic neuronal plate, which may further induce muscle paralysis and lead to diaphragmatic dysfunction, respiratory failure and death. Muscarinic receptors are G protein-coupled acetylcholine receptors, expressed on the plasma membranes of certain muscle strips (e.g., bladder, colon) and exocrine glandular cells, including lacrimal and salivary glands. Autoantibodies against M3 muscarinic receptor (M3R) are frequently detected in patients with SS, which target the extracellular domains of salivary epithelial cells. Anti-M3R IgG can block cholinergic activation-mediated calcium influx and signaling transduction that promote water transportation in the epithelial cells, hence resulting in hypofunction of salivary and lacrimal glands and clinical manifestations of dry mouth and dry eyes, respectively, suggesting a pathophysiological function of anti-M3R IgG during SS progression (Fayyaz et al. 2016).

In 1977, Donath and colleague reported 349 patients with Küttner's tumor (now known as "IgG4-related sialadenitis") (Seifert and Donath 1977). Later, in 2001, Kiyosawa and colleagues used serum protein electrophoresis and identified a noninvasive biomarker to distinguish autoimmune pancreatitis from pancreatic cancer, namely IgG4 (Schuurman et al. 2001). Consequently, IgG4-related disease (IgG4-RD) is characterized by high serum levels of IgG4, massive lymphocytic infiltration with a large number of IgG4-positive plasma cells in tumefactive lesions. Various degrees of tissue fibrosis are usually accompanied by IgG4-RD, while immunosuppressive agents such as corticosteroids are effectively used in the clinical applications. IgG4-RD has a broad clinicopathologic spectrum and is often organ-specific including autoimmune pancreatitis, autoimmune hepatitis, thyroiditis, rhinosinusitis, glomerulonephritis, pneumonia, Mikulicz's disease, etc. (Obiorah et al. 2018). Interestingly, IgG4-related Mikulicz's disease with sialoadenitis was previously considered to be a subset of SS, while further studies reveal the absence of anti-SSA/SSB and antinuclear autoantibodies in these patients, revealing the diagnostic discrepancies from patients with SS. Similar to other autoantibody isotypes, IgG4 can serve as serological markers or elicit various biological functions during inflammations. Pemphigus is a family of autoimmune blistering disorders of the skin and mucous membranes. Autoantibodies of the IgG4 isotype in pemphigus vulgaris and pemphigus foliaceus predominantly target the antigenic epitopes of desmogleins, which has been reported to mediate intra-epidermal blistering in epitope-binding manner. Given the conserved epitopes between mouse and human, passive transfer of IgG4 autoantibodies from pemphigus patients can induce the disease pathology in BALB/c mice, showing histological features similar to humans (Trampert et al. 2018).

It has been reported that anti-glomerular basement membrane (GBM) IgG also elicits pathogenic effect in Goodpasture's syndrome, a rare but serious autoimmune disease with target organs of kidney and lung. Anti-GBM IgG binds to the $\alpha3$ chain of type IV collagen expressed in the basement membranes, leading to glomerulonephritis and pulmonary hemorrhage, respectively, which further contribute to the renal failure. This was supported by the attenuated disease symptoms upon pathogenic antibodies removal and plasma exchange (Cui and Zhao 2011). Therefore, both pathogenic and non-pathogenic autoantibodies have supported a key role of B cells in autoimmune pathogenesis.

Although BCR consists of membrane-bound IgM, the secreted form of IgM is found produced during the primary immune response. Secreted IgM (sIgM) can be categorized as natural and immune IgM, while the immune IgM is referred to the BCR engagement upon antigen-specific stimulation as mentioned above. Natural IgM, however, is polyreactive and often responds to endogenous antigens (Haury et al. 1997). Natural IgM can also be detected at normal quantities in the peripheral blood of mice under germ-free conditions. Unlike conventional (B2) B cells, natural IgM is mainly produced by B1 B cells from body cavities. The polyreactivity of natural IgM allows its binding to diverse epitopes of antigens, hence resulting in the neutralization of foreign pathogens during infections. Notably, sIgM is also strongly involved in autoimmunity. It is reported that mice with sIgM deficiency are more prone to develop autoimmune diseases and spontaneously predisposed to atherosclerosis (Tsiantoulas et al. 2017). Although the underlying mechanisms are not fully understood, reduced capacity of apoptotic cell clearance may contribute to the autoimmune etiology. Since apoptotic cells are persistently releasing autoantigens during inflammations, the removal of antigenic compartment is crucial in maintaining the immune tolerance. sIgM, including natural IgM, can recognize various autoantigens, such as phospholipids, the products from apoptotic cascade, and mediate opsonization of apoptotic cells, thereby enhancing the clearance by phagocytic cells (Peng et al. 2005). Consistently, declined serum IgM levels are detected in patients with SLE. Moreover, reduction or deficiency of sIgM may also increase the risk of infection, which leads to chronic inflammations and consequent autoimmunity. There are also other possible mechanisms involved in sIgM deficiency and autoimmunity. MZ B cells are well known for their T cell-independent immune response and capacity of producing large amount of IgM. In addition to their antibody productions, MZ B cells also secret anti-inflammatory cytokines, e.g., IL-10, when encountering apoptotic cells. Early studies have demonstrated that MZ B cell serves as a major producer of IL-10. Moreover, MZ B cell-derived IL-10 could significantly ameliorate disease pathology of collagen-induced arthritis in mice (Yang et al. 2010). Interestingly, IL-10-producing capacity was found diminished in the absence of sIgM in mice, which are more prone to autoimmune development. Consistently, increased susceptibility of infection and autoimmune diseases is observed in patients with selective IgM deficiency (Gupta and Gupta 2017).

During inflammatory responses, sIgM may also elicit pathogenic effects. Recent studies have revealed a potential role of sIgM in the gout pathogenesis by enhancing the precipitation of urate crystals, while natural IgM that binds to urate crystals can promote the phagocytosis of urate crystals, as well as chemotaxis of neutrophils to the affected tissues, boosting local inflammatory reactions within the microenvironment (Kanevets et al. 2009).

The pathogenicity of antibodies in the autoimmune pathogenesis is not only dependent on their bindings to the antigenic epitope, but also varied concurrently, including forming an immune complex that induces complement and Fc receptor activation. Immune complexes are commonly found deposited in variety of tissues and organs in autoimmune diseases (e.g., exocrine glands, blood vessels, kidney, lung, etc.), which induces tissue hypofunction and damage. In SLE patients, glomerular immune complexes can be detected in the renal biopsies, mainly in the mesangium or the subendothelial and subepithelial spaces, which cause renal damage via binding to nucleosomes. This observation is further supported by the findings in humanized mouse model that renal damage can be induced in immunodeficient mice upon serum transfer from patients with lupus nephritis. In addition to tissue cells, immune complexes also activate macrophages and dendritic cells in the target organ that produce pro-inflammatory cytokines, including IFN-α and IFN-β.

Furthermore, immune complexes also elicit pathogenic function through activating complement system. Activated complements generate three types of effector molecules: (1) anaphylatoxins that mediate lymphocytes chemotaxis; (2) opsonins that enhance phagocytosis of antigens via covalent bonding to immune complexes; (3) forming complexes that lyse target cells. Complement components can form complex structure via its subunits, e.g., C1q binding to antigen-associated IgG at the Fc fragments. Dysregulated complement system is involved in the pathogenesis and clinical manifestations of several autoimmune diseases including SLE, SS, RA, anti-phospholipid syndrome, MS and dermatomyositis (Ballanti et al. 2013). RA patients have increased levels of circulating and synovial immune complexes. It appears that autoantigens from cartilage such as fibromodulin can induce complement activation by binding to the globular head of C1q. In addition, the activated complement product C5a is also elevated in the synovial fluids of RA patients. C5a serves as a potent chemoattractant for neutrophils, monocytes and eosinophils, which may lead to the activation of pro-inflammatory cascade in situ. Notably, anti-C5 monoclonal antibody exerts therapeutic effects in mice with collagen-induced arthritis (Wang et al. 1995).

The FcγR is a group of surface glycoproteins that binds to the Fc portion of IgG, *i.e.*, FcγRI (also known as CD64) with high affinity, FcγRII (also known as CD32) and FcγRIII (also known as CD16) with low affinity. Genetic polymorphism of FcγR is strongly associated with autoimmunity. For instance, engagement of FcγRIIb cross-links BCR complex and transduces inhibitory signals that negatively regulate B cell activation. Indeed, mice deficient for FcγRIIb exhibited exacerbated lupus-like symptoms, but can be rescued when FcγRIIb expression is partially restored by B cells (McGaha et al. 2005). Likewise, mutation and decreased expression FcγRIIb in memory B cells have also been detected in patients with SLE, RA and MS (Smith and Clatworthy 2010), indicating a close involvement of FcγRIIb in regulating B cell response in autoimmune pathogenesis. Furthermore, Fc receptors are also expressed by monocytes and dendritic cells. Since IgG can significantly reduce the threshold of antigen concentration for dendritic cell activation by binding with its Fc receptors, autoantibodies produced by B cells can indirectly promote the autoreactive T cell responses. Consistently, mice deficient for FcγRIIb are resistant to T cell-dominant autoimmune disorders including myelin oligodendrocyte glycoprotein-induced experimental autoimmune encephalomyelitis (EAE).

11.5 Antibody-Independent B Cell Functions in Autoimmune Diseases

11.5.1 Antigen Presentation

Central T cell tolerance is mainly induced by thymic dendritic cells and medullary thymic epithelial cells (mTECs). As mentioned above, thymus also harbors substantial numbers of B cells that may arise via intrathymic B lymphopoiesis or chemotaxis from the periphery. Highly expressed co-stimulatory molecules on thymic B cells may promote central tolerance of T cells. While early studies have identified a central role of Aire-expressing mTECs in the thymus, recent findings that a novel subset of thymic B cells express Aire gene suggest a previously unappreciated role of B cells in T cell tolerance induction.

Memory B cells are long-lived and can persist in the body for decades. As the antibodies of switched isotypes are generated from germinal centers with high affinity, it has been thought that upon secondary antigen challenges, memory B cells are functionally important to rapidly produce antibodies, mainly IgA and IgG isotypes. The antigen-mediated cross-linking of membrane IgA or IgG provides stronger activation signals than IgM, which may explain the significant lower antigen concentration required for memory B cell activation and prompt differentiation into a plasma cell. Consequently, with extremely low threshold for antigen activation, memory B cells also serve as powerful antigen-presenting cells, and hence could be crucial in promoting autoreactive T cell responses during chronic inflammatory immune response, in particular autoimmune progression (Schrezenmeier et al. 2018). Indeed, the memory BCR repertoire is shaped by abnormal selection during autoimmune development, with exaggerated somatic hypermutation and BCR editing. Remarkably, peripheral blood of patients with SLE and RA consists of mainly activated $CD27^{+}IgD^{-}$ memory B cells and only a low percentage of naïve B cells, which is associated with a proportional increase of autoantibody-producing plasma cells. In addition, the accumulation of $CD27^{+}$ memory B cells in the lymphocytic foci is detected in inflamed tissues of patients with SS and SLE. A monoclonal antibody (clone 9G4) has been discovered to detect an idiotype rising from heavy chains encoded by the VH4-21 gene segment in disease-specific fashion of SLE, while $9G4^{+}$ memory B cells are generated unimpeded through immune checkpoints (Cappione et al. 2005), hence serving as a promising indicator for disease diagnosis and prognosis. B cells in the tonsils of patients with SLE are found to circumvent negative selection and subsequently differentiate into memory B cells and plasma cells with the capacity to produce anti-dsDNA antibodies, which are positively correlated with the disease activities. Although the role of memory B cell dysregulation in disease pathogenesis is not fully understood, viral infection has been considered as a risk factor including Epstein–Barr virus (EBV). Since the complement C2 receptor expressed by $CD27^+$ B cells is a co-receptor for EBV, memory B cells become a major reservoir of EBV. In patients with MS, latent EBV infection can drive the expansion of $CD27^+$ B cells and cause the augmented memory B cell response, which may possibly contribute to exacerbated disease activities. $CD27^+$ memory B cells are known to be resistant to the treatment of immunosuppressive drugs although the underlying mechanisms remain elusive.

11.5.2 Pro-inflammatory Cytokine Productions by B Cells

LTα1β2. Increasing evidence indicates a vital role of B cells in forming the secondary and tertiary lymphoid structures. The production of $LT\alpha1\beta2$ and TNF-α by B cells is found essential for FDCs development. FDCs in turn organize the follicular structures and recruit B cells by B cell-attracting chemokine 1 (BCA-1), also known as CXCL13. Reciprocally, FDC-derived CXCL13 further promotes $LT\alpha1\beta2$ production by B cells (Ansel et al. 2000). In the context of this positive feedback loop, B cells and their produced cytokines are considered as potential therapeutic targets for the therapy of autoimmune diseases.

IL-6. B cells are also a major source for IL-6 production under pathologic conditions. Increased IL-6-producing B cells are frequently observed in both patients and mouse models with autoimmune diseases. Remarkably, a significant elevation of IL-6-producing B cells was detected in the mice with EAE, in which B cell-derived IL-6 is critical in regulating Th1 and Th17 cell response during disease development (Barr et al. 2012). Consistently, B cell depletion therapy of patients with SS resulted in decreased circulating Th17 cells, supporting a role of B cells in regulating Th17 cell response. Recently, therapeutic strategies of targeting IL-17A have shown promising effects in attenuating the clinical symptoms of MS and psoriasis patients, which include secukinumab and brodalumab against IL-17 and IL-17 receptor A, respectively. IL-17-targeting therapy has been further found beneficial in patients with RA and Crohn's disease.

Among various effector T cell subsets, T follicular helper (Tfh) cells have been shown to play a pivotal role in autoimmune pathogenesis since Tfh cell-deficient mice exhibit diminished autoantibody production and attenuated disease pathology upon autoimmune induction (Fu et al. 2018). Clinical studies have reported significant increase of circulating Tfh cells, as well as their presence in the ELS within the target organs of patients with SLE and RA (Tangye et al. 2013). Tfh cells possess the chemotactic capacity to migrate into the B cell follicles and provide robust B cell help for autoantibody production. Notably, B cells can also reciprocally promote Tfh cell differentiation by IL-6 production and antigen presentation (Arkatkar et al. 2017).

GM-CSF. Granulocyte-macrophage colony-stimulating factor (GM-CSF) is first characterized in mice that triggers the proliferation of bone marrow-derived macrophages and granulocytes. Mice with a B cell-specific deficiency of GM-CSF are more susceptible to bacterial and viral infections with increased morbidity and mortality (Rauch et al. 2012). Recently, GM-CSF has also been implicated in the pathogenesis of autoimmunity as elevated titers of serum GM-CSF are detected in patients with autoimmune diseases. GM-CSF-producing B cells, in particular memory B cells, have been reported in patients with RA and SLE, which are positively correlated with disease activities. Notably, these memory B cells showed enhanced transcriptional signatures including upregulated STAT5 and STAT6 activities in B cells. In addition, B cell-derived GM-CSF can modulate the inflammatory phenotype of myeloid cells in cultures. MS patients treated with dimethyl fumarate have shown ameliorated disease pathology by targeting GM-CSF-producing B cells. Accordingly, B cell depletion therapy is also accompanied by dampened pro-inflammatory myeloid cell responses.

IFN-γ. B cell-derived IFN-γ has been reported to participate in cartilage proteoglycan-induced arthritis in mice (Bao et al. 2014). Remarkably, mice with B cell-specific deficiency of IFN-γ are almost completely resistant to the induction of arthritis, showing significantly reduced serum autoantibodies, decreased autoreactive Th1 cells and increased Treg cells. Although the exact mechanism is not fully understood, B cell-derived IFN-γ has been shown to suppress Treg cell differentiation (Olalekan et al. 2015). Moreover, IFNγ-producing B cells can promote cognate Th1 cell response during *Salmonella typhimurium* infection and enhance macrophage activation upon *Listeria monocytogenes* infection. Cao and colleagues have demonstrated that IFN-γ-producing B cells exhibit $CD19^{+}CD11a^{hi}Fc\gamma RIII^{hi}$ phenotype with their unique transcriptional signatures compared with conventional B cells (Bao et al. 2014). Thus, these findings suggest that B cell-derived IFN-γ may participate in the autoimmune pathogenesis by orchestrating autoreactive T cell subsets or innate immune cells. In addition to IFN-γ, B cells can produce other cytokines including IL-2, IL-4 and IL-13 upon stimulation of pattern recognition receptors. However, the roles of these cytokines-producing B cells in the autoimmune pathogenesis and their clinical implications require further investigations.

11.5.3 Regulatory B Cells

Although numerous studies indicate a pathogenic role of B cells in the development of autoimmunity, there is compelling evidence that a subpopulation of B cells negatively regulates immune responses, namely regulatory B (Breg) cells (Katz et al. 1974; Mizoguchi and Bhan 2006). The dynamic changes of Breg cells are reported to be associated with the progression of human diseases. It has been recognized that Breg cells can exert their inhibitory functions with different mechanisms in various mouse models of disease, including inflammation, cancer and autoimmunity (Yang et al. 2013). A suppressive role of B cells is first supported by exacerbated disease pathology in an EAE mouse model with B cell deficiency, followed by findings that B cells exert their suppressive function in an IL-10-dependent manner. Consistently, spontaneous intestinal inflammation is also observed when T cell receptor alpha (TCRα)-/- mice crossbreed with B cell-deficient mice, which can be controlled by a subpopulation of $CD1d^{+}$ B cells. Remarkably, IL-10 is found diminished in those CD1d-/- mice, indicating that CD1d may directly induce IL-10 production by B cells. Further studies reveal that $CD1d^{hi}$ B cells produce a higher amount of IL-10 when compared with $CD1d^{lo}$ B cells upon lipopolysaccharide (LPS) stimulation. Tedder and colleagues have identified a subset of IL-10-producing Breg cells in mice with a unique phenotype $CD1d^{hi}CD5^{+}$ (Yanaba et al. 2008). Similar to Treg cells, Breg cells-derived IL-10 was found to suppress effector T cell response in mouse disease models by inhibiting STAT3 activation in T cells. In addition to TLRs, CD40 and MHC class II molecules are also involved in enhancing IL-10 transcription in B cells. Although BAFF has been suggested to be pathogenic and overexpressed in the autoimmune diseases, recent findings have identified a novel function of BAFF at low concentrations in promoting IL-10 transcription by MZ B cells via AP-1 binding to the promoter region of *il10* (Yang et al. 2010). Importantly, by combining stimulations of CD40, BAFF, BCR and IL-21, Tedder and colleagues have succeeded in expanding Breg cells in culture by four million times than the initial cell numbers (Yoshizaki et al. 2012). In humans, Mauri and colleagues have identified a subset of $CD19^{+}CD24^{+}CD38^{hi}$ as the major population of IL-10 production in the peripheral blood from healthy individuals (Blair et al. 2010), which is associated with the phenotype of immature transitional B cells. These human Breg cells also respond to CD40 stimulation but exhibit impaired IL-10 production in patients with SLE, possibly owing to an altered STAT3 activation in Breg cells. Moreover, Tedder and colleagues reported that human $CD24^{hi}CD27^{+}$ B cells possess a strong capacity of IL-10 production (Iwata et al. 2011). Interestingly, since CD27 serves as a marker for human memory B cells, these Breg cells may not be newly migrated subsets from bone marrow. Although both $CD24^{+}CD38^{hi}$ and $CD24^{hi}CD27^{+}$ Breg cells have been found increased in patients with various autoimmune diseases, including SLE, RA, autoimmune skin disease and MS, we have revealed significantly impaired IL-10-producing capacity in these human Breg cells upon disease progression (Lin et al. 2019), suggesting a close involvement of Breg cells in the autoimmune pathogenesis. Using mouse models of autoimmunity, including experimental arthritis, SLE and MS, extensive investigations have demonstrated a critical role of endogenous IL-10 production by B cells in restraining Th1 and Th17 cells while promoting Treg cell expansion during disease development. Mechanistic studies reveal that IL-10/IL-10 receptor signaling potently inhibits the expression of t-bet and RORγt, the signature transcription factors of Th1 and Th17 cells, respectively. Using an experimental SS model, we have demonstrated a role of IL-10-producing B cells in controlling humoral autoimmunity by suppressing Tfh cell response via STAT5 activation (Lin et al. 2019). Moreover, adoptive transfer of Breg cells elicits therapeutic effects in diseased mice with T1D, experimental SS, CIA and EAE, while IL-10-/- Breg cells fail to exhibit such protective functions. Although B cell depletion therapy attenuates ongoing EAE in mice, B cell depletion prior to EAE induction accelerates the disease onset and exacerbates the severity, supporting a notion that Breg cells are critically involved in maintaining T cell tolerance during autoimmune development.

In addition to IL-10, emerging evidence has suggested a potent regulatory function of IL-35 in orchestrating autoreactive T cell responses. IL-35 is first identified (Collison et al. 2007) as a heterodimeric cytokine of the IL-12 family, consisting of IL-12p35 and Epstein–Barr virus-induced gene 3 (EBi3). Similar to *Il10*, IL-35 is unregulated upon CD40 and BCR engagement. Using EAE mouse model, Fillatreau and colleagues have demonstrated a pivotal role of IL-35-producing B cells in controlling effector T cell responses and disease development (Shen et al. 2014). Moreover, B cell-derived IL-35 can exert an autocrine function by activating IL-35 receptor (IL-12Rβ2 and IL-27Rβ) to induce IL-10-producing Breg cells, which in turn elicit immunosuppressive function on autoreactive T cells. Interestingly, Breg cells can also produce TGF-β that promotes IL-10-producing T cells and $Foxp3^{+}$ Treg cells, as revealed by recent findings that B cell-specific TGF-β mutant donor cells result in much less IL-10 secretion and enhanced effector T cell responses during allogenic grafts (Lee et al. 2014).

It has been reported that IL-21 can promote the expression of lytic granules such as granzyme B (GrB), by tumor-infiltrating B cells. Further characterization of these GrB-producing Breg revealed a $CD19^{+}CD38^{+}CD1d^{+}IgM^{+}CD147^{+}$ phenotype (Lindner et al. 2013). Notably, GrB-expressing Breg cells can suppress T cell response in GrB-dependent manner, together with IL-10 and indoleamine-2,3-dioxygenase. Consistently, $CD5^{+}$ B cells from SLE patients, but not $CD5^{-}$ B cells, express high levels of IL-21 receptor and produce GrB (Hagn et al. 2010), suggesting the diverse mechanism of Breg cells in the immunomodulation during autoimmunity.

In EAE mice with transgenic TCR for myelin basic protein, transfer of wild-type or IL-10-/- B cells elicits comparable immunoregulatory functions, suggesting the existence of heterogenous subpopulations of Breg cells. In these EAE mice, B cells that express glucocorticoid-induced TNFR ligand (GITRL) could promote Treg cell expansion, which was abolished upon GITRL blockage of B cells (Ray et al. 2012). Moreover, a population of B cells in both human and mouse is found to express CD73 and CD39 with potent immunosuppressive function. Indeed, $CD73^{+}CD39^{+}$ B cells can inhibit $CD4^{+}$ T cell proliferation in cocultures. Apart from secreting cytokines, Breg cells also modulate immune responses in a cell contact-dependent manner. Thrombospondin 1 (TSP1), an adhesive glycoprotein, is detected in a small population of $CD35^{+}CD80^{-}$ B cells, which not only inhibits the expression of co-stimulatory molecules CD80 and CD86 by dendritic cells, but also promotes $Foxp3^{+}$ Treg cells as TSP1 is reported to activate TGF-β1. By contrast, anti-TGF-β, but not anti-IL-10, neutralizing antibody abolishes $CD35^{+}CD80^{-}$ B cell-mediated Treg cell expansion. Recent studies also identify a novel Breg cell subset expressing a high level of PD-L1. $PD\text{-}L1^{hi}$ Breg cells can suppress $PD\text{-}1^{+}$ Tfh cells both in vitro and in vivo. Interestingly, high-cholesterol diet activates a homeostatic and anti-inflammatory program in MZB cells, in particular PD-L1, thereby suppressing Tfh cells and disease development in a mouse model of atherosclerosis (Nus et al. 2017). Notably, these $PD\text{-}L1^{hi}$ Breg cells are resistant to anti-CD20 therapy due to their high expression levels of BAFF receptors.

11.6 Targeting B Cells in Autoimmune Diseases

11.6.1 B Cell Depletion Therapy

The biological therapies against B cells have been initially developed against B cell cancers, using anti-CD20 monoclonal antibodies (mAb). Both relative safety and good tolerance of anti-CD20 mAb have been shown in patients with both chronic lymphocytic lymphoma (CLL) and autoimmune disorders (Franks et al. 2016). For B cell-targeting approach, the mechanisms of mAb-mediated cell death such as antibody-dependent cell-mediated cytotoxicity (ADCC) have been suggested. Type I mAb recognizes CD20 in the lipid rafts and enables complement-dependent cytotoxicity (CDC), while type II mAb directly binds the region of CD20 outside the lipid raft, with little CDC effect but strongly induces programmed cell death in B cells (Meyer et al. 2018). In addition, mAb can also recruit innate effector cells via Fc/FcγR axis and serve as a potent therapeutic candidate. FcγRs are expressed on a wide range of innate immune cells including FcγRIII on NK cells. Upon IgG binding to the FcγR, stimulated NK cells can release a large amount of cytotoxic molecules from their granules to achieve the killing effect on B cell subset, including malignant B cells.

Rituximab (RTX), as the representative type I mAb against CD20, is the first drug approved by US Food and Drug Administration (FDA) for medical use in 1997. RTX is well-tolerated and most widely used in B cell depletion therapy. Peripheral B cells are rapidly diminished upon the RTX administration, accompanied by reduced total IgG levels in patients with MS, RA, SLE and SS, which is further synergized with immunosuppressive drugs such as glucocorticoids (Didona et al. 2019). On the contrary, the clinical outcomes of RTX therapy may vary among different studies with differential results. For example, severe infections such as recurrent pneumonia and sinusitis have been reported in patients with relapsing-remitting multiple sclerosis following RTX treatment (Chisari et al. 2019), while in some cases patients with primary progressive MS even show worsened clinical outcomes. In addition, following the withdrawal of RTX treatment, B cell subsets can repopulate within 6–20 months, which also serve as a predictor of disease relapse. Obinutuzumab, the type II anti-CD20 mAb, has shown beneficial efficacies in recent clinical trials for patients with follicular B cell lymphoma, exhibiting longer progression-free survival than rituximab-based therapy (Marcus et al. 2017). With more potent capacity for B cell depletion than RTX on patients with RA and SLE, obinutuzumab at phase 2 clinical trial has reached both primary and key secondary endpoints, showing improved overall renal responses and serological markers of disease activity in patients when compared with those placebo-treated subjects.

During the terminal differentiation of B cell maturation, CD20 expression is downregulated at plasma cell stage, rendering their insusceptibility of anti-CD20 therapy. Given the highly efficient autoantibody production, patients with autoreactive plasma cells are more likely refractory to RTX therapy. In patients with SS, the serum levels of IgG are significantly reduced upon RTX treatment but anti-M3R IgG titers are unaltered, together with hypofunctions of salivary and lacrimal glands, suggesting that long-lived plasma cells may account for anti-M3R autoantibody production. Furthermore, recent cohort studies showed reduced IgG levels in only 11 out of 32 SLE patients with IgG hypergammaglobulinemia after 12 months of treatment with RTX (Reddy et al. 2017). Consistently, the reduction of anti-dsDNA levels varies, in serum titers and isotypes of IgG among different individuals. However, those "memory" antibodies, such as vaccination-mediated anti-tetanus, anti-rubella and anti-measles antibodies have sustained after RTX therapy (Teng et al. 2012), suggesting that RTX may not affect the early generation of protective antibodies by plasma cells. Moreover, RTX may also benefit autoantibody-negative patients by affecting antibody-independent functions of B cells. There is evidence indicating that B cell depletion therapy is also associated with a reduction of effector T cell subsets and pro-inflammatory cytokines. In patients with RA and SS, those "good responders," who exhibiting significantly improved clinical manifestations, are strongly associated with lower serum levels of IFN-γ and Th17 cell response. However, among those "non-responders" with less efficacy or even worsened disease severity, it is proposed that anti-CD20 mAb may also lead to the depletion of Breg cells (Mauri and Menon 2017), a notion further supported by the positive correlation between efficient repopulation of functional Breg cells and long-term remission with improved clinical outcomes in SLE patients.

In some cases, B cells can be resistant to anti-CD20 treatment in organ-specific manner. For example, the peritoneal cavity provides survival niches for both B1 and B2 B cells upon anti-CD20 administration in mice, as revealed by the increased survival rates of intraperitoneal transfer of splenic B cells. Moreover, liver-resident B cells are also refractory to anti-CD20-mediated depletion, as the saturated phagocytosis of Kupffer cells exhibits downregulated Fc receptor and impaired killing capacity against IgG-opsonized B cells (Gong et al. 2005). Since B cell depletion is more efficient in eliminating peripheral B cells, B cells in the target organs such as synovium, are less affected upon anti-CD20 treatment. In addition, during chronic inflammations, B cells in the ELS of target organs that form a survival niche are found to more resistant to cell death induction, suggesting that biological treatment against total B cells in patients with autoimmune diseases remains challenging. Remarkably, upon the development of new technologies, multicenter clinical trials of anti-CD19 chimeric antigen receptor (CAR) T cell therapy that depletes B cells have shown promising clinical outcomes and long-term remissions in patients with B cell lymphomas (Mardiana et al. 2019). With relative safety and good tolerance, adoptive cell therapy could be further extended for the treatment of autoimmune diseases. Indeed, recent study has suggested that anti-CD19 CAR-T cells significantly attenuated disease pathology in two mouse models of SLE (Kansal et al. 2019).

11.6.2 Targeting Immune Checkpoints

More recent therapeutic attempts have been directed at the manipulation of B cell immune checkpoints including B cell activation, differentiation and survival. For example, using local delivery of therapeutic vectors for BAFF gene silencing, we have demonstrated the significant amelioration of joint pathology in mice with collagen-induced arthritis (Lai Kwan Lam et al. 2008). Further, clinical trials with Belimumab, the human monoclonal anti-BAFF IgG1λ antibody have been extensively conducted in patients with SLE, RA and SS. Based on its effectiveness in treating SLE patients, Belimumab has been approved by FDA in the treatment of refractory SLE.

Upon BCR stimulation, the signaling transduction in the cytoplasmic domains is mainly involved in phosphatidylinositol 3-kinase (PI3K) pathways, which recruit Bruton's tyrosine kinase (BTK) and protein kinase B (also known as AKT) to elicit the cascade of B cell activation. Currently, multiple forms of small molecule drug targeting PI3K, BTK and AKT have been developed in treating B cell lymphomas and autoimmunity. Ibrutinib, a representative inhibitor of BTK, has been shown to attenuate patients with B cell malignancies and even serves as combinational therapy with RTX. Compelling studies also demonstrate that ibrutinib can elicit therapeutic effects in animal models of arthritis and lupus, suggesting its therapeutic potentials in treating human autoimmune diseases (Norman 2016).

It has been reported that proteasome, a non-lysosomal protein complex critically regulates protein secretion at cellular levels. Bortezomib is the first FDA approved proteasome inhibitor for treating patients with multiple myeloma by targeting plasma cells. Early studies by Voll and colleagues reported that Bortezomib treatment efficiently depletes both short-lived and long-lived plasma cells in mouse model of lupus nephritis (Neubert et al. 2008), which has led to the subsequent clinical trials in humans. Indeed, increasing evidence shows beneficial effects of patients with refractory SS, refractory SLE and thrombotic thrombocytopenic purpura.

Together, there are multiple mechanisms underlying the contributions of B cells to autoimmune development, as revealed by the complex interplay between their pathogenic and regulatory functions. Therefore, future investigations of precision medicine with fine-tuned strategies against B cell functions may shed new light on the treatment of autoimmune diseases.

Acknowledgements This work is supported by grants from the National Natural Science Foundation of China (81771761 and 91842304); General Research Fund, Hong Kong Research Grants Council (17114515 and 17149716) and Hong Kong Croucher Foundation (260960116).

References

Ansel KM et al (2000) A chemokine-driven positive feedback loop organizes lymphoid follicles. Nature 406(6793):309–314

Arkatkar T et al (2017) B cell-derived IL-6 initiates spontaneous germinal center formation during systemic autoimmunity. J Exp Med 214(11):3207–3217

Ballanti E et al (2013) Complement and autoimmunity. Immunol Res 56(2–3):477–491

Bao Y et al (2014) Identification of IFN-gamma-producing innate B cells. Cell Res 24(2):161–176

Barr TA et al (2012) B cell depletion therapy ameliorates autoimmune disease through ablation of IL-6-producing B cells. J Exp Med 209(5):1001–1010

Batten M et al (2004) TNF deficiency fails to protect BAFF transgenic mice against autoimmunity and reveals a predisposition to B cell lymphoma. J Immunol 172(2):812–822

Blair PA et al (2010) CD19(+)CD24(hi)CD38(hi) B cells exhibit regulatory capacity in healthy individuals but are functionally impaired in systemic lupus erythematosus patients. Immunity 32(1):129–140

Buyon JP, Clancy RM (2003) Neonatal lupus: review of proposed pathogenesis and clinical data from the US-based Research Registry for Neonatal Lupus. Autoimmunity 36(1):41–50

Cappione A 3rd et al (2005) Germinal center exclusion of autoreactive B cells is defective in human systemic lupus erythematosus. J Clin Invest 115(11):3205–3216

Cepeda S et al (2018) Age-associated decline in thymic B cell expression of aire and aire-dependent self-antigens. Cell Rep 22(5):1276–1287

Chisari CG et al (2019) An update on the safety of treating relapsing-remitting multiple sclerosis. Expert Opin Drug Saf

Collison LW et al (2007) The inhibitory cytokine IL-35 contributes to regulatory T-cell function. Nature 450 (7169):566–569

Corsiero E et al (2016) Ectopic lymphoid structures: powerhouse of autoimmunity. Front Immunol 7:430

Cui Z, Zhao MH (2011) Advances in human antiglomerular basement membrane disease. Nat Rev Nephrol 7 (12):697–705

Cyster JG (1999) Chemokines and cell migration in secondary lymphoid organs. Science 286(5447):2098–2102

Didona D et al (2019) Pemphigus: current and future therapeutic strategies. Front Immunol 10:1418

Fayyaz A, Kurien BT, Scofield RH (2016) Autoantibodies in Sjogren's Syndrome. Rheum Dis Clin North Am 42(3):419–434

Franks SE et al (2016) Targeting B cells in treatment of autoimmunity. Curr Opin Immunol 43:39–45

Fu W et al (2018) Deficiency in T follicular regulatory cells promotes autoimmunity. J Exp Med 215(3):815–825

Gong Q et al (2005) Importance of cellular microenvironment and circulatory dynamics in B cell immunotherapy. J Immunol 174(2):817–826

Groom J et al (2002) Association of BAFF/BLyS overexpression and altered B cell differentiation with Sjogren's syndrome. J Clin Invest 109(1):59–68

Gupta S, Gupta A (2017) Selective IgM deficiency—an underestimated primary immunodeficiency. Front Immunol 8:1056

Hagn M et al (2010) CD5+B cells from individuals with systemic lupus erythematosus express granzyme B. Eur J Immunol 40(7):2060–2069

Hasegawa M et al (2001) A CD19-dependent signaling pathway regulates autoimmunity in Lyn-deficient mice. J Immunol 167(5):2469–2478

Haury M et al (1997) The repertoire of serum IgM in normal mice is largely independent of external antigenic contact. Eur J Immunol 27(6):1557–1563

Higuchi T et al (2002) Cutting edge: Ectopic expression of CD40 ligand on B cells induces lupus-like autoimmune disease. J Immunol 168(1):9–12

Hokazono Y et al (2003) Inhibitory coreceptors activated by antigens but not by anti-Ig heavy chain antibodies install requirement of costimulation through CD40 for survival and proliferation of B cells. J Immunol 171(4):1835–1843
Humby F et al (2009) Ectopic lymphoid structures support ongoing production of class-switched autoantibodies in rheumatoid synovium. PLoS Med 6(1):e1
Isaacson PG, Norton AJ, Addis BJ (1987) The human thymus contains a novel population of B lymphocytes. Lancet 2(8574):1488–1491
Iwata Y et al (2011) Characterization of a rare IL-10-competent B-cell subset in humans that parallels mouse regulatory B10 cells. Blood 117(2):530–541
Jonsson R et al (2013) Autoantibodies present before symptom onset in primary Sjogren syndrome. JAMA 310(17):1854–1855
Kanevets U et al (2009) A role of IgM antibodies in monosodium urate crystal formation and associated adjuvanticity. J Immunol 182(4):1912–1918
Kansal R et al (2019) Sustained B cell depletion by CD19-targeted CAR T cells is a highly effective treatment for murine lupus. Sci Transl Med 11(482)
Katz SI, Parker D, Turk JL (1974) B-cell suppression of delayed hypersensitivity reactions. Nature 251(5475): 550–551
Kleindienst P et al (2000) Functional comparison of thymic B cells and dendritic cells in vivo. Blood 95(8):2610–2616
Lai Kwan Lam Q et al (2008) Local BAFF gene silencing suppresses Th17-cell generation and ameliorates autoimmune arthritis. Proc Natl Acad Sci USA 105(39): 14993–14998
Leadbetter EA et al (2002) Chromatin-IgG complexes activate B cells by dual engagement of IgM and Toll-like receptors. Nature 416(6881):603–607
Lee KM et al (2014) TGF-beta-producing regulatory B cells induce regulatory T cells and promote transplantation tolerance. Eur J Immunol 44(6):1728–1736
Lin X et al (2019) IL-10-producing regulatory B cells restrain the T follicular helper cell response in primary Sjogren's syndrome. Cell Mol Immunol
Lindner S et al (2013) Interleukin 21-induced granzyme B-expressing B cells infiltrate tumors and regulate T cells. Cancer Res 73(8):2468–2479
Marcus R et al (2017) Obinutuzumab for the first-line treatment of follicular lymphoma. N Engl J Med 377 (14):1331–1344
Mardiana S et al (2019) Supercharging adoptive T cell therapy to overcome solid tumor-induced immunosuppression. Sci Transl Med 11(495)
Mauri C, Menon M (2017) Human regulatory B cells in health and disease: therapeutic potential. J Clin Invest 127(3):772–779
McGaha TL, Sorrentino B, Ravetch JV (2005) Restoration of tolerance in lupus by targeted inhibitory receptor expression. Science 307(5709):590–593
Meyer S et al (2018) New insights in Type I and II CD20 antibody mechanisms-of-action with a panel of novel CD20 antibodies. Br J Haematol 180(6):808–820
Mizoguchi A, Bhan AK (2006) A case for regulatory B cells. J Immunol 176(2):705–710
Moritoki Y et al (2006) B cells and autoimmune liver diseases. Autoimmun Rev 5(7):449–457
Neubert K et al (2008) The proteasome inhibitor bortezomib depletes plasma cells and protects mice with lupus-like disease from nephritis. Nat Med 14(7):748–755
Ng LG et al (2004) B cell-activating factor belonging to the TNF family (BAFF)-R is the principal BAFF receptor facilitating BAFF costimulation of circulating T and B cells. J Immunol 173(2):807–817
Norman P (2016) Investigational Bruton's tyrosine kinase inhibitors for the treatment of rheumatoid arthritis. Expert Opin Investig Drugs 25(8):891–899
Nus M et al (2017) Marginal zone B cells control the response of follicular helper T cells to a high-cholesterol diet. Nat Med 23(5):601–610
Obiorah IE, Henao Velasquez A, Ozdemirli M (2018) The clinicopathologic spectrum of IgG4-related disease. Balkan Med J 35(4):292–300
Olalekan SA et al (2015) B cells expressing IFN-gamma suppress Treg-cell differentiation and promote autoimmune experimental arthritis. Eur J Immunol 45(4): 988–998
Pelka K et al (2016) Nucleic acid-sensing TLRs and autoimmunity: novel insights from structural and cell biology. Immunol Rev 269(1):60–75
Peng Y et al (2005) The role of IgM antibodies in the recognition and clearance of apoptotic cells. Mol Immunol 42(7):781–787
Perera J et al (2013) Autoreactive thymic B cells are efficient antigen-presenting cells of cognate self-antigens for T cell negative selection. Proc Natl Acad Sci USA 110(42):17011–17016
Pitzalis C et al (2014) Ectopic lymphoid-like structures in infection, cancer and autoimmunity. Nat Rev Immunol 14(7):447–462
Rauch PJ et al (2012) Innate response activator B cells protect against microbial sepsis. Science 335(6068): 597–601
Ray A et al (2012) A novel IL-10-independent regulatory role for B cells in suppressing autoimmunity by maintenance of regulatory T cells via GITR ligand. J Immunol 188(7):3188–3198
Reddy V et al (2017) Pragmatic treatment of patients with systemic lupus erythematosus with rituximab: long-term effects on serum immunoglobulins. Arthritis Care Res (Hoboken) 69(6):857–866
Rubin SJS, Bloom MS, Robinson WH (2019) B cell checkpoints in autoimmune rheumatic diseases. Nat Rev Rheumatol 15(5):303–315
Sato S et al (2000) Quantitative genetic variation in CD19 expression correlates with autoimmunity. J Immunol 165(11):6635–6643
Schrezenmeier E, Jayne D, Dorner T (2018) Targeting B cells and plasma cells in glomerular diseases: translational perspectives. J Am Soc Nephrol 29(3):741–758
Schuurman J et al (2001) The inter-heavy chain disulfide bonds of IgG4 are in equilibrium with intra-chain disulfide bonds. Mol Immunol 38(1):1–8

Seifert G, Donath K (1977) On the pathogenesis of the Kuttner tumor of the submandibular gland—analysis of 349 cases with chronic sialadenitis of the submandibular (author's transl). HNO 25(3):81–92

Shen P et al (2014) IL-35-producing B cells are critical regulators of immunity during autoimmune and infectious diseases. Nature 507(7492):366–370

Smith KG, Clatworthy MR (2010) FcgammaRIIB in autoimmunity and infection: evolutionary and therapeutic implications. Nat Rev Immunol 10(5):328–343

Steri M et al (2017) Overexpression of the Cytokine BAFF and autoimmunity risk. N Engl J Med 376(17):1615–1626

Tangye SG et al (2013) The good, the bad and the ugly—TFH cells in human health and disease. Nat Rev Immunol 13(6):412–426

Teng YK et al (2012) Induction of long-term B-cell depletion in refractory rheumatoid arthritis patients preferentially affects autoreactive more than protective humoral immunity. Arthritis Res Ther 14(2):R57

Theander E et al (2011) Lymphoid organisation in labial salivary gland biopsies is a possible predictor for the development of malignant lymphoma in primary Sjogren's syndrome. Ann Rheum Dis 70(8):1363–1368

Trampert DC et al (2018) On the role of IgG4 in inflammatory conditions: lessons for IgG4-related disease. Biochim Biophys Acta Mol Basis Dis 1864 (4 Pt B):1401–1409

Tsiantoulas D et al (2017) Increased plasma IgE accelerate atherosclerosis in secreted IgM deficiency. Circ Res 120(1):78–84

Vincent FB et al (2014) The BAFF/APRIL system in SLE pathogenesis. Nat Rev Rheumatol 10(6):365–373

Wang Y et al (1995) Anti-C5 monoclonal antibody therapy prevents collagen-induced arthritis and ameliorates established disease. Proc Natl Acad Sci USA 92(19):8955–8959

Wardemann H et al (2003) Predominant autoantibody production by early human B cell precursors. Science 301(5638):1374–1377

Ware CF (2005) Network communications: lymphotoxins, LIGHT, and TNF. Annu Rev Immunol 23:787–819

Yanaba K et al (2008) A regulatory B cell subset with a unique CD1dhiCD5+ phenotype controls T cell-dependent inflammatory responses. Immunity 28(5):639–650

Yang M et al (2013) Regulatory B cells in autoimmune diseases. Cell Mol Immunol 10(2):122–132

Yang M et al (2010) Novel function of B cell-activating factor in the induction of IL-10-producing regulatory B cells. J Immunol 184(7):3321–3325

Yoshizaki A et al (2012) Regulatory B cells control T-cell autoimmunity through IL-21-dependent cognate interactions. Nature 491(7423):264–268

B Cell Lymphoma

12

Xin Meng, Qing Min, and Ji-Yang Wang

Abstract

B cell development and activation are accompanied by dynamic genetic alterations including V(D)J rearrangements and immunoglobulin-gene somatic hypermutation and class-switch recombination. Abnormalities in these genetic events can cause chromosomal translocations and genomic mutations, leading to altered expression and function of genes involved in B cell survival or proliferation and consequently B lymphomagenesis. In fact, B cell lymphoma accounts for 95% of the lymphomas. In this chapter, we summarize the morphology, immunophenotypes, clinical features, genetic defects that cause the malignancies, treatments, and prognosis of the most prevalent types of B cell lymphomas, including typical precursor B cell malignance (B-ALL/LBL) and mature B cell lymphoma (Hodgkin lymphoma and B cell non-Hodgkin lymphoma).

X. Meng · Q. Min · J.-Y. Wang (✉)
Department of Immunology, School of Basic Medical Sciences, Fudan University, Shanghai, China
e-mail: wang@fudan.edu.cn

Keywords

B lymphoblastic leukemia/lymphoma · Hodgkin lymphoma · B cell non-Hodgkin lymphoma · Chromosomal translocation · Molecular target therapy

12.1 Introduction

Lymphomas represent a diverse group of neoplastic disorders of lymphocytes. Lymphoid neoplasms rank 4th in frequency (93,420 incident cases) among all cancers and are the 6th most common cause of cancer death (38,000 cases) in the United States in 2005. Around 20/100,000 people are diagnosed as lymphomas every year in other westernized countries (Fisher and Fisher 2004; Teras et al. 2016). Surprisingly, 95% of the lymphomas are of B cell origin in spite of the similar frequency of B and T cells in vivo.

The challenge of lymphoma classification is the difference between biologically rational classification and clinically useful classification. Biologically rational classification distinguishes diseases by morphology, immunophenotype, and genetic features, but clinically useful classification prefers to distinguish them by clinical features, natural history, prognosis, and treatment. The World Health Organization (WHO) classification of lymphoma neoplasms established guidelines for the diagnosis of malignant

J.-Y. Wang (ed.), *B Cells in Immunity and Tolerance*, Advances in Experimental Medicine and Biology 1254, https://doi.org/10.1007/978-981-15-3532-1_12

Table 12.1 Human B cell lymphomas

Lymphoma	Feature	Frequency (%)[a]	Proposed cellular origin	Risk and prognosis
B-ALL/LBL	B cell precursor acute lymphoblastic leukemia. B-lymphoblasts present positive expression in CD19, cytoplasmic CD79a, PAX-5, TdT, CD10, and cytoplasmic CD22; Two B-ALL categories: B-ALL with iAMP21 and *BCR-ABL1*-like ALL; TP53 and ATM pathways suppressed	<1	Memory B	Poor, B-ALL patients with iAMP21 are assigned into very high-risk group
Hodgkin lymphoma	Two types of malignant cells: HRS cells in cHL; LP cells in NLPHL	10.5	GCB	NLPHL is good; cHL is uniquely sensitive to PD-1 blockade
CLL/SLL	Indolent; Small mature lymphocytes in PB with CD5 expression; Lymphadenopathy in SLL; *TP53*-related mutations: most frequent del (13q14) and the strongest poor prognostic factor del (17p); Hyper-mutated *IGHV*, and lack of SOX11 expression	7	Memory B/Naïve B/Marginal-zone B?	Good
FL	Indolent; Nodal lymphoma with a follicular growth pattern; Lymphoma cells resemble GCB; t(14;18)(q32;q21) translocation	20	GCB	Good, but histologic transformation into an aggressive lymphoma may occur at a rate of 2–3% each year
MCL	Aggressive NHL; *BCL1-IgH* translocation; t(11:14) (q13; 32) leads to the overexpression of cyclin D1; Overexpression of SOX11 has been described as a diagnostic marker; A high Ki-67 proliferation index or *p53* mutations and p16 deletions are closely related to the more aggressive MCL subtypes	5	Naïve B	Poor
DLBCL	Large B cells arranged in a diffuse pattern; Germinal center B cell-like (GCB) and activated B cell-like (ABC) are two molecular subgroups; GCB subtype usually has the histone methyl transferase *EZH2* mutations, *BCL2* translocations and *GNA13* mutation; ABC subtype has mutations in genes associated with activation of the BCR/TLR and NF-kB pathways; t(14;18)(q21;q32)/ *IGH-BCL2*; Translocations involving *MYC*, *BCL2*, *BCL6*; More prevalent in elderly	30–40	GC or post-GC B cell	GCB DLBCL is associated with a better prognosis; ABC DLBCL is associated with a worse prognosis

(continued)

Table 12.1 (continued)

Lymphoma	Feature	Frequency (%)[a]	Proposed cellular origin	Risk and prognosis
Burkitt lymphoma	Mostly extranodal; *MYC-Ig* translocation; Endemic form is EBV$^+$; Three subtypes of BL: endemic BL, immunodeficiency-associated BL and sporadic BL; *MYC* gene activation; 14q32, κ light-chain gene (*2p11*) and the λ light-chain gene (*22q11*) breakpoint; Decreased expression of genes from NF-κB pathway and *MYC*-targeted genes highly expressed.	2	GCB	Fast growing, aggressive but highly curable in children and young adults
HGBL	Two new categories: (1) HGBL, with *MYC* and *BCL2* and/or *BCL6* translocations; (2) HGBL, not otherwise specified; *MYC/BCL6* double hit lymphoma	2–4	GCB	Very poor, aggressive clinical course with rapid progression and poor response to standard chemotherapy regimens

[a]These numbers refer to the frequencies among lymphoma in Europe and North America (Kuppers 2005). B-ALL/LBL, B-lymphoblastic leukemia/lymphoma; CLL/SLL, chronic lymphocytic leukemia/small lymphocytic lymphoma; FL, follicular lymphoma; MCL,mantle cell lymphoma; DLBCL, diffuse large B cell lymphoma; BL, Burkitt lymphoma; HGBL, high-grade B cell lymphoma; HRS cells, Hodgkin and Reed–Sternberg cells; LP, lymphocyte-predominant; cHL, classical Hodgkin lymphoma; NLPHL, nodular lymphocyte-predominant Hodgkin lymphoma; GCB, germinal center B cell; iAMP21, intrachromosomal amplification of chromosome 21; BCR-ABL1-like ALL, B-ALL with tanslocations involving tyrosine kinases or cytokine receptors

lymphomas and revised based on these major advances with significant clinical and biologic implications subsequently. Mature B cell neoplasms are divided into 42 types according to the WHO classification (2016), which is a refinement of Revised European–American Lymphoma classification (REAL) (Table 12.1). This review will emphasize on B cell lymphomas including Hodgkin lymphoma and B cell non-Hodgkin lymphoma with rare involvement of T and NK cell neoplasms or histiocytic- and dendritic-cell neoplasms. To date, over forty types of mature B cell neoplasms and Hodgkin lymphoma are distinguished in the WHO lymphoma classification in 2016 (Swerdlow et al. 2016).

12.2 B-acute Lymphoblastic Leukemia/Lymphoblastic Lymphoma (B-ALL/LBL)

B-acute lymphoblastic leukemia/lymphoblastic lymphoma (B-ALL/LBL) accounts for the majority of cases of ALL in both children and adults but only accounts approximately for 10% cases of LBL, in which T-LBL predominates (Dong et al. 2018). B-lymphoblasts express CD19, cytoplasmic CD79a, PAX-5, TdT, CD10, and cytoplasmic CD22, variable levels of CD20, CD34, and CD24, and a low/negative level of CD45 (Wenzinger et al. 2018). The WHO classification incorporated two important new entities with recurrent genetic abnormalities, "B-ALL with intrachromosomal amplification of chromosome 21" and "B-ALL with translocations involving tyrosine kinases or cytokine receptors" (Arber et al. 2016). In addition, association between low hypodiploid ALL and constitutional *TP53* mutations was highlighted in the classification of hypodiploid B-ALL (Muhlbacher et al. 2014).

Intrachromosomal amplification of chromosome 21 (iAMP21) is a distinct cytogenetic subgroup of B cell precursor acute lymphoblastic leukemia. Characteristically, B-ALL with iAMP21 is detected for the amplification of *RUNX1* gene located on chromosome 21 by fluorescence in situ hybridization (FISH). It is the only reliable detection method, with the existence of 5 or more *RUNX1* signals per cell through a probe for this gene (Heerema et al. 2013). This new entity is associated with an adverse prognosis and occurs in about 2% of children with ALL, especially older children with low white blood cell (WBC) counts, but is uncommon in adults. B-ALL patients with iAMP21 are assigned into very high-risk group and should be treated with more aggressive therapy due to poor prognosis in pediatric patient population (Harrison 2015; Moorman et al. 2007). In addition, B-ALL with iAMP21 is now considered as a distinct cytogenetic subgroup of B-ALL because cytogenetic change of iAMP21 has been confirmed to be a primary genetic event (Rand et al. 2011).

B-ALL with translocations involving tyrosine kinases or cytokine receptors (BCR-ABL1-like ALL, or Ph-like ALL) is a subgroup of B-ALL with poor prognosis and high risk for relapse (Boer et al. 2015; Moorman 2016). Originally, it was described as a subgroup of childhood B-ALL that lacks chromosomal rearrangement of *BCR-ABL1* but exhibits a similar gene expression profile (Den Boer et al. 2009). Latter studies show that BCR-ABL1-like ALL occurs in all age groups and is associated with event-free and overall survival (OS) rates equal or inferior to high-risk ALL subtypes, including BCR-ABL1 positive and *KMT2A/MLL*-rearranged B-ALL (Roberts et al. 2014, 2017). Many different genetic alterations are involved in BCR-ABL1-like ALL, for example, translocations involving tyrosine kinases, translocation involving cytokine receptor genes such as *CRLF2*, activating mutations or deletions of tyrosine kinase genes (*ABL1*, *JAK2*, etc.), and activating mutations or deletions of Ras signaling pathway genes (Roberts et al. 2014). More importantly, patients with BCR-ABL1-like ALL have improved clinical outcome with remarkable responses to tyrosine kinases inhibitor therapy, especially those with translocations involving tyrosine kinases (Weston et al. 2013).

12.3 Hodgkin Lymphoma

Hodgkin lymphoma (HL) is a rare B cell malignant neoplasm affecting approximately 9000 new patients annually in the United States. This disease represents approximately 11% of all lymphomas seen in the United States and comprises 2 discrete disease entities, classical Hodgkin lymphoma (cHL) and nodular lymphocyte-predominant Hodgkin lymphoma (NLPHL) (Ansell 2015). In cHL, the malignant cells are referred to as Hodgkin and Reed–Sternberg (HRS) cells, and in NLPHL, they are lymphocyte-predominant (LP) cells. Clinically, NLPHL has localized peripheral lymphadenopathy without associated B-symptoms or mediastinal involvement but 5–10% of cases have an increased risk for progression to diffuse large B cell lymphoma (DLBCL). In contrast, cHL of nodular sclerosis (NS) subtype usually has an involvement of a mediastinal mass, with or without cervical lymphadenopathy, and a tendency to spread in lymphatic drainage pathways. However, it is associated with various forms of B cell lymphoma at a lower rate (Song et al. 2011).

12.3.1 Classical Hodgkin Lymphoma

cHL is an unusual B cell-derived malignancy in which few tumor cells were surrounded by immune cells, fibroblasts, specialized mesenchymal stromal cells and endothelial cells (Fig. 12.1A). HRS tumor cells derived from mature B cells are the typical cells in HL. HRS cells have largely lost their B cell phenotypes and express many unusual markers of other hematopoietic cell lineages. This feature not only helps the differential diagnosis between cHL and NLPHL but also helps in distinguishing cHL from all other hematopoietic malignancies. Many signaling pathways are dysregulated in HRS cells. It is partly mediated by cellular interactions in the lymphoma microenvironment and partly by genetic lesions involving members of the nuclear factor-κB (NF-κB), JAK/STAT pathways and genes involved in the major histocompatibility complex (MHC) expression. However, there are less than 2% HRS cells in cHLs; the remainder includes macrophages, eosinophils, neutrophils, mast cells, and T cells (Mathas et al. 2016). Thus, the tumor microenvironment is important in cHL. cHL was further classified as nodular sclerosis cHL, lymphocyte-rich cHL, mixed cellularity cHL, lymphocyte-depleted cHL in 2016 WHO classification. Staging of this disease is essential for the choice of optimal therapy. In recent years, many new therapeutic agents that target molecular hallmarks of Hodgkin lymphoma have emerged, including the aberrant phenotype of the tumor cells, deregulated oncogenic pathways, and immune escape. Among them, immune checkpoint inhibitors targeting PD-1 or PD-L1 in this disease have achieved remarkable success (Borchmann and Engert 2017). The genetic basis for immune evasion in cHL could be near-uniform copy number alterations of chromosome 9p24.1 and the associated PD-1 ligand loci, CD274/PD-L1, and PDCD1LG2/PD-L2. HRS cells also express PD-1 ligands which induce PD-1 signaling and associated immune evasion, which is the genetic bases why cHL is uniquely sensitive to PD-1 blockade (Liu and Shipp 2017).

12.3.2 Nodular Lymphocyte-Predominant Hodgkin Lymphoma

NLPHL is a rare subtype of Hodgkin lymphoma with distinct pathological and clinical features compared with cHL. Histologically, NLPHL is defined with the presence of lymphocyte predominant (LP) cells (Fig. 12.1B), which express CD20 but lack CD15 and CD30 expression that are positive in HRS cells (Fig. 12.1C and D). These LP cells are found scattered amongst small B-lymphocytes arranged in a nodular pattern (Savage et al. 2016). The early-stage NLPHL has an excellent prognosis, with progression-free survival and overall survival rates exceeding 90% (Chen et al. 2010). However, some cases with frequent and often late or multiple relapses could be transformed into aggressive B cell non-Hodgkin lymphoma (NHL) despite more aggressive first-line treatment (Xing et al. 2014). The inherent risk of secondary aggressive NHL is highest in those with splenic involvement at presentation (Savage et al. 2016). Fortunately, salvage therapies, ranging from single-agent anti-CD20 antibody treatment to high-dose chemotherapy followed by autologous stem-cell transplantation are successfully responded in multiple relapse NLPHL cases (Schulz et al. 2008).

12.4 B Cell Non-Hodgkin Lymphomas

12.4.1 Monoclonal B Cell Lymphocytosis (MBL), Chronic Lymphocytic Leukemia (CLL), and Small Lymphocytic Lymphoma (SLL)

Monoclonal B cell lymphocytosis (MBL) is characterized by monoclonal B cell populations under 5×10^9/L in the peripheral blood (PB) in the absence of clinical signs or symptoms of a B cell lymphoproliferative disorder (2008 WHO classification). Monoclonal B cell could be

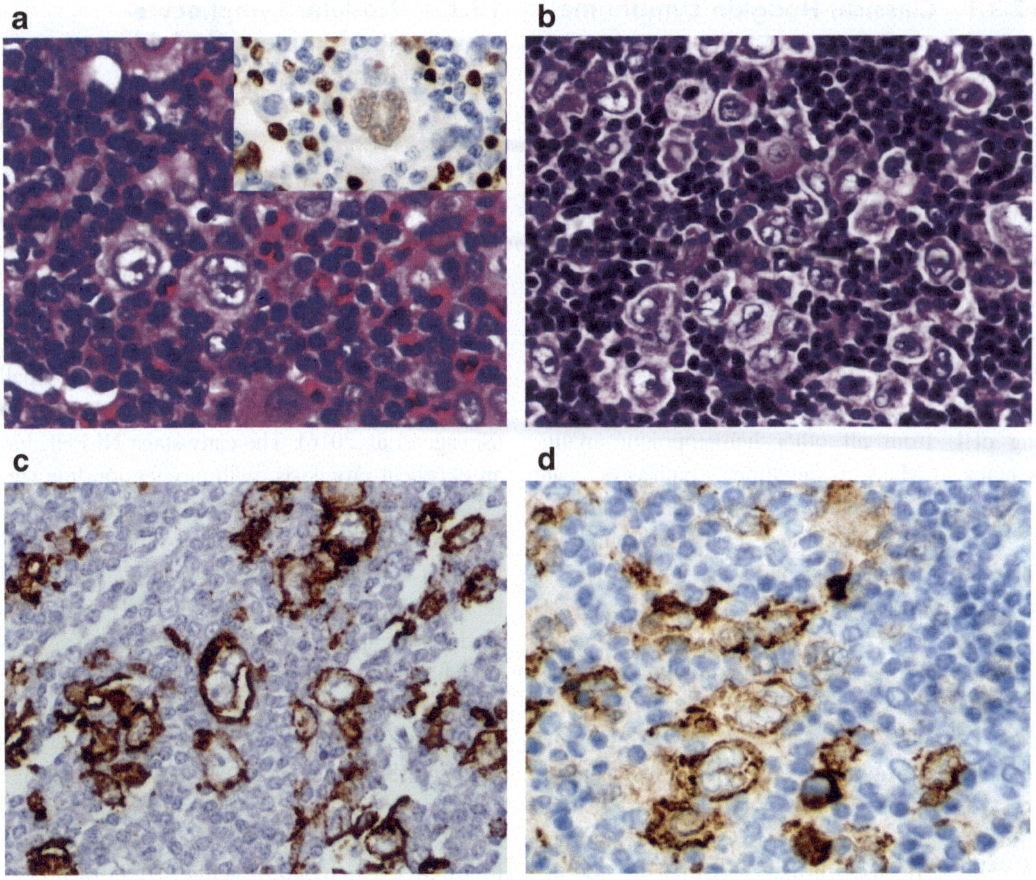

Fig. 12.1 Hodgkin lymphoma. (**A**) HRS cells are scattered against a mixed infiltrate (H&E, 40×). These cells were weakly positive for PAX5 (inset). (**B**) Characteristic LP cells with multilobulated and "popcorn" nuclei (H&E, 40×). (**C** and **D**) HRS cells are positive for CD30 and CD15, respectively (Immunoperoxidase stain, 40×). Adopted from Song et al. 2011

detected in 12% healthy individuals and is associated with a lymphocytosis that precedes virtually chronic lymphocytic leukemia (CLL)/ small lymphocytic lymphoma (SLL) in a prospective cohort study (Campo et al. 2011; Landgren et al. 2009; Nieto et al. 2009). Considering prognostic significance, low-count MBL should be distinguished from high-count MBL. Low-count MBL (a clonal CLL cell count <0.5 10^9/L) does not require routine follow-up outside of standard medical care since its extremely low chance of progression. In contrast, high-count MBL has very similar phenotypic and genetic/molecular features as Rai stage 0 CLL and progresses to CLL at a rate of 1–2% per year which means the requirement of routine/yearly follow-up (Morabito et al. 2013).

CLL and SLL are recognized as two faces of the same disease. Both of them are considered as indolent lymphocytic malignancies which mean more requirement of active surveillance rather than intervention (Tees and Flinn 2017). Diagnosis of CLL is dependent on blood counts, bone marrow (BM) smear, a blood smear, and immunophenotyping. WHO classification describes CLL as leukemic, lymphocytic lymphoma, being only distinguishable from SLL by its leukemic appearance. In SLL, lymphadenopathy may often be the first manifestation identified by the patients. Usually, SLL patients presenting only with lymphadenopathy are diagnosed by an excisional lymph node biopsy. Despite the slight differences in presentation, CLL and SLL remain united as one disease entity in the 2016 revision of WHO classification.

CLL is a clonal lymphoproliferative disorder characterized by >5 × 10^9/L peripheral B-lymphocytes for the duration of at least 3 months. CLL is the most common type of leukemia in western countries. The median age at diagnosis lies between 67 and 72 years and more male than female patients (1.7:1) are affected (Molica 2006). CLL/SLL cells express CD5, CD19 and CD23, and low levels of surface immunoglobulin (Ig), CD20 and CD79b as revealed by flow cytometry (Ginaldi et al. 1998; Moreau et al. 1997). Characteristically, the CLL cells found in the blood smear are small, mature lymphocytes with a narrow border of cytoplasm, and a dense nucleus lacking discernible nucleoli and having partially aggregated chromatin. These cells may comprise up to 55% of the blood lymphocytes admixed with larger or atypical cells, cleaved cells, or prolymphocytes (Melo et al. 1986). In proliferation centers, the survival and growth of CLL cells require a permissive microenvironment comprising T cells, macrophages, and stromal cells. FISH analysis has revealed that almost 80% of CLL cases carry chromosomal abnormalities including the most frequent del (13q14) and the strongest poor prognostic factor del (17p), both related to *TP53* mutations. A large cohort genomic landscape study indicates that CLL may be initiated by the loss or addition of large chromosomal material (e.g. deletion 13q, deletion 11q, and trisomy 12) and the subsequent additional mutations may render the leukemia more aggressive (Landau et al. 2015).

Prognostication in CLL has witnessed the development from the addition of mutational status of variable region of Ig heavy chain (*IGHV*) and chromosomal analyses using FISH in late 90s to the stereotype of BCR (B cell receptor) and specific mutations (such as *NOTCH1*, *TP53*, *SF3B1*, *XPO-1*, *BIRC3*, *ATM*, and *RPS15*) based on whole exome sequencing (WES) (Rai and Jain 2016). In therapy, the field of CLL has gone through several stages. In the beginning, oral chlorambucil and steroids are prior choices in 1980s and chemo-immunotherapy (CIT) with fludarabine, cyclophosphamide, and rituximab (FCR) followed. Later the patients were orally administered with targeted therapeutic agents inhibiting kinases in the BCR signaling pathway such as Ibrutinib (BTK inhibitor) and Idelalisib (p110 PI3Kδ inhibitor) and novel anti-CD20 monoclonal antibodies (mAbs) such as obinutuzumab, which is continued with other targeted therapeutics such as BCL2 antagonists (Venetoclax or ABT-199). Finally, chimeric antigen receptor T cells (CAR-T) is in the process of being developed (Rai and Jain 2016).

Rai and Binet staging systems are two widely accepted clinical staging systems containing the risk, stratification, staging, and indication for treatment. The Rai classification was later modified to reduce the number of prognostic groups from 5 to 3 (Rai et al. 1975). The modified Rai staging system defines low-risk, intermediate-risk, and high-risk disease according to lymphocytosis, enlarged nodes in any site, splenomegaly, hepatomegaly, disease-related anemia or thrombocytopenia, lymphocytosis with leukemia cells in the blood and/or BM (lymphoid cells >30%). The Binet staging system is based on the number of involved areas with enlarged lymph nodes of >1 cm in diameter or organomegaly, and on whether there is anemia or thrombocytopenia. Recently, a potentially most relevant prognostic score has been developed by an international consortium of study groups based on a meta-analysis of individual patient data and is called the CLL International Prognostic Index (CLL-IPI) (2016).

12.4.2 Follicular Lymphoma (FL)

Follicular Lymphoma (FL) is a heterogeneous disease arising from malignant transformation of normal germinal center B cells (GCB). It is the second most common type of non-Hodgkin lymphoma. While it belongs to indolent lymphomas, histologic transformation into an aggressive lymphoma may occur at a rate of 2–3% each year, leading to rapid progression, treatment resistance, and poor prognosis (Fischer et al. 2018). Approximately 85% of cases harbor the t(14;18)(q32;q21) translocation, resulting in an inability to down-regulate expression of anti-apoptotic protein B cell lymphoma 2 (BCL2), which is absent in normal GCB (Fig. 12.2) (Roulland et al. 2011). The microenvironment of FL is composed of a mixture of neoplastic centrocytes and centroblasts along with various non-neoplastic cells mirroring the formation of secondary lymphoid follicles,including T cells, follicular dendritic cells, and macrophages that have relevance in the prognosis of FL patients (Sugimoto and Watanabe 2016). Meanwhile, mutations in key genes, such as *EZH2, ARID1A, MEF2B, EP300, FOXO1, CREBBP,* and *CARD11*, are also the important prediction factor of the prognosis.

FL can be divided into many different subgroups based on the age of onset, affected organ, and genetic abnormality. There are three variants included in the 2016 WHO classification, namely pediatric follicular lymphoma, duodenal-type follicular lymphoma, and in situ follicular lymphoma (Swerdlow et al. 2016). Pediatric FL is now known as a rare nodal disease. Although predominantly occurring in children, they can manifest in the adult population as well. It is characterized by large expansile highly proliferative follicles in the nodals filled with prominent blastoid follicular center cells rather than classic centroblasts (or centrocytes) (Liu et al. 2013). In situ follicular neoplasia (ISFN) is known as a precursor lesion of FL with low risk of progression to manifest FL but is often associated with prior or synchronous overt lymphomas. Immunohistochemically, ISFN have accumulations of strongly $BCL2^{+}$, $CD10^{+}$, $t(14;18)^{+}$ clonal B cells in reactive lymph nodes. These clonal B cells are confined only to GC and the BCL2 staining in the abnormal follicles is notable for its high-level and uniform intensity (Carbone et al. 2012).

12.4.3 Mantle Cell Lymphoma (MCL)

Mantle cell lymphoma (MCL) is an aggressive NHL with a particularly poor clinical outcome.

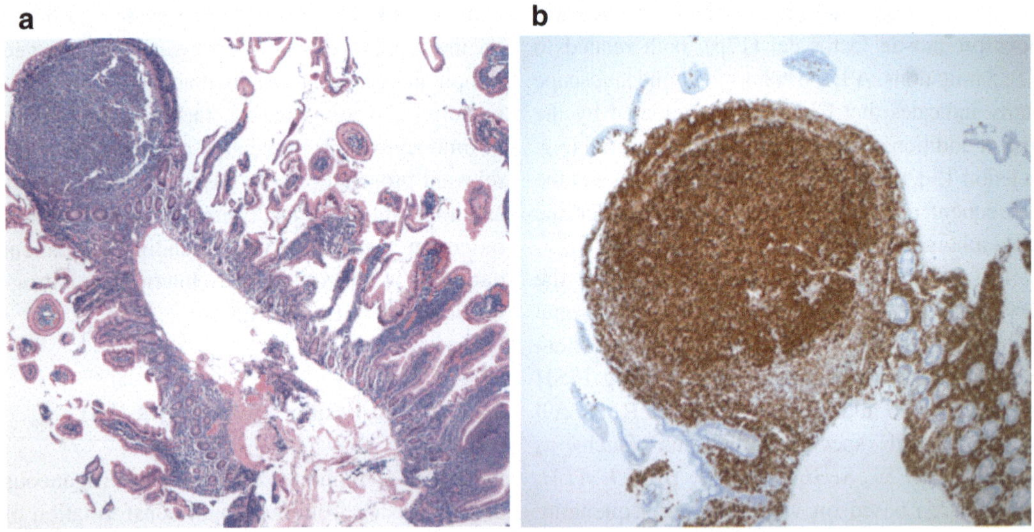

Fig. 12.2 Follicular lymphoma in the duodenum. (**A**) Follicular lymphoma (H&E, 40×). (**B**) Follicular lymphoma stained with antibody to BCL2 (Immunoperoxidase stain,100×). Adopted from Graham et al. 2015

Patients generally have stage III/IV disease and present with lymph nodes, spleen, blood, and BM involvement with a short-remission duration to standard therapies and a median overall survival (OS) of 4–5 years. The median age of MCL patients is 60 and more males are influenced than females (2:1). MCL cells, developed from naive B cell lineage, are identified with $CD3^+$, $CD20^+$, $CD5^+$, and Cyclin $D1^+$ while $CD10^-$ and BCL6 (Fig. 12.3). The chromosomal translocation t (11:14) (q13; 32) is the molecular hallmark of MCL (Bertoni et al. 2006). This translocation leads to the overexpression of cyclin D1 which is not typically expressed in normal lymphocytes and can be detected in 98% of MCL cases immunohistochemically (Rosenwald et al. 2003). Overexpression of SOX11 has been described as a diagnostic marker for MCL and the absence of SOX11 or a low Ki-67 may correlate with indolent MCL (Fernandez et al. 2010). A high Ki-67 proliferation index or *p53* mutations and p16 deletions are closely related to the more aggressive MCL subtypes (Bernard et al. 2001). As an aggressive NHL, the prognosis of patients with MCL is generally poor. Conventional chemotherapy response is temporary and relapses at last. A rituximab-containing chemotherapy regimen as a primary treatment option is administered for patients with untreated MCL according to their eligibility for high-dose chemotherapy followed by autologous stem-cell transplantation (ASCT) (Izutsu 2017). Recently, ibrutinib, an inhibitor of Bruton tyrosine kinase, has been approved for relapsed/refractory MCL. Recent advances in the management of MCL will improve the prognosis of patients with MCL.

Two types of clinically indolent variants are now recognized, which developed along two very different pathways (Jares et al. 2012). In classical MCL, *IGHV* is unmutated or minimally mutated and SOX11 is usually expressed in B cells, and lymph nodes together with other extranodal sites are typically involved. When additional molecular/cytogenetic abnormalities were acquired, MCL can lead to even more aggressive variants. Meanwhile, other MCL developed from B cells with mutated *IGHV* and negative for SOX11 expression leads to leukemic nonnodal MCL that involves the PB, BM and spleen. They are frequently clinically indolent, but when secondary abnormalities occur, usually *TP53* and other oncogenic abnormalities, may lead to very aggressive disease. In situ mantle cell neoplasia (ISMCN) characterized by the presence of cyclin $D1^+$ cells in the inner mantle zones of follicles is more conservative with a low rate of progression (Carvajal-Cuenca et al. 2012). ISMCN should be distinguished from overt MCL with a mantle zone growth pattern because it may also be relatively indolent as well as other classical MCL with a low proliferative fraction.

Heterogeneous MCL evolution course may be related to the different biological characteristics of conventional MCL and the distinct subgroup of leukemic nonnodal MCL (nnMCL). Recently, a novel molecular assay to distinguish cMCL and nnMCL was described in a cohort study. They found that conventional MCL and nnMCL differed in nodal presentation, lactate dehydrogenase, Ig heavy chain gene mutational status, management options, genomic complexity, and *CDKN2A/ATM* deletions (Clot and Jares 2018).

12.4.4 Diffuse Large B Cell Lymphoma (DLBCL)

DLBCL is the most common type of non-Hodgkin lymphoma worldwide, counting for approximately 30–40% of all cases around the world. DLBCL is defined as a neoplasm of large B cells arranged in a diffuse pattern in WHO classification. The large size means that the lymphoma cells are larger than the nuclei of benign histiocytes in the same tissue section.

DLBCL is subdivided into groups with the advance and application of gene expression profiling (GEP). GCB cell-like and activated B cell-like (ABC) are two molecular subgroups of DLBCL based on their cell-of-origin determinded by GEP, but 10–15% of the cases are unclassifiable. The GCB and ABC subgroups differed in many aspects, such as chromosomal alterations, activation of BCR signaling pathways, and clinical

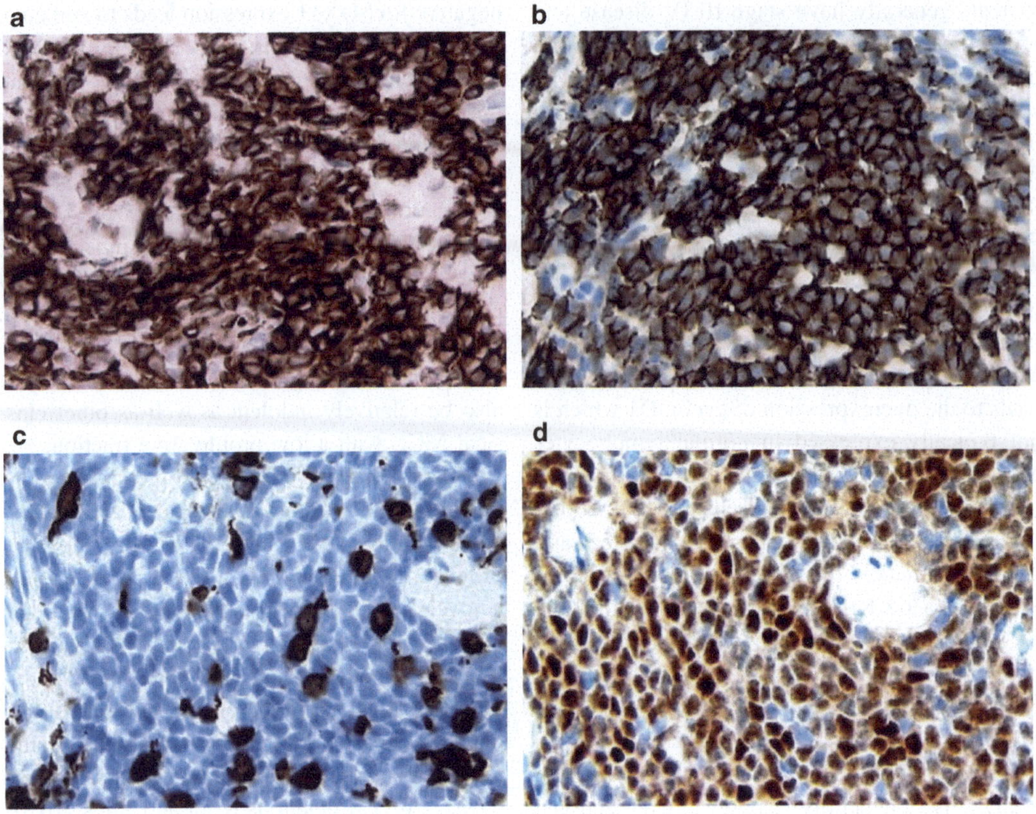

Fig. 12.3 Mantle cell lymphoma. Positive for CD5 (**A**), CD20 (**B**), CD3 (**C**) and cyclin D1 (**D**) (Immunoperoxidase stain, 40x). Adopted from Rajput et al. 2014

outcome (Havranek et al. 2017). GCB neoplasms proved to have a better survival rate than ABC tumors in patients treated with standard therapy (Rosenwald et al. 2002). GCB subtype usually has the histone methyl transferase *ZEH2* mutation, *BCL2* translocations such as t(14;18)(q32;q21)/*IGH-BCL2* and mutations in the cell motility regulator *GNA13*, but ABC subtype have mutations in *MYD88*, *CD79A*, *CARD11*, and *TNFAIP3* genes, which is associated with activation of the BCR/TLR and NF-kB pathways (Pasqualucci and Dalla-Favera 2015).

There are three major translocations that occur in DLBCL. *BCL6* is the most common one and occurs in about 30% of the cases. It is often juxtaposed with *IGH* and many potential partner loci t(14;18)(q21;q32)/IGH-BCL2 is observed in 20–30% of DLBCL cases (Kramer et al. 1998). Translocations involving *MYC*, juxtaposed with *IGH, IGK, IGL* or non-Ig-gene loci, occur in 10–15% of DLBCL cases and the rearrangement of MYC is associated with high-grade morphological features, a complex karyotype and poor prognosis (Barrans et al. 2010). Recent next generation sequencing studies have identified common somatic mutations in all subgroups of DLBCL. They are inactivating mutations of *TP53* and genes involved in immunosurveillance (*B2M, CD58*), alterations in epigenetic regulators (*CREBBP/EP300, KMT2D/C, MEF2B*), and oncogenic activation of *BCL6*. It is believed that these mutations will become important in guiding future targeted therapies although the clinical implications are not fully understood (Intlekofer and Younes 2014; Roschewski et al. 2014).

DLBCL is more prevalent in elderly patients with a median age in the 7th decade, although it and also occurs in young adults but rarely in children. Clinically, most patients present with a rapidly growing tumor mass involving one or more lymph nodes and extranodal sites (Martelli et al. 2013). In 1994, the international prognostic index (IPI) containing five variables was developed to stratify risk for patients with DLBCL, including age, Eastern Cooperative Oncology Group performance status, serum LDH level, number of extranodal sites, and stage. The IPI has been popular for many years but it still has some limitations. For example, it over-simplifies the spectrum of some patient abnormalities as categorical variables. Later the National Cancer Center Network (NCCN) proposed an enhanced IPI system that is more proper to be used in DLBCL patients receiving chemo-immunotherapy. In this enhanced IPI, age and serum LDH level were further stratified and specific extranodal sites prognostic importance was emphasized (Zhou et al. 2014). Besides, CD5 expression and co-expression of MYC/BCL2 or MYC/BCL2/BCL6 appear to have prognostic value and should be assessed by immunohistochemistry (Fig. 12.4) (Ting et al. 2019).

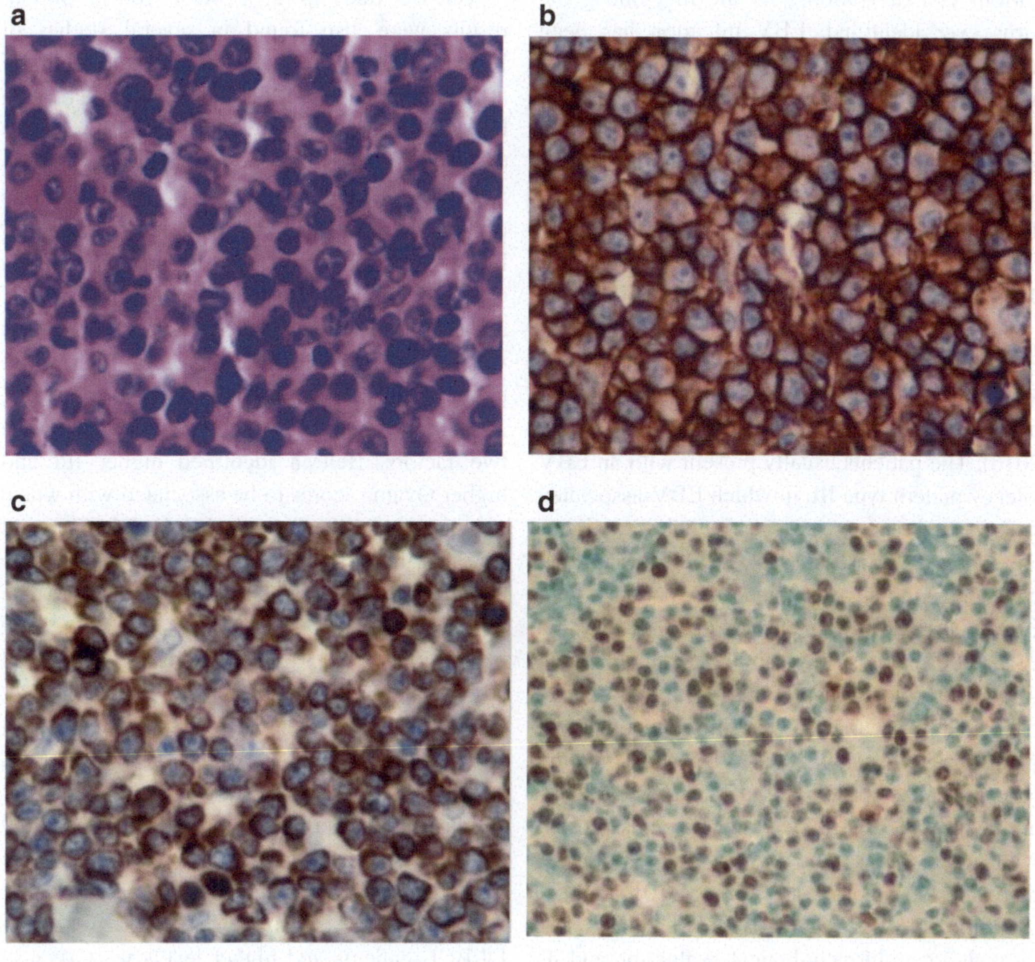

Fig. 12.4 Diffuse large B cell lymphoma (DLBCL). (**A**) DLBCL tissue microarray (H&E 400×). (**B**) CD20 expression in a tissue core of DLBCL(400×). (**C**) BCL2 expression in a tissue core of DLBCL (Immunoperoxidase stain 400×). (**D**) BCL6 expression in a tissue core of DLBCL (Immunoperoxidase stain 200×). Adopted from Tzankov et al. 2003

12.4.5 EBV$^+$ Diffuse Large B Cell Lymphomas and EBV$^+$ Mucocutaneous Ulcer

The Epstein–Barr virus is a ubiquitous organism, achieving asymptomatic lifelong carrier status in a large proportion of the world's population. The pathophysiology of this latent infection is due to the interaction of EBV with the memory B cells of a healthy, immunocompetent individual. Disruptions in the balance of this interaction are believed to result in the lymphoproliferation of various cell derivations. As the first oncogenic virus ever identified, EBV infection has been associated with a number of malignancies, such as nasopharyngeal carcinoma and Burkitt lymphoma. EBV infection has been related to immunosuppression and chronic antigenic of the neoplastic process (Rowe et al. 2014; Tsao and Tsang 2017).

12.4.5.1 EBV$^+$ Diffuse Large B Cell Lymphomas

Epstein–Barr virus-positive (EBV$^+$) DLBCL is an entity included in the 2016 WHO classification of lymphoid neoplasms (Swerdlow et al. 2016). The patients usually present with an EBV latency pattern type III, in which EBV-associated latent membrane proteins and nuclear antigens are expressed (Castillo et al. 2011). Oyama and colleagues initially described 22 patients with EBV$^+$ DLBCL in the elderly in 2003 (Oyama et al. 2003). Later this tumor is defined as an EBV$^+$ monoclonal large B cell lymphoproliferative disorder arising in immunocompetent patients >50 years in 2008 WHO classification (Campo et al. 2011). This age cutoff is clearly arbitrary. EBV$^+$ DLBCL young patients present with nodal disease and have a good prognosis than elderly (Nicolae and Pittaluga 2015).

Clinically, EBV$^+$ DLBCL is diagnosed through a careful pathological evaluation and its differential diagnosis includes infectious mononucleosis (specifically in younger patients), lymphomatoid granulomatosis, HL, and gray zone lymphoma, among others. Standard for diagnosis is the detection of EBV-encoded RNA (EBER) but there is no defined clear cutoff for positivity (Castillo et al. 2016). Several groups have shown that patients with EBV$^+$ DLBCL have worse prognosis when compared with patients with EBV$^-$ DLBCL. A Japanese study compared the outcomes between 96 patients with EBV$^+$ and 107 with EBV$^-$ DLBCL (Oyama et al. 2007). Approximately 60% of the EBV$^+$ patients achieved CR (complete response) after chemotherapy, in contrast with 90% in EBV$^-$ patients. EBV$^+$ DLBCL patients had worse survival than EBV$^-$ DLBCL patients with estimated 5-year OS rates of 25% versus 65%. Similar results were also found in several studies of Korean (Park et al. 2007) and Peruvian (Morales et al. 2010) patients. IPI and the Oyama score can be used for risk-stratification. The IPI score is one of the most commonly used risk-stratification tools in DLBCL but appears to be of limited prognostic value in patients with EBV$^+$ DLBCL, as shown in an early report (Oyama et al. 2007). A prognostic index that consisted of age (>70 years old) and B cell-related symptoms was designed. In this index, median OS times in patients showed 56 months with zero factor, 25 months with one factor, and 9 months with two factors. Beltran identified higher IPI and higher Oyama scores to be associated with worse outcome in patients with EBV$^+$ DLBCL and revealed that lymphopenia (absolute lymphocyte count of $<1.0 \times 10^9$/L) is a notable adverse prognostic factor (Beltran et al. 2011). The expression of CD30 is emerging as a potential adverse and targetable prognostic factor. EBER$^+$/CD30$^+$ DLBCL patients had worse outcome than EBER$^+$/CD30$^-$ or EBER$^-$/CD30$^+$ DLBCL patients (Ok et al. 2014). Survivin can affect cellular apoptosis through inhibition of caspase 9 and high serum survivin levels were associated with poor outcomes (Ambrosini et al. 1997). Serum levels of survivin were high in 12% of DLBCL patients and higher levels were seen in EBV$^+$ than in EBV$^-$ cases (Hong et al. 2017). High expression of survivin in DLBCL treated with R-CHOP was related to poor prognosis, especially in the ABC subtype (Liu et al. 2015).

12.4.5.2 EBV$^+$ Mucocutaneous Ulcer

EBV positive B cell lymphoproliferative disorders (LPDs) are a spectrum of diseases that range from self-limiting, localized conditions to aggressive lymphomas (Dojcinov et al. 2018). EBV$^+$ mucocutaneous ulcer (EBVMCU) is an indolent condition on this spectrum of LPDs, which localizes to the skin and mucosal surfaces (Satou et al. 2019). It is a rare lymphoproliferation that gained recognition as a new entity in the 2016 revisions to the World Health Organization classifications. EBVMCU typically presents with isolated, sharply well-circumscribed ulcerations on the oropharyngeal mucosa (52%), on the skin (29%), or in the gastrointestinal tract (19%). Other symptoms shown in patients include weight loss, odynophagia, and abdominal emergencies but lack of systemic symptoms, lymphadenopathy, organomegaly, or BM involvement (Roberts et al. 2015). Diagnostic challenges of EBVMCU included distinguishing it from DLBCL, post-transplant lymphoproliferative disorder, or cHL. Its clinical course is typically fluctuant with worsening of lesion-associated tissue damage when maintaining or increasing iatrogenic immunosuppression (Dojcinov et al. 2018).

Many commonly used immunosuppressive drugs have correlations with the development of EBVMCU, including methotrexate, cyclosporin A, azathioprine, tacrolimus, TNF inhibitors, mycophenolate, and topical steroid treatment (Dojcinov et al. 2018). Reports also suggest that immunosenescence is a significant predisposing factor for patients who are also on immunomodulating drugs (Roberts et al. 2015). The pathogenesis of EBVMCU in immunosuppressed patients is thought to correlate with a diminished T cell repertoire. This suppression leads to a reduced ability to target all EBV-associated antigens and results in a proliferation of restricted clones of EBV-specific T cells when infected with EBV. These cytotoxic T cells can manage the EBV-induced B cell proliferation and keep the virus in the dormant state in the immunocompetent individual. Once exposure to a site-restricted immune-modulating factor, a localized EBV-driven lymphoproliferation will occur, since the immune system of EBVMCU patients is only able to keep the virus in a dormant state systemically (Gali et al. 2018; Natkunam et al. 2017).

Biopsies of EBVMCU surface ulceration found an infiltrate of atypical lymphoid cells appeared as DLBCL, cHL, or as atypical immunoblasts. Often there is a rim of reactive T cells around the EBV$^+$ B cell areas. The lesional B cell expresses B cell markers PAX5, CC79a, OCT2, and BOB1. CD20 was down-regulated in a proportion of cases reported and CD30, CD15, and MUM1 are similar to the phenotype of classic Hodgkin lymphoma. In contrast to cHL where only large cells are EBV$^+$, EBER in situ hybridization is positive in many cells with a variety of cell sizes (Roberts et al. 2015; Willemze et al. 2019). Most EBVMCU cases have a benign course and respond well to conservative management. Complete remission received either spontaneously, or in response to reduction of their immunosuppressive therapies. Reports exist of CD20 or CD30 directed antibody therapy, local radiation, surgical excision, chemotherapy or a combination of these treatments with excellent response. However, there are reports of more persistent and debilitating cases that required more aggressive treatment (Magalhaes et al. 2015).

12.4.6 Burkitt Lymphoma

Burkitt's lymphoma (BL) is a rare, aggressive B cell lymphoma that is highly curable in children and young adults. BL was thought to be a sarcoma of the jaw when first described by Denis Burkitt in African children in 1958 (O'Conor and Davies 1960). Then pathologist George O'Connor described it as a lymphoma and it was recognized to be associated with EBV several years later (Epstein et al. 1964). There are three subtypes of BL, endemic BL, immunodeficiency-associated BL and sporadic BL. Nearly 30–50% of childhood cancers in equatorial Africa and most cases of NHL are endemic BL, affecting 3–6 cases/100,000 children (Orem et al. 2007).

EBV infection, as a risk factor, is found in nearly 100% of patients with endemic BL and it is also linked geographically with *Plasmodium falciparum* infection (de-The et al. 1978; Geser et al. 1989). *P. falciparum* may cause the deregulated expression of activation-induced cytidine deaminase (AID) which can promote *C-MYC* translocation in EBV latent infecting cells, thereby facilitating endemic BL oncogenesis (Torgbor et al. 2014). The immunodeficiency-associated form of BL is found in patients infected with human immunodeficiency virus (HIV) but is rarely seen with other immunodeficient states, and its frequency has no correlation with CD4 count and is often EBV negative. Besides, antiretroviral therapy has not changed its incidence (Kalter et al. 1985). Sporadic BL is uncommon, accounting for 1–2% of NHL diagnoses in adults and between 30 and 40% of NHL in children (Morton et al. 2006) and exhibits a bimodal age distribution with two incidence peaks at approximately 10 and 75 years of age (Mbulaiteye et al. 2010).

MYC gene activation is the hallmark of Burkitt lymphoma. *MYC* is activated at 8q24 where it is overexpressed constitutively under the control of transcriptional enhancers through one of three possible translocations in the Ig heavy- or light-chain locus. The translocations present in BL involving *MYC* can be detected by FISH and are helpful to confirm the diagnosis. The 14q32 breakpoint occurring in 80% of the cases is at the class-switch region. Other breakpoints include the κ light-chain gene (2p11) and the λ light-chain gene (22q11) but there are no translocations involving *BCL2* or *BCL6* since it origins from GC (Casulo and Friedberg 2015). Decreased expression of genes from NF-κB pathway and highly expressed target genes of *MYC*, as well as markers of GCB were revealed through gene expression profiling studies (Dave et al. 2006). BL can be distinguished from DLBCL and other high-grade NHL by low karyotypic complexity and the lack of non-Ig partners (Hummel et al. 2006). In addition to mutations in *MYC*, as many as 70 additional gene mutations have been found in BL, and some may contribute to its pathogenesis, such as mutations in *TCF3, ID3,* and *CCND3* (Love et al. 2012). They are involved in BL survival and differentiation or G1 to S-phase transition in the cell cycle (Richter et al. 2012; Schmitz et al. 2012). BL is composed of intermediate-sized cells with round nuclei, multiple nucleoli pathologically (Fig. 12.5A). Its high proliferation can cause spontaneous apoptosis characterized with "starry sky" pattern observed in marrow and lymph nodes. Immunophenotypically, BL tumor cells origin from GCB and express CD10, BCL6, CD20, CD79a, and CD45 except for CD5, CD23 and BCL2 (Fig. 12.5B–F) (Dunleavy 2018; Nakamura et al. 2002).

Clinically, BL is very chemosensitive even though belonging to highly aggressive lymphoma. Excellent results such as long-term remission rates and long-term survival were achieved in several intensive multiagent chemotherapeutic programs especially in children and younger adults (Magrath et al. 1996; Rizzieri et al. 2004; Soussain et al. 1995). Specific chemotherapy regimens have been developed to treat BL, the first of these was the CODOX-M-IVAC regimen, conceived by Magrath and colleagues (Magrath et al. 1996). In later iterations of the regimen, confirmatory studies and modification to the Magrath regimen were conducted for older adults (Mead et al. 2002, 2008). The addition of the anti-CD20 monoclonal antibody rituximab in Magrath regimen demonstrated superior outcomes compared with historical controls in several researches (Barnes et al. 2011; Corazzelli et al. 2012; Evens et al. 2013). Based upon these findings and extrapolating from histologies of other lymphoma studies, rituximab should be incorporated in the treatment algorithms of BL routinely. In addition, a multiagent lower-intensity chemotherapy program had excellent results as published by the National Cancer Institute (Dunleavy et al. 2013). A phase 2 multiinstitution trial of an intensive but short-duration regimen was designed by the Cancer and Leukemia Group B (CALGB) (Rizzieri et al. 2014).

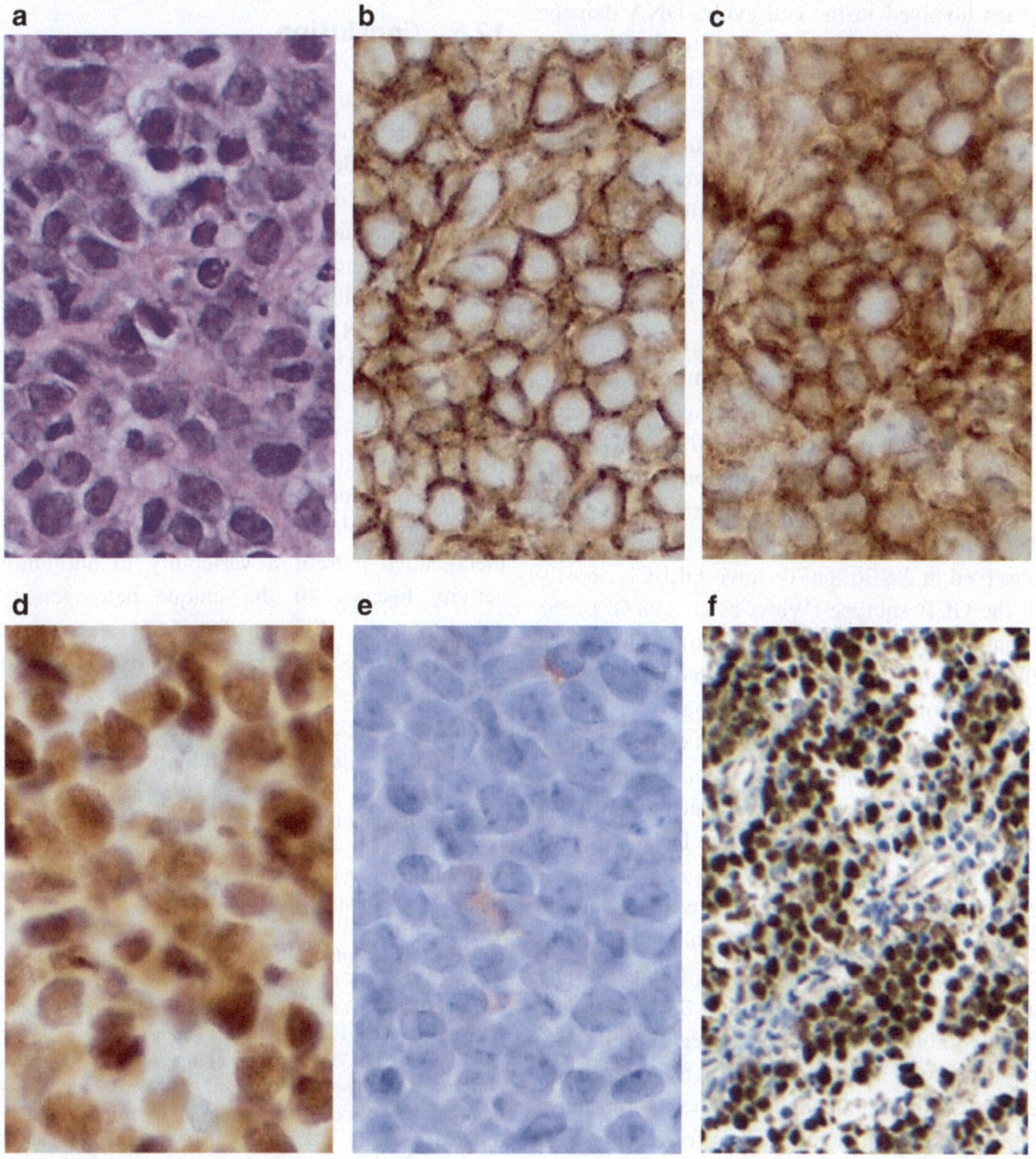

Fig. 12.5 Burkitt lymphoma. (**A**) Burkitt lymphoma is composed of intermediate-sized cells with round nuclei, multiple nucleoli pathologically (H&E 40×). Immunohistochemistry shows strong homogenous staining for CD20 (**B**) (40×), CD10 (**C**) (40×), BCL6 (**D**) (40×), and MYC (**F**) (20×). Tumor cells are negative for BCL2 (**E**) (40×). Adopted from Vishnu et al. 2015

12.4.7 High-Grade B Cell Lymphomas

In 2016 WHO classification, the B cell lymphoma, unclassifiable, with features intermediate between DLBCL and Burkitt lymphoma (BCLU) category that included in the 2008 WHO classification is eliminated and replaced by two new categories: (1) High-grade B cell lymphoma, with *MYC* and *BCL2* and/or *BCL6* translocations; (2) High-grade B cell lymphoma, not otherwise specified.

MYC gene located on chromosome 8 (8q24) encodes c-MYC oncogenic protein which is a transcription factor regulating the expression of genes involved in the cell cycle, DNA damage repair, metabolism, protein synthesis, and response to stress (Dang et al. 2006). In humans, mutations involving regulatory or promoter regions, chromosomal translocation, and copy number increase activate MYC (Meyer and Penn 2008). Physiologically, MYC induces apoptosis of normal cells through activating the TP53 pathway. However, tumor cells with *MYC* translocations accompanied by *TP53* inactivating mutations allow them to escape apoptosis. *BCL2* and/or *BCL6* translocations presenting in DLBCL with *MYC* translocations confers aggressive clinical behavior. Approximately 10% of DLBCL harbors *MYC* translocation, predominantly in the subset of GCB subtype (Rosenthal and Younes 2017). Similarly, *BCL2* translocations are observed in 20–30% of de novo DLBCL, mostly in the GCB subtype (Weiss et al. 1987). In the event of a t(14; 18), the anti-apoptotic function of BCL2 is constitutively dysregulated due to *BCL2* transcription, thereby providing a survival advantage in affected B cells. As a transcription repressor, BCL6 is expressed in mature GCB cells. When overexpressed, it can prevent p53-mediated apoptosis in response to DNA damage.

Double hit lymphoma (DHL) is a type of B cell NHL characterized by rearrangements in both *MYC* and *BCL2* genes. While DHL overexpresses both MYC and BCL2 proteins, it only accounts for a small subset of the cases with double protein expression. Other B cell lymphomas, such as a fraction of ABC, also overexpress both proteins although they do not have dual gene rearrangements. Therefore, analysis of chromosomal translocations using FISH or immunohistochemistry is needed to confirm the diagnosis of DHL. A fraction of DLBCL have rearrangements in both *MYC* and *BCL2* genes and are thus categorized as DHL. The incidence of double protein expressing DLBCL is estimated to be 19–34%, and is associated with worse prognosis compared to patients with c-Myc protein alone or no proteins expression (Rosenthal and Younes 2017). Clinically, double protein expressing lymphoma has an outcomes intermediate between DLBCL NOS and DHL when treated with RCHOP (Green et al. 2012).

12.5 Conclusion

Studies thus far have uncovered many genetic defects that cause different types of B cell lymphomas. In addition to standard regiment of chemotherapy, recently immune checkpoint PD-1 blockade achieved marvelous success in cHL (Borchmann and Engert 2017). Molecular target therapy using Ibrutinib (BTK inhibitor), Idelalisib (p110 PI3Kδ inhibitor), obinutuzumab (novel anti-CD20 mAb), and BCL2 antagonists (Venetoclax or ABT-199) has improved clinical outcome with remarkable responses in patients (Rai and Jain 2016). Besides, personalized therapy for the treatment of B cell lymphoma is being rapidly developed. However, these novel therapeutics present a variability to antitumor activity because of the unique heterogeneity existed among different lymphoma types and within subtypes. Further studies are required to understand the pathogenesis of B cell lymphomas and the roles of gene mutations/translocations in lymphomagenesis.

Acknowledgements We thank Luming Zhang for secretarial assistance, Fudan University Animal Facility for maintaining the mice and the members in Wang Lab for helpful suggestions. This work was supported by the Major Research Plan of the National Natural Science Foundation of China (91942302 to J.Y.W.), the National Key R & D Plan of the Ministry of Science and Technology (SQ2019YFE0100600 to J.Y.W.), the National Natural Science Foundation of China (81571529 and 31870898 to J.Y.W), Projects of International Cooperation and Exchanges NSFC (81811540035 to J.Y.W.), a grant-in-aid for scientific research (C) from Japan Society for the Promotion of Science (17K08878 to J.Y.W) and a grant for the Innovative Research Team of High-Level Local Universities in Shanghai.

References

Ambrosini G, Adida C, Altieri DC (1997) A novel anti-apoptosis gene, survivin, expressed in cancer and lymphoma. Nat Med 3:917–921

Ansell SM (2015) Hodgkin lymphoma: diagnosis and treatment. Mayo Clin Proc 90:1574–1583

Arber DA, Orazi A, Hasserjian R, Thiele J, Borowitz MJ, Le Beau MM, Bloomfield CD, Cazzola M, Vardiman JW (2016) The 2016 revision to the World Health

Organization classification of myeloid neoplasms and acute leukemia. Blood 127:2391–2405
Barnes JA, Lacasce AS, Feng Y, Toomey CE, Neuberg D, Michaelson JS, Hochberg EP, Abramson JS (2011) Evaluation of the addition of rituximab to CODOX-M/IVAC for Burkitt's lymphoma: a retrospective analysis. Ann Oncol Off J Eur Soc Med Oncol 22:1859–1864
Barrans S, Crouch S, Smith A, Turner K, Owen R, Patmore R, Roman E, Jack A (2010) Rearrangement of MYC is associated with poor prognosis in patients with diffuse large B-cell lymphoma treated in the era of rituximab. J Clin Oncol Off J Am Soc Clin Oncol 28:3360–3365
Beltran BE, Castillo JJ, Morales D, de Mendoza FH, Quinones P, Miranda RN, Gallo A, Lopez-Ilasaca M, Butera JN, Sotomayor EM (2011) EBV-positive diffuse large B-cell lymphoma of the elderly: a case series from Peru. Am J Hematol 86:663–667
Bernard M, Gressin R, Lefrere F, Drenou B, Branger B, Caulet-Maugendre S, Tass P, Brousse N, Valensi F, Milpied N et al (2001) Blastic variant of mantle cell lymphoma: a rare but highly aggressive subtype. Leukemia 15:1785–1791
Bertoni F, Rinaldi A, Zucca E, Cavalli F (2006) Update on the molecular biology of mantle cell lymphoma. Hematol Oncol 24:22–27
Boer JM, Koenders JE, van der Holt B, Exalto C, Sanders MA, Cornelissen JJ, Valk PJ, den Boer ML, Rijneveld AW (2015) Expression profiling of adult acute lymphoblastic leukemia identifies a BCR-ABL1-like subgroup characterized by high non-response and relapse rates. Haematologica 100: e261–264
Borchmann S, Engert A (2017) The genetics of Hodgkin lymphoma: an overview and clinical implications. Curr Opin Oncol 29:307–314
Campo E, Swerdlow SH, Harris NL, Pileri S, Stein H, Jaffe ES (2011) The 2008 WHO classification of lymphoid neoplasms and beyond: evolving concepts and practical applications. Blood 117:5019–5032
Carbone A, Gloghini A, Santoro A (2012) In situ follicular lymphoma: pathologic characteristics and diagnostic features. Hematol Oncol 30:1–7
Carvajal-Cuenca A, Sua LF, Silva NM, Pittaluga S, Royo C, Song JY, Sargent RL, Espinet B, Climent F, Jacobs SA et al (2012) In situ mantle cell lymphoma: clinical implications of an incidental finding with indolent clinical behavior. Haematologica 97:270–278
Castillo JJ, Beltran BE, Miranda RN, Paydas S, Winer ES, Butera JN (2011) Epstein–Barr virus—positive diffuse large B-cell lymphoma of the elderly: what we know so far. Oncologist 16:87–96
Castillo JJ, Beltran BE, Miranda RN, Young KH, Chavez JC, Sotomayor EM (2016) EBV-positive diffuse large B-cell lymphoma of the elderly: 2016 update on diagnosis, risk-stratification, and management. Am J Hematol 91:529–537
Casulo C, Friedberg J (2015) Treating Burkitt lymphoma in adults. Curr Hematol Malignancy Rep 10:266–271
Chen RC, Chin MS, Ng AK, Feng Y, Neuberg D, Silver B, Pinkus GS, Stevenson MA, Mauch PM (2010) Early-stage, lymphocyte-predominant Hodgkin's lymphoma: patient outcomes from a large, single-institution series with long follow-up. J Clin Oncol Off J Am Soc Clin Oncol 28:136–141
Clot G, Jares P (2018) A gene signature that distinguishes conventional and leukemic nonnodal mantle cell lymphoma helps predict outcome. Blood 132:413–422
Corazzelli G, Frigeri F, Russo F, Frairia C, Arcamone M, Esposito G, De Chiara A, Morelli E, Capobianco G, Becchimanzi C et al (2012) RD-CODOX-M/IVAC with rituximab and intrathecal liposomal cytarabine in adult Burkitt lymphoma and 'unclassifiable' highly aggressive B-cell lymphoma. Br J Haematol 156:234–244
Dang CV, O'Donnell KA, Zeller KI, Nguyen T, Osthus RC, Li F (2006) The c-Myc target gene network. Semin Cancer Biol 16:253–264
Dave SS, Fu K, Wright GW, Lam LT, Kluin P, Boerma EJ, Greiner TC, Weisenburger DD, Rosenwald A, Ott G et al (2006) Molecular diagnosis of Burkitt's lymphoma. New Engl J Med 354:2431–2442
Den Boer ML, van Slegtenhorst M, De Menezes RX, Cheok MH, Buijs-Gladdines JG, Peters ST, Van Zutven LJ, Beverloo HB, Van der Spek PJ, Escherich G et al (2009) A subtype of childhood acute lymphoblastic leukaemia with poor treatment outcome: a genome-wide classification study. Lancet Oncol 10:125–134
de-The G, Geser A, Day NE, Tukei PM, Williams EH, Beri DP, Smith PG, Dean AG, Bronkamm GW, Feorino P, Henle W (1978) Epidemiological evidence for causal relationship between Epstein–Barr virus and Burkitt's lymphoma from Ugandan prospective study. Nature 274:756–761
Dojcinov SD, Fend F, Quintanilla-Martinez L (2018) EBV-positive lymphoproliferations of B- T- and NK-cell derivation in non-immunocompromised hosts. Pathogens 7:28
Dong M, Zhang X, Yang Z, Wu S, Ma M, Li Z, Chang Y, Wang X, Li L, Li X et al (2018) Patients over 40 years old with precursor T-cell lymphoblastic lymphoma have different prognostic factors comparing to the youngers. Sci Rep 8:1088
Dunleavy K (2018) Approach to the diagnosis and treatment of adult Burkitt's lymphoma. J Oncol Pract 14:665–671
Dunleavy K, Pittaluga S, Shovlin M, Steinberg SM, Cole D, Grant C, Widemann B, Staudt LM, Jaffe ES, Little RF, Wilson WH (2013) Low-intensity therapy in adults with Burkitt's lymphoma. New Engl J Med 369:1915–1925
Epstein MA, Achong BG, Barr YM (1964) Virus particles in cultured lymphoblasts from Burkitt's lymphoma. Lancet (London, England) 1:702–703
Evens AM, Carson KR, Kolesar J, Nabhan C, Helenowski I, Islam N, Jovanovic B, Barr PM, Caimi PF, Gregory SA, Gordon LI (2013) A multicenter phase II study incorporating high-dose rituximab and liposomal doxorubicin into the CODOX-

M/IVAC regimen for untreated Burkitt's lymphoma. Ann Oncol Off J Eur Soc Med Oncol 24:3076–3081
Fernandez V, Salamero O, Espinet B, Sole F, Royo C, Navarro A, Camacho F, Bea S, Hartmann E, Amador V et al (2010) Genomic and gene expression profiling defines indolent forms of mantle cell lymphoma. Can Res 70:1408–1418
Fischer T, Zing NPC, Chiattone CS, Federico M, Luminari S (2018) Transformed follicular lymphoma. Ann Hematol 97:17–29
Fisher SG, Fisher RI (2004) The epidemiology of non-Hodgkin's lymphoma. Oncogene 23:6524–6534
Gali V, Bleeker JS, Lynch D (2018) Epstein–Barr virus positive mucocutaneous ulcer: a case report. S Dakota Med J S Dakota State Med Assoc 71:252–255
Geser A, Brubaker G, Draper CC (1989) Effect of a malaria suppression program on the incidence of African Burkitt's lymphoma. Am J Epidemiol 129:740–752
Ginaldi L, De Martinis M, Matutes E, Farahat N, Morilla R, Catovsky D (1998) Levels of expression of CD19 and CD20 in chronic B cell leukaemias. J Clin Pathol 51:364–369
Graham RL, Mardones MA, Krause JR (2015) Primary follicular lymphoma of the duodenum. Proc (Bayl Univ Med Cent) 28:381–383
Green TM, Young KH, Visco C, Xu-Monette ZY, Orazi A, Go RS, Nielsen O, Gadeberg OV, Mourits-Andersen T, Frederiksen M et al (2012) Immunohistochemical double-hit score is a strong predictor of outcome in patients with diffuse large B-cell lymphoma treated with rituximab plus cyclophosphamide, doxorubicin, vincristine, and prednisone. J Clin Oncol Off J Am Soc Clin Oncol 30:3460–3467
Harrison CJ (2015) Blood Spotlight on iAMP21 acute lymphoblastic leukemia (ALL), a high-risk pediatric disease. Blood 125:1383–1386
Havranek O, Xu J, Kohrer S, Wang Z, Becker L, Comer JM, Henderson J, Ma W, Man Chun Ma J, Westin JR et al (2017) Tonic B-cell receptor signaling in diffuse large B-cell lymphoma. Blood 130:995–1006
Heerema NA, Carroll AJ, Devidas M, Loh ML, Borowitz MJ, Gastier-Foster JM, Larsen EC, Mattano LA Jr, Maloney KW, Willman CL et al (2013) Intrachromosomal amplification of chromosome 21 is associated with inferior outcomes in children with acute lymphoblastic leukemia treated in contemporary standard-risk children's oncology group studies: a report from the children's oncology group. J Clin Oncol Off J Am Soc Clin Oncol 31:3397–3402
Hong JY, Ryu KJ, Park C, Hong M, Ko YH, Kim WS, Kim SJ (2017) Clinical impact of serum survivin positivity and tissue expression of EBV-encoded RNA in diffuse large B-cell lymphoma patients treated with rituximab-CHOP. Oncotarget 8:13782–13791
Hummel M, Bentink S, Berger H, Klapper W, Wessendorf S, Barth TF, Bernd HW, Cogliatti SB, Dierlamm J, Feller AC et al (2006) A biologic definition of Burkitt's lymphoma from transcriptional and genomic profiling. New Engl J Med 354:2419–2430
International CLL-IPI Working Group (2016) An international prognostic index for patients with chronic lymphocytic leukaemia (CLL-IPI): a meta-analysis of individual patient data. Lancet Oncol 17:779–790
Intlekofer AM, Younes A (2014) Precision therapy for lymphoma—current state and future directions. Nat Rev Clin Oncol 11:585–596
Izutsu K (2017) Treatment for mantle cell lymphoma [Rinsho ketsueki]. Japan J Clin Hematol 58:2026–2032
Jares P, Colomer D, Campo E (2012) Molecular pathogenesis of mantle cell lymphoma. J Clin Investig 122:3416–3423
Kalter SP, Riggs SA, Cabanillas F, Butler JJ, Hagemeister FB, Mansell PW, Newell GR, Velasquez WS, Salvador P, Barlogie B et al (1985) Aggressive non-Hodgkin's lymphomas in immunocompromised homosexual males. Blood 66:655–659
Kramer MH, Hermans J, Wijburg E, Philippo K, Geelen E, van Krieken JH, de Jong D, Maartense E, Schuuring E, Kluin PM (1998) Clinical relevance of BCL2, BCL6, and MYC rearrangements in diffuse large B-cell lymphoma. Blood 92:3152–3162
Kuppers R (2005) Mechanisms of B-cell lymphoma pathogenesis. Nat Rev Cancer 5:251–262
Landau DA, Tausch E, Taylor-Weiner AN, Stewart C, Reiter JG, Bahlo J, Kluth S, Bozic I, Lawrence M, Bottcher S et al (2015) Mutations driving CLL and their evolution in progression and relapse. Nature 526:525–530
Landgren O, Albitar M, Ma W, Abbasi F, Hayes RB, Ghia P, Marti GE, Caporaso NE (2009) B-cell clones as early markers for chronic lymphocytic leukemia. New Engl J Med 360:659–667
Liu Q, Salaverria I, Pittaluga S, Jegalian AG, Xi L, Siebert R, Raffeld M, Hewitt SM, Jaffe ES (2013) Follicular lymphomas in children and young adults: a comparison of the pediatric variant with usual follicular lymphoma. Am J Surg Pathol 37:333–343
Liu WR, Shipp MA (2017) Signaling pathways and immune evasion mechanisms in classical Hodgkin lymphoma. Blood 130:2265–2270
Liu Z, Xu-Monette ZY, Cao X, Manyam GC, Wang X, Tzankov A (2015) Prognostic and biological significance of survivin expression in patients with diffuse large B-cell lymphoma treated with rituximab-CHOP therapy. Mod Pathol 28:1297–1314
Love C, Sun Z, Jima D, Li G, Zhang J, Miles R, Richards KL, Dunphy CH, Choi WW, Srivastava G et al (2012) The genetic landscape of mutations in Burkitt lymphoma. Nat Genet 44:1321–1325
Magalhaes M, Ghorab Z, Morneault J, Akinfolarin J, Bradley G (2015) Age-related Epstein–Barr virus-positive mucocutaneous ulcer: a case report. Clin Case Rep 3:531–534
Magrath I, Adde M, Shad A, Venzon D, Seibel N, Gootenberg J, Neely J, Arndt C, Nieder M, Jaffe E et al (1996) Adults and children with small non-

cleaved-cell lymphoma have a similar excellent outcome when treated with the same chemotherapy regimen. J Clin Oncol Off J Am Soc Clin Oncol 14:925–934
Martelli M, Ferreri AJ, Agostinelli C, Di Rocco A, Pfreundschuh M, Pileri SA (2013) Diffuse large B-cell lymphoma. Crit Rev Oncol/hematol 87:146–171
Mathas S, Hartmann S, Kuppers R (2016) Hodgkin lymphoma: pathology and biology. Semin Hematol 53:139–147
Mbulaiteye SM, Anderson WF, Bhatia K, Rosenberg PS, Linet MS, Devesa SS (2010) Trimodal age-specific incidence patterns for Burkitt lymphoma in the United States, 1973–2005. Int J Cancer 126:1732–1739
Mead GM, Sydes MR, Walewski J, Grigg A, Hatton CS, Pescosta N, Guarnaccia C, Lewis MS, McKendrick J, Stenning SP, Wright D (2002) An international evaluation of CODOX-M and CODOX-M alternating with IVAC in adult Burkitt's lymphoma: results of United Kingdom lymphoma group LY06 study. Ann Oncol Off J Eur Soc Med Oncol 13:1264–1274
Mead GM, Barrans SL, Qian W, Walewski J, Radford JA, Wolf M, Clawson SM, Stenning SP, Yule CL, Jack AS (2008) A prospective clinicopathologic study of dose-modified CODOX-M/IVAC in patients with sporadic Burkitt lymphoma defined using cytogenetic and immunophenotypic criteria (MRC/NCRI LY10 trial). Blood 112:2248–2260
Melo JV, Catovsky D, Galton DA (1986) The relationship between chronic lymphocytic leukaemia and prolymphocytic leukaemia. I. Clinical and laboratory features of 300 patients and characterization of an intermediate group. Br J Haematol 63:377–387
Meyer N, Penn LZ (2008) Reflecting on 25 years with MYC. Nat Rev Cancer 8:976–990
Molica S (2006) Sex differences in incidence and outcome of chronic lymphocytic leukemia patients. Leuk Lymphoma 47:1477–1480
Moorman AV (2016) New and emerging prognostic and predictive genetic biomarkers in B-cell precursor acute lymphoblastic leukemia. Haematologica 101:407–416
Moorman AV, Richards SM, Robinson HM, Strefford JC, Gibson BE, Kinsey SE, Eden TO, Vora AJ, Mitchell CD, Harrison CJ (2007) Prognosis of children with acute lymphoblastic leukemia (ALL) and intrachromosomal amplification of chromosome 21 (iAMP21). Blood 109:2327–2330
Morabito F, Mosca L, Cutrona G, Agnelli L, Tuana G, Ferracin M, Zagatti B, Lionetti M, Fabris S, Maura F et al (2013) Clinical monoclonal B lymphocytosis versus Rai 0 chronic lymphocytic leukemia: a comparison of cellular, cytogenetic, molecular, and clinical features. Clin Cancer Res Off J Am Assoc Cancer Res 19:5890–5900
Morales D, Beltran B, De Mendoza FH, Riva L, Yabar A, Quinones P, Butera JN, Castillo J (2010) Epstein–Barr virus as a prognostic factor in de novo nodal diffuse large B-cell lymphoma. Leuk Lymphoma 51:66–72
Moreau EJ, Matutes E, A'Hern RP, Morilla AM, Morilla RM, Owusu-Ankomah KA, Seon BK, Catovsky D (1997) Improvement of the chronic lymphocytic leukemia scoring system with the monoclonal antibody SN8 (CD79b). Am J Clin Pathol 108:378–382
Morton LM, Wang SS, Devesa SS, Hartge P, Weisenburger DD, Linet MS (2006) Lymphoma incidence patterns by WHO subtype in the United States, 1992–2001. Blood 107:265–276
Muhlbacher V, Zenger M, Schnittger S, Weissmann S, Kunze F, Kohlmann A, Bellos F, Kern W, Haferlach T, Haferlach C (2014) Acute lymphoblastic leukemia with low hypodiploid/near triploid karyotype is a specific clinical entity and exhibits a very high TP53 mutation frequency of 93%. Genes Chromosom Cancer 53:524–536
Nakamura N, Nakamine H, Tamaru J, Nakamura S, Yoshino T, Ohshima K, Abe M (2002) The distinction between Burkitt lymphoma and diffuse large B-cell lymphoma with c-myc rearrangement. Mod Pathol Off J US Can Acad Pathol Inc 15:771–776
Natkunam Y, Goodlad JR, Chadburn A, de Jong D, Gratzinger D, Chan JK, Said J, Jaffe ES (2017) EBV-positive B-cell proliferations of varied malignant potential: 2015 SH/EAHP workshop report—part 1. Am J Clin Pathol 147:129–152
Nicolae A, Pittaluga S (2015) EBV-positive large B-cell lymphomas in young patients: a nodal lymphoma with evidence for a tolerogenic immune environment. Blood 126:863–872
Nieto WG, Almeida J, Romero A, Teodosio C, Lopez A, Henriques AF, Sanchez ML, Jara-Acevedo M, Rasillo A, Gonzalez M et al (2009) Increased frequency (12%) of circulating chronic lymphocytic leukemia-like B-cell clones in healthy subjects using a highly sensitive multicolor flow cytometry approach. Blood 114:33–37
O'Conor GT, Davies JN (1960) Malignant tumors in African children: with special reference to malignant lymphoma. J Pediatr 56:526–535
Ok CY, Li L, Xu-Monette ZY, Visco C, Tzankov A, Manyam GC, Montes-Moreno S, Dybkaer K, Chiu A, Orazi A et al (2014) Prevalence and clinical implications of Epstein–Barr virus infection in de novo diffuse large B-cell lymphoma in Western countries. Clin Cancer Res Off J Am Assoc Cancer Res 20:2338–2349
Orem J, Mbidde EK, Lambert B, de Sanjose S, Weiderpass E (2007) Burkitt's lymphoma in Africa, a review of the epidemiology and etiology. Afr Health Sci 7:166–175
Oyama T, Ichimura K, Suzuki R, Suzumiya J, Ohshima K, Yatabe Y, Yokoi T, Kojima M, Kamiya Y, Taji H et al (2003) Senile EBV+ B-cell lymphoproliferative disorders: a clinicopathologic study of 22 patients. Am J Surg Pathol 27:16–26
Oyama T, Yamamoto K, Asano N, Oshiro A, Suzuki R, Kagami Y, Morishima Y, Takeuchi K, Izumo T, Mori S et al (2007) Age-related EBV-associated B-cell lymphoproliferative disorders constitute a distinct clinicopathologic group: a study of 96 patients. Clin

Cancer Res Off J Am Assoc Cancer Res 13:5124–5132

Park S, Lee J, Ko YH, Han A, Jun HJ, Lee SC, Hwang IG, Park YH, Ahn JS, Jung CW et al (2007) The impact of Epstein–Barr virus status on clinical outcome in diffuse large B-cell lymphoma. Blood 110:972–978

Pasqualucci L, Dalla-Favera R (2015) The genetic landscape of diffuse large B-cell lymphoma. Semin Hematol 52:67–76

Rai KR, Jain P (2016) Chronic lymphocytic leukemia (CLL)—then and now. Am J Hematol 91:330–340

Rai KR, Sawitsky A, Cronkite EP, Chanana AD, Levy RN, Pasternack BS (1975) Clinical staging of chronic lymphocytic leukemia. Blood 46:219–234

Rajput AB, Burns B, Gerridzen R, van der Jagt R (2014) Coexisting mantle cell lymphoma and prostate adenocarcinoma. Case Rep Med 2014:247286

Rand V, Parker H, Russell LJ, Schwab C, Ensor H, Irving J, Jones L, Masic D, Minto L, Morrison H et al (2011) Genomic characterization implicates iAMP21 as a likely primary genetic event in childhood B-cell precursor acute lymphoblastic leukemia. Blood 117:6848–6855

Richter J, Schlesner M, Hoffmann S, Kreuz M, Leich E, Burkhardt B, Rosolowski M, Ammerpohl O, Wagener R, Bernhart SH et al (2012) Recurrent mutation of the ID3 gene in Burkitt lymphoma identified by integrated genome, exome and transcriptome sequencing. Nat Genet 44:1316–1320

Rizzieri DA, Johnson JL, Niedzwiecki D, Lee EJ, Vardiman JW, Powell BL, Barcos M, Bloomfield CD, Schiffer CA, Peterson BA et al (2004) Intensive chemotherapy with and without cranial radiation for Burkitt leukemia and lymphoma: final results of cancer and leukemia group B study 9251. Cancer 100:1438–1448

Rizzieri DA, Johnson JL, Byrd JC, Lozanski G, Blum KA, Powell BL, Shea TC, Nattam S, Hoke E, Cheson BD, Larson RA (2014) Improved efficacy using rituximab and brief duration, high intensity chemotherapy with filgrastim support for Burkitt or aggressive lymphomas: cancer and leukemia group B study 10 002. Br J Haematol 165:102–111

Roberts TK, Chen X, Liao JJ (2015) Diagnostic and therapeutic challenges of EBV-positive mucocutaneous ulcer: a case report and systematic review of the literature. Experimental Hematol Oncol 5:13

Roberts KG, Gu Z, Payne-Turner D, McCastlain K, Harvey RC, Chen IM, Pei D, Iacobucci I, Valentine M, Pounds SB et al (2017) High frequency and poor outcome of philadelphia chromosome-like acute lymphoblastic leukemia in adults. J Clin Oncol Off J Am Soc Clin Oncol 35:394–401

Roberts KG, Li Y, Payne-Turner D, Harvey RC, Yang YL, Pei D, McCastlain K, Ding L, Lu C, Song G et al (2014) Targetable kinase-activating lesions in Ph-like acute lymphoblastic leukemia. New Engl J Med 371:1005–1015

Roschewski M, Staudt LM, Wilson WH (2014) Diffuse large B-cell lymphoma-treatment approaches in the molecular era. Nat Rev Clin Oncol 11:12–23

Rosenthal A, Younes A (2017) High grade B-cell lymphoma with rearrangements of MYC and BCL2 and/or BCL6: double hit and triple hit lymphomas and double expressing lymphoma. Blood Rev 31:37–42

Rosenwald A, Wright G, Chan WC, Connors JM, Campo E, Fisher RI, Gascoyne RD, Muller-Hermelink HK, Smeland EB, Giltnane JM et al (2002) The use of molecular profiling to predict survival after chemotherapy for diffuse large-B-cell lymphoma. N Engl J Med 346:1937–1947

Rosenwald A, Wright G, Wiestner A, Chan WC, Connors JM, Campo E, Gascoyne RD, Grogan TM, Muller-Hermelink HK, Smeland EB et al (2003) The proliferation gene expression signature is a quantitative integrator of oncogenic events that predicts survival in mantle cell lymphoma. Cancer Cell 3:185–197

Roulland S, Faroudi M, Mamessier E, Sungalee S, Salles G, Nadel B (2011) Early steps of follicular lymphoma pathogenesis. Adv Immunol 111:1–46

Rowe M, Fitzsimmons L, Bell AI (2014) Epstein–Barr virus and Burkitt lymphoma. Chin J Cancer 33:609–619

Satou A, Banno S, Hanamura I, Takahashi E, Takahara T, Nobata H, Katsuno T, Takami A, Ito Y, Ueda R et al (2019) EBV-positive mucocutaneous ulcer arising in rheumatoid arthritis patients treated with methotrexate: single center series of nine cases. Pathol Int 69:21–28

Savage KJ, Mottok A, Fanale M (2016) Nodular lymphocyte-predominant Hodgkin lymphoma. Semin Hematol 53:190–202

Schmitz R, Young RM, Ceribelli M, Jhavar S, Xiao W, Zhang M, Wright G, Shaffer AL, Hodson DJ, Buras E et al (2012) Burkitt lymphoma pathogenesis and therapeutic targets from structural and functional genomics. Nature 490:116–120

Schulz H, Rehwald U, Morschhauser F, Elter T, Driessen C, Rudiger T, Borchmann P, Schnell R, Diehl V, Engert A, Reiser M (2008) Rituximab in relapsed lymphocyte-predominant Hodgkin lymphoma: long-term results of a phase 2 trial by the German Hodgkin lymphoma study group (GHSG). Blood 111:109–111

Song JY, Eberle FC, Xi L, Raffeld M, Rahma O, Wilson WH, Dunleavy K, Pittaluga S, Jaffe ES (2011) Coexisting and clonally identical classic Hodgkin lymphoma and nodular lymphocyte predominant Hodgkin lymphoma. Am J Surg Pathol 35:767–772

Soussain C, Patte C, Ostronoff M, Delmer A, Rigal-Huguet F, Cambier N, Leprise PY, Francois S, Cony-Makhoul P, Harousseau JL et al (1995) Small noncleaved cell lymphoma and leukemia in adults: a retrospective study of 65 adults treated with the LMB pediatric protocols. Blood 85:664–674

Sugimoto T, Watanabe T (2016) Follicular lymphoma: the role of the tumor microenvironment in prognosis. J Clin Exp hematopathol JCEH 56:1–19

Swerdlow SH, Campo E, Pileri SA, Harris NL, Stein H, Siebert R, Advani R, Ghielmini M, Salles GA (2016) The 2016 revision of the World Health Organization classification of lymphoid neoplasms. Blood 127:2375–2390

Tees MT, Flinn IW (2017) Chronic lymphocytic leukemia and small lymphocytic lymphoma: two faces of the same disease. Expert Rev Hematol 10:137–146

Teras LR, DeSantis CE, Cerhan JR, Morton LM, Jemal A, Flowers CR (2016) 2016 US lymphoid malignancy statistics by World Health Organization subtypes. CA: A Cancer J Clin 66:443–459

Ting CY, Chang KM, Kuan JW, Sathar J, Chew LP, Wong OJ, Yusuf Y, Wong L, Samsudin AT, Pana M et al (2019) Clinical significance of BCL2, C-MYC, and BCL6 genetic abnormalities, Epstein–Barr virus infection, CD5 protein expression, germinal center B cell/non-germinal center B-cell subtypes, co-expression of MYC/BCL2 proteins and co-expression of MYC/BCL2/BCL6 proteins in diffuse large B-cell lymphoma: a clinical and pathological correlation study of 120 patients. Int J Med Sci 16:556–566

Torgbor C, Awuah P, Deitsch K, Kalantari P, Duca KA, Thorley-Lawson DA (2014) A multifactorial role for P. falciparum malaria in endemic Burkitt's lymphoma pathogenesis. PLoS Pathog 10:e1004170

Tsao SW, Tsang CM (2017) Epstein–Barr virus infection and nasopharyngeal carcinoma. Philos Trans R Soc B Biol Sci 372

Tzankov A, Pehrs AC, Zimpfer A, Ascani S, Lugli A, Pileri S, Dirnhofer S (2003) Prognostic significance of CD44 expression in diffuse large B cell lymphoma of activated and germinal centre B cell-like types: a tissue microarray analysis of 90 cases. J Clin Pathol 56:747–752

Vishnu P, Dorer RP, Aboulafia DM (2015) Immune reconstitution inflammatory syndrome-associated Burkitt lymphoma after combination antiretroviral therapy in HIV-infected patients. Clin Lymphoma Myeloma Leuk 15:e23–29

Weiss LM, Warnke RA, Sklar J, Cleary ML (1987) Molecular analysis of the t(14;18) chromosomal translocation in malignant lymphomas. N Engl J Med 317:1185–1189

Wenzinger C, Williams E, Gru AA (2018) Updates in the pathology of precursor lymphoid neoplasms in the revised fourth edition of the WHO classification of tumors of hematopoietic and lymphoid tissues. Curr Hematol Malignancy Rep 13:275–288

Weston BW, Hayden MA, Roberts KG, Bowyer S, Hsu J, Fedoriw G, Rao KW, Mullighan CG (2013) Tyrosine kinase inhibitor therapy induces remission in a patient with refractory EBF1-PDGFRB-positive acute lymphoblastic leukemia. J Clin Oncol Off J Am Soc Clin Oncol 31:e413–416

Willemze R, Cerroni L, Kempf W, Berti E, Facchetti F (2019) The 2018 update of the WHO-EORTC classification for primary cutaneous lymphomas. Blood 133:1703–1714

Xing KH, Connors JM, Lai A, Al-Mansour M, Sehn LH, Villa D, Klasa R, Shenkier T, Gascoyne RD, Skinnider B, Savage KJ (2014) Advanced-stage nodular lymphocyte predominant Hodgkin lymphoma compared with classical Hodgkin lymphoma: a matched pair outcome analysis. Blood 123:3567–3573

Zhou Z, Sehn LH, Rademaker AW, Gordon LI, Lacasce AS, Crosby-Thompson A, Vanderplas A, Zelenetz AD, Abel GA, Rodriguez MA et al (2014) An enhanced international prognostic index (NCCN-IPI) for patients with diffuse large B-cell lymphoma treated in the rituximab era. Blood 123:837–842

The manufacturer's authorised representative in the EU is Springer Nature Customer Service Centre GmbH, Europaplatz 3, 69115 Heidelberg, Germany. If you have any concerns regarding our products, please contact ProductSafety@springernature.com

Printed and bound by CPI Group (UK) Ltd, Croydon, CR0 4YY
05/10/2026
02228120-0020